Eldercare

Positioning Your Hospital for the Future

Nancy Alfred Persily, Editor

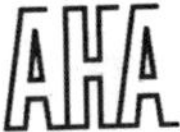

books are published by
American Hospital Publishing, Inc.,
an American Hospital Association company

The views expressed in this publication are strictly those of the authors and do not necessarily represent official positions of the American Hospital Association.

Library of Congress Cataloging-in-Publication Data

Eldercare : positioning your hospital for the future / Nancy Alfred Persily, editor.
p. cm.
Includes bibliographical references.
ISBN 1-55648-062-8
1. Aged–Medical care–United States–Planning.
2. Aged–Hospital care–United States–Planning.
3. Hospitals–United States–Planning. I. Persily, Nancy A. (Nancy Alfred).
[DNLM: 1. Health Services for the Aged–organization & administration–United States. 2. Hospitals–organization & administration–United States. WT 27 AA1 E3]
RA564.8.E35 1991
362.1'9897'00973–dc20
DNLM/DLC
for Library of Congress

90-14473
CIP

Catalog no. 130102

Printed in the USA

AHA is a service mark of the American Hospital Association used under license by American Hospital Publishing, Inc.

Text set in Palatino
3M–02/91–0282

Marlene Chamberlain, Project Editor
Linda Conheady, Manuscript Editor
Lawrence Denne, Editorial Assistant
Marcia Bottoms, Managing Editor
Peggy DuMais, Production Coordinator
Marcia Vecchione, Designer
Brian Schenk, Books Division Director

Contents

About the Editor

Nancy Alfred Persily, M.P.H., is vice-president, Lewin/ICF, a policy research and management consulting firm specializing in health care and economic analysis in Washington, DC. Former president of Nancy Alfred Persily Associates, Inc., consultants to health care organizations, she also was president of the Caregivers Network, a case-management firm and licensed home health agency. Prior to that, she was director of planning and marketing at Mount Sinai Medical Center, Miami Beach. Over the years Ms. Persily has been involved with the planning and development of acute-care hospitals, rehabilitation hospitals, nursing homes, home health agencies, hospices, older adult housing programs, and retirement communities. She lectures extensively on health care topics and has served on the faculties of the Mount Sinai School of Medicine, the University of Miami School of Medicine, The University of South Florida, and Florida International University. She is coauthor of *Hospitals and the Aged: The New Old Market* (Aspen Publishers, 1984).

List of Figures

List of Tables

Contributors

Sonya R. Albury, M.S.W., is senior health planner, Health Council of South Florida, Inc., a health planning and policy-making organization in Miami. She spent four years as a consultant at Nancy Alfred Persily Associates in Coral Gables, Florida, where she conducted market research and related health care planning activities. She has coauthored several articles on long-term care and assisted in the establishment of the Southeast Florida Center on Aging at Florida International University.

Ron J. Anderson, M.D., is president and chief executive officer, Parkland Memorial Hospital in Dallas County, Texas, the primary teaching hospital for the University of Texas Southwestern Medical Center at Dallas. He previously served as medical director for ambulatory care and emergency services at Parkland. Dr. Anderson has remained on the faculty of the medical school as professor of internal medicine and continues to see patients and teach house staff physicians at Parkland. From 1983 to 1987, Dr. Anderson was chairman of the Texas Board of Health. He is a member of the Executive Committee of the Board of the National Association of Public Hospitals.

John C. Beck, M.D., Ph.D., is center director, Long-Term Care National Resource Center; director, California Geriatric Education Center; and director, Academic Geriatric Resource Center at the University of California, Los Angeles. He has served as professor of medicine at the University of California, San Francisco; director of the Robert Wood Johnson Clinical Scholar Program; and senior consultant, Robert Wood Johnson Foundation, Princeton, New Jersey.

Robert N. Butler, M.D., is Brookdale professor and chairman of the Gerald and May Ellen Ritter Department of Geriatrics and Adult Development of the Mount Sinai Medical Center, New York City. Dr. Butler was founding director of the National Institute on Aging of the National Institutes of Health from 1975 to 1982. In 1976, Dr. Butler won the Pulitzer Prize for his book *Why Survive? Being Old in America.* He is a member of the Institute of Medicine and has served as a consultant to the U.S. Senate Special Committee on Aging, the Commonwealth Fund, the Brookdale Foundation, and numerous other organizations. He helped found the Alzheimer's Disease Association, the American Federation of Aging Research, the American Association of Geriatrics Psychiatry, and the Alliance for Aging Research.

David R. Cornell, Ph.D., F.A.C.H.E., is president and chief executive officer of Western Reserve Care System, a multihospital system located in Youngstown, Ohio. From 1979 to 1988, he was president and chief executive officer of Montana Deaconess Medical Center in Great Falls, Montana. Dr. Cornell is a past delegate to the American Hospital Association's Section for Aging and Long-Term Care Services and is currently an alternate delegate for the Section for Health Care Systems. Since 1975 he has been involved in the design and implementation of senior membership programs.

Linda J. Cragin, M.S., is director of geriatrics and long-term care programs of Beverly Hospital and its parent company, Northeast Health Systems, Inc., both in Beverly, Massachusetts, where she is responsible for implementing all programs and services related to eldercare. She serves on the boards of several of the subsidiary corporations of Northeast Health Systems, including boards for hospice, home health agency, nursing home, and substance abuse treatment programs, and on several community boards providing services for the elderly. Previously Ms. Cragin worked at the Massachusetts Executive Office of Elder Affairs and Perkins School for the Blind.

Robert B. Culbertson, M.S., is former director, Center for Geriatric Care, Morristown Memorial Hospital, Morristown, New Jersey. He was responsible for the development and implementation of the Geriatric Center under a Robert Wood Johnson Foundation grant, and he continued to administer the program after the grant period. He was also director of community services for the Rehabilitation Institute of Morristown Memorial Hospital, where he directed marketing and admissions activities. Mr. Culbertson served on the Governor's Conference on Aging Task Force on Long-Term Care in New Jersey.

Linda Cutler, M.A., is education coordinator, Geriatrics Institute of Sinai Samaritan Medical Center, a subsidiary of Aurora Health Care in Milwaukee. She is responsible for coordination of community and professional education programs in geriatrics and gerontology.

Eugene E. Dawson, Jr., Ph.D., is coordinator of the Health Care Management Program and director of the Institute for Gerontology at Metropolitan State College of Denver. Previously he served for 4½ years as director of Swedish Gerontology Center, Swedish Medical Center, Englewood, Colorado. He is presently a faculty associate with the American College of Healthcare Executives.

JoAnna "Jody" DeMeyer, R.N., M.N., is a consultant with DeMeyer and Associates, Boise, Idaho, providing consultation on nursing and quality assurance programs in hospitals and on hospital senior programs. Her past experience includes serving as vice-president, patient care services, for St. Luke's Regional Medical Center, Boise. She developed the medical center's first home care program and its first programs for older adults. She planned and implemented for St. Luke's the Robert Wood Johnson Foundation grant, *Hospital Initiatives in Long-Term Care.* She has served on the School of Nursing faculty at the University of California at San Francisco, the University of Oregon, the University of Washington, and on national, regional, and local health care–related commissions and committees.

Carolee A. DeVito, Ph.D., M.P.H., is associate professor and vice-chairperson, Department of Family Medicine and Community Health, University of Miami; and director, Department of Community Health Services, South Shore Hospital and Medical Center, Miami Beach. Dr. DeVito has directed program development and research efforts in long-term care, including the Geriatric Assessment and Planning Program at South Shore Hospital and Medical Center, funded by the Robert Wood Johnson Foundation; the Service Credit Banking Program; and the Study to Assess Falls among the Elderly (SAFE), funded by the Centers for Disease Control. She has published numerous materials and spoken extensively about long-term care and the care of the frail elderly.

Robert R. Fanning, Jr., M.B.A., joined Beverly Hospital in Beverly, Massachusetts, as president and chief executive officer in 1980. He is also president of Northeast Health Systems, Inc., Beverly Hospital's parent corporation, and chairman of the board of the Massachusetts Hospital Association. Previously Mr. Fanning was executive vice-president and chief operating officer of the Children's Hospital Medical Center, Boston, and held various administrative positions at the Burbank Hospital, Fitchburg, Massachusetts. A Fellow in the American College of Healthcare Executives and past governor for District One, he won the 1979 Recognition Award of the Health Care Management Association and was selected "CEO of the Year" in 1989 by the Massachusetts members of the American College of Healthcare Executives. He serves as vice-chairman of the board of the Massachusetts Health and Educational Facilities Authority.

Kathleen J. Farkas, Ph.D., is an assistant professor of social work at the Mandel School of Applied Social Sciences, Case Western Reserve University, Cleveland, where she is also responsible for research in gerontology and substance abuse. She is a licensed independent social worker and consultant and board member for addiction treatment and long-term care organizations. Dr. Farkas has served as program coordinator for the Geriatric Program at Cleveland's MetroHealth Medical Center.

Elaine M. Frank, M.H.S., is a planner at the Human Services Council in Lebanon, New Hampshire. Previously she was vice-president for Program and Human Development at the Greater Southeast Community Center for the Aging, a subsidiary of the Greater Southeast Community Hospital Foundation. While employed at the Center, she developed and implemented a number of innovative gerontological programs, including the Service Credit Volunteer System.

J. Dermot Frengley, M.D., was born, educated, and trained in New Zealand and did graduate studies in medicine at the University of London, England, and at Case Western Reserve University, Cleveland. He was on the faculty in the Department of Medicine, St. George's Hospital Medical School, University of London. In 1975, he joined the Department of Medicine of Case Western's School of Medicine at Cleveland Metropolitan General Hospital. In 1980, he began development of a comprehensive multilevel program of geriatric care. As director of geriatric medicine for the MetroHealth Hospital System, he was principal investigator of the Robert Wood Johnson Foundation's *Hospital Initiatives in Long-Term Care* program. Dr. Frengley also was associate director of the Office of Geriatric Medicine at Case Western Reserve.

Judith L. Howe, M.A., M.P.A., is administrator, the Gerald and May Ellen Ritter Department of Geriatrics and Adult Development, the Mount Sinai Medical Center, New York City. She has been with the department since it was established in 1982 and has participated in a wide variety of program development and planning activities. Previously Ms. Howe served as an adviser for the United National World Assembly on Aging (1982). From 1977 to 1982, she was with the National Institute on Aging, U.S. Department of Health and Human Services, where she was involved in program evaluation, planning, and legislative activities.

Paul J. Lanzikos, M.B.A., is secretary, Executive Office of Elder Affairs, Commonwealth of Massachusetts. Previously he was vice-president of Beverly Hospital and its not-for-profit parent corporation, Northeast Health Systems, Inc., both in Beverly, Massachusetts. He directed the development of a comprehensive geriatric service system including a nursing home, assisted housing, home health agency, and other community-based programs.

Peter J. Levin, Sc.D., is the founding dean of the College of Public Health at the University of South Florida in Tampa. He chaired the Florida Hospital Cost Containment Board from 1985 to 1988, was dean of the College of Public Health at the University of Oklahoma, and served as executive director of the Stanford University Hospital. He writes and lectures on health care in Japan and on how American health care will be managed in the future.

Marie Bolduc Liston, M.S.W., M.S.G., is a consultant at the University of Southern California's Andrus Gerontology Center in Los Angeles. Her responsibilities include writing and editing training manuals for care givers of people with senile dementia. Ms. Bolduc Liston was previously employed at the UCLA Multicampus Division of Geriatric Medicine and Gerontology for nine years, where she collaborated on numerous long-term care projects with hospital personnel, including administrators, emergency room personnel, and discharge planners. She also served as a contributor to "On Aging," a nationally syndicated column for the *Washington Post* Writers Group.

Paula A. Loftis, M.S., R.N., is director of the Department of Geriatrics at Parkland Memorial Hospital in Dallas. She has developed, directed, and managed the activities of the Department of Geriatrics since its inception in 1984 and continues in active practice as a clinical nurse specialist. Prior to her present appointment, she practiced in and directed the home care/discharge planning program and established the nurse-managed health care clinic concept at Parkland Hospital. Ms. Loftis is adjunct faculty and clinical associate with the University of Texas at Arlington and Texas Woman's University graduate and undergraduate nursing program. She has participated on several home health care professional advisory boards and service committees with community health care organizations.

Edward jj Olson, M.S., is president of E jj Olson & Associates in Milwaukee, a health care and human services consulting firm. Previously he was administrator of the Geriatrics Institute of Mount Sinai Medical Center, Milwaukee, which was a designated site for the Robert Wood Johnson Foundation's *Hospital Initiatives in Long-Term Care* program. He served as the chairman of the Milwaukee County Commission on Aging from 1974 to 1989 and was a board member of the American Society on Aging and the National Urban Elderly Coalition. Mr. Olson has served as an adjunct professor at the School of Architecture and Urban Planning at the University of Wisconsin-Milwaukee. He has done postgraduate work at Roosevelt University and the University of Chicago, authored numerous articles, and lectured extensively nationally and internationally.

Maria Garza Reynolds, C.S.W., is associate executive director of Senior Citizens of Greater Dallas, a United Way agency. She is responsible for programming and direct supervision of the agency's five programs, which are the Retired Senior Volunteer Program, the Foster Grandparent Program, "Off Our Rockers," the Advocacy Group for the Elderly, and the Nursing Home Ombudsman Program. Her previous experience at Dallas's Parkland Memorial Hospital is in the area of geriatric social work and case management. She has also served as community resource consultant for the Dallas County Department of Human Service Nutrition Program's 34 senior centers.

Craig D. Rubin, M.D., F.A.C.P., is medical director of the Geriatric Assessment Team at Parkland Memorial Hospital in Dallas. He is an assistant professor of internal medicine at the University of Texas Southwestern Medical Center and is chief of the Section on Clinical Geriatrics in the Department of Internal Medicine.

Elyse Salend, M.S.W., is a lecturer at the University of California, Los Angeles (UCLA) School of Medicine and the deputy director of the Long-Term Care National Resource Center at UCLA/University of Southern California in Los Angeles. She was project director of two programs at UCLA, the *Emergency Medicine Center: Improved Geriatric Care and Caring* program, and the Robert Wood Johnson Foundation's *Hospital Initiatives in Long-Term Care* program. Ms. Salend writes and lectures on aging issues for professional and consumer audiences. She is the originator of "On Aging," a nationally syndicated newspaper column geared toward older readers. She is also coauthor of *PG 50: A Consumer's Guide to Growing Older,* a comprehensive book for older people and their families (Simon & Schuster, 1990).

Mark T. Sizemore, Ph.D., is an assistant professor at the University of Texas Southwestern Medical Center at Dallas. He was principal investigator of a grant from the National Institute on Aging to develop Spanish-language educational videotapes on Alzheimer's disease. He has also assessed the effectiveness of an outpatient geriatric assessment program with data files available from the Health Care Financing Administration.

Michael Gordon Sorohan, B.A., is marketing/communications manager for the Greater Southeast Management Company in Washington, D.C., a private, not-for-profit health care system that includes Greater Southeast Community Hospital, the Greater Southeast Center for the Aging, and several other health ventures. Before joining Greater Southeast in 1984, Mr. Sorohan worked in the community relations department of Community General Osteopathic Hospital in Harrisburg, Pennsylvania. He is the author of several free-lance articles in the health care and education fields.

Susan Taylor, B.S., is vice-president of marketing and development and senior housing operations for the Ebenezer Society in Minneapolis. She was formerly with the Health One Corporation, where she was responsible for senior housing and home care operations as well as planning, developing, and implementing new programs for older adults. She has been active in many professional organizations, has published several articles on marketing older adult services, and has made numerous presentations around the country on this topic.

Rein Tideiksaar, Ph.D., is an assistant professor of geriatrics in the Gerald and May Ellen Ritter Department of Geriatrics and Adult Development, the Mount Sinai Medical Center, New York City, and director of its Falls and Immobility Program. He is on the geriatric faculty at the Jewish Home and Hospital for Aged, New York City, where he participates in a falls consulting service. He is also a visiting clinical assistant professor in the Department of Geriatric Medicine, the New York College of Osteopathic Medicine, Long Island.

Anne H. Williams, R.N., is manager of the Patient and Family Services Department at Craven Regional Medical Center, New Bern, North Carolina. The department's responsibilities include CAP case management, discharge planning, social services, utilization review, private case management, personal care, an information and referral case-management pilot program, and a Gold Care membership program. Mrs. Williams is a board member of the North Carolina Association of Continuity of Care. Her past experience includes conducting a research program for the University of North Carolina on older adults.

Jay Wolfson, Dr.P.H., is director of the Florida Public Health Information Center and associate professor of Health Care Finance and Policy at the College of Public Health, University of South Florida in Tampa, where he also has served as acting department chairman for the Department of Health Policy and Management. He is a trustee of the Tampa General Hospital and is vice-president of Health Cost Management, Inc., a consulting and technical assistance firm. He has published extensively on topics ranging from the evaluation of managed health care systems to the financing of health services in Japan. He was a W. K. Kellogg Fellow in Health Care Finance and a Senior Fulbright Fellow at the University of Tokyo and the National Institute of Public Health in Japan. He has been on the faculties of the University of Texas, the University of South Carolina, the University of Oklahoma, and the University of Tokyo.

William Zubkoff, Ph.D., M.P.H., is chief executive officer, South Shore Hospital and Medical Center, Miami Beach, and professor, Department of Family Medicine and Community Health, University of Miami.

Under Dr. Zubkoff's leadership, South Shore Hospital and Medical Center has become a model for the care of the elderly. Dr. Zubkoff has numerous publications in hospital literature and has spoken at various national conferences and teleconferences regarding hospitals and the elderly.

Preface

Stanley J. Brody and I wrote *Hospitals and the Aged: The New Old Market* in 1984, because we believed that hospitals had a role to play in ensuring the well-being of older Americans that went beyond the acute-care medical model. We attempted to prove the thesis that the general hospital has a central role in the long-term care system. With thoughtful reevaluation of their mission within the greater social evolution of their communities, hospitals can take their rightful place as leaders in the health care system that offers a continuum of services: preventive, acute, transitional, and long-term care.

Now, years later, *Eldercare: Positioning Your Hospital for the Future* further develops this thesis to respond to recent changes in the health care marketplace. Since the development of DRGs, a myriad of changes have had a profound effect on the way hospitals and physicians conduct their business. Both government restrictions and developments among third-party payers continue to force hospitals and other health care organizations to evaluate their markets and make choices. Health care choices for the consumer are being changed by insurance companies and employers, and competition in the health care market continues to increase as new players provide services formerly offered exclusively in the hospital setting. During this same time, the demand for inpatient care has declined for all but the elderly–making them a prime market for all health care providers.

Demographics continue to reinforce the fact that older adults are today's market–and even more so–tomorrow's. This book addresses the hospital's new old responsibility: to care for older adults through the health care continuum. As disability rather than age becomes the calibration for determining health status of the chronically ill, new definitions of long-term services for the aging population are provided within the context of continuity of care.

Part One of this book presents three elements of discussion regarding the future of eldercare. The first element describes the changing profile of the older population and its impact on hospital care. It further reviews the changing nature of medicine and eldercare services and discusses the process of moving the acute care hospital toward continuity of care. The second element discusses service options for providing continuity of care for the elderly and organizational structures for developing these marketing initiatives. This section also reviews the importance of patient assessment and case management and examines its role as the linchpin around which all services for the elderly are provided. The third element discusses the financing of eldercare services, thus providing a practical orientation to the process and a rationale for developing innovative programming. An in-depth discussion of the corporate response to aging America and the hospital's role in interfacing with corporations to provide services for the elderly and their care givers also is included.

Part Two presents 14 case studies of institutions that not only have already addressed their roles in providing health care services to the elderly but have gone far beyond the acute-care model in providing a continuum of care. These case studies represent rural and urban hospitals under private and public auspices. Some are small independent facilities whereas others are members of larger systems. Several of the case examples were sites of the Robert Wood Johnson Foundation's *Program for Hospital Initiatives in Long-Term Care.* Others were facilities that received no initial grants to develop their eldercare programming but were just as committed to providing integrated services for their elderly citizens.

Finally, the authors have included a bibliography for the reader's use. This, we hope, can further aid you in the process of understanding the impact of the older adult market and the potential for eldercare services.

Acknowledgments

Each institution represented by the case studies has attempted to share its developmental process with the reader and has freely discussed its marketing successes and frustrations. These institutions and authors were chosen because of their keen recognition of the hospital's role as a health care center, not just an acute-care provider. I am very grateful to all of those who generously shared their experiences with us.

I am grateful also to my colleagues Drs. Carolee DeVito, William Zubkoff, Peter Levin, and Jay Wolfson for their contributions to this text in providing innovative approaches to programming and financing.

A very special thanks and recognition must go to my former associate, Sonya R. Albury, whose work has been integral to the completion of this book. In her role as office manager and administrative assistant, Nancy Hallford typed numerous drafts of the manuscript. Her work was critical and much appreciated.

Finally I want to thank four people to whom this book is dedicated: My mother, who always taught me that a woman could accomplish anything she wished. My children, Meredith and Nathaniel, who have been a source of great pride and encouragement. With their support I was able to complete this book as well as continue my commitment to my career and dedication to the elderly and disabled. Above all I shall always be grateful to my late husband Andrew, who believed in the value of my work and the importance of my writing and teaching. He filled my life with love and laughter.

Part One

Hospitals and the Elderly: The Future in Eldercare

Chapter 1

Tomorrow's Eldercare Challenges

Nancy Alfred Persily

In his book *Seed for Thought* (1949) Charles Franklin Kettering said, "We should all be concerned about the future because we will have to spend the rest of our lives there." Concern about the future is nothing new. What is truly a cause for concern is that health care planners and administrators are having more difficulty than ever in predicting the health care scene of the 1990s and beyond. As Tom Peters said in *Thriving on Chaos,* "Predictability is a thing of the past."[1] For example, no one would have predicted the backlash by some older adults that forced Congress to repeal the Medicare Catastrophic Coverage Act in 1989. Although Congress has become somewhat gun-shy after this repeal, according to a congressional staffer it recognized that "No politician can afford to ignore an important interest group that votes like crazy."[2] And no health care institution, regardless of restrictions on Medicare and shrinking reimbursement, can ignore older Americans, the one group that uses health care services "like crazy."

Hospitals today face many challenges. They can grow, stay the same size, reevaluate the nature of the services they provide, joint venture with physicians and other groups, merge with another institution, go out of business, or change their business to respond to change within their community and competition from other hospitals that provide better, more cost-effective service.

What will be profitable for hospitals in the 1990s are programs that also will profit the patient. Entrepreneurial programs that take a fresh look at ways to serve people may be risky, but they have a greater opportunity for success than the "me-too" programs that follow the nearest hospital for no reason other than to "keep up with the Joneses."

The elderly market is the largest group of health care consumers. Throughout many civilized cultures it has been said often that the way a people treat their elderly is a reflection on their society. In health care, how effectively hospitals care for the elderly reflects how effectively they care for all patients. Hospitals that pay attention to the individual, to continuity of care, to quality, to service, and to their reputations and those who can make or break them can do well in any market.

The 1990s will not tolerate business as usual. Hospitals that want to be around at the turn of the century or next year must begin *now* to explore their potential to change with the environment—to survive and thrive. They must examine the elderly market and reevaluate their service options in order to capture that market. For example, because tomorrow's older adults did not experience the economic turmoil or losses of a Great Depression, they will not have the same fear of poverty as previous generations and generally will be better off. Consequently, they will be willing to spend money for their health, happiness, and welfare.[3]

As a growing market for health care services, these older consumers will play a major role in every hospital's economic viability. However, the rush to capture that market without appropriate research and a strategic plan could lead to fragmented services, lack of continuity of care, and—perhaps most important to the consumer—a downslide in quality. To succeed in the 1990s, hospitals will need to develop a multiple strategy. That is, health care institutions of the future must be sensitive to the need for service and high-quality care, maintain a strong reputation, operate proactively and innovatively, and respond to community needs.

Be Service- and Quality-Conscious

People of the 1990s will be more service-conscious and want providers to be more responsive to their general needs and wants. This decade's bywords will be *sharing* and *caring*. Although patients know that hospitals will provide high-tech services, they also will expect them to be equally concerned with "high touch."

Due to competition in the health care marketplace, hospitals are forced to promise the consumer "service." However, this concern often is underrated when hospitals plan their strategies, and administration would do well to treat the older person as an "appreciating asset."[4] Because people need more health care as they age, hospital administrators and care givers must recognize that the elderly (along with their families) are potential "repeat customers." This view can and should carry over into the practice of hiring appropriate personnel and training them properly to care for elderly patients. It also redefines each element of the caring process to determine which facilities and services the hospital should provide and how they should be delivered.

Quality, measured by more than just the professional competence of care providers, reaches across all levels of care and requires continuity.

For instance, if an older person receives state-of-the-art acute care and then is discharged without proper supportive aftercare services, clearly there is a gap in quality of care.

High-quality medical care also requires personal acceptability. Patients and/or families will not cooperate effectively if they are not involved in the decision-making process. Hospitals must involve patients and families in the treatment process, and that process does not end at the hospital door. This people-centered care relies on a continuous relationship with providers who coordinate care within the hospital and with providers outside in the community once a patient is discharged. Thus, within the context of high-quality health care for older persons, a complete range of personal health and support services should be provided. By responding to older persons' needs, you also meet the needs of family members, who often are the ultimate determiners of quality of care for older persons and other family members.

Maintain a Strong Reputation

Referring to a particular hospital as "the hospital that cares" may sound old-fashioned, but a hospital's reputation is paramount. Hospitals have overrelied on the mass media to advertise their products and underrelied on informal word of mouth to promote their institutions and services. However, word of mouth allows hospitals to rely on patients and families who have had positive experiences from their prehospital care. Their testimonials provide the best chance of gaining long-term recognition for providing these services. Such reputational "campaigns" are the keystone for launching any real promotional effort. Targets for a reputational campaign include the elderly patient, the family, physicians, employees, governing board members, affiliated and networking organizations, and corporations.

The Elderly Patient

Older people are very concerned with their health and often discuss their health care experiences with friends and family. Their assessment of high-quality care goes beyond simply noticing a hospital's state-of-the-art technology and is based on their total experience, from preadmission to discharge and postdischarge. Older adults want to be treated with dignity while they are hospitalized and enjoy amenities such as special dinners, patient relations visitations, medical claims assistance, and other services that can reduce their anxiety during and following hospitalization.

The Family

Because the family often is involved with the care of an older relative, responding to family needs as well as those of the patient can provide positive spin-offs. A hospital that cares well for older adults is recognized as a facility that cares for everyone, not as a "hospital for old people," and will attract patients from a broad age spectrum.

Physicians

Physicians have been in the driver's seat lately in successfully competing with hospitals to provide a significant share of health care services. Like hospitals, however, they are challenged by new reimbursement systems–many of which are connected to caring for their older patients. As hospitals work with physicians in partnership and provide them with the tools and support needed to manage their older patients, the physicians will be more likely to refer patients to the hospital and will be vital to enhancing the hospital's image and reputation. Thus, the hospital must engage physicians in the management process–both in caring for patients as well as in managing patient care.

Employees

Just as the medical staff affects morale, reputation, and the bottom line, so can hospital employees. As hospitals provide educational opportunities and integrate the staff into the care management process and the continuum of care, employees will become energized by the opportunity to provide high-quality care. The work force is the hospital's key marketing agent both internally and externally. Staff who feel appreciated and personally fulfilled will be more sensitive to patient needs and more likely to promote the hospital's programs to their friends in the community. Special staff training in eldercare will enhance understanding and appreciation of this growing market. Furthermore, providing the employee with information–both clinical data and social data on patients–will help employees who are closest to the patient manage their care more appropriately. Employees' contribution to the bottom line can be tracked by improvements they make in helping to streamline operations, reduce employee burnout and turnover, and foster a positive community image.

Governing Board Members

Often, the governing board is closely linked to the greater community. Educating board members in continuity of care can be a positive force for spreading the word to outside groups. Board members also are important in garnering legislative and other political support for programming, zoning, and reimbursement. Most important, the board should be involved in the hospital as an effective ally. When board members are provided with appropriate information and kept abreast of new programming initiatives, they can be an effective force in promoting continuity of care—within the hospital as well as in developing linkages with aftercare programs or supporting the development of such programs by the hospital itself.

Affiliated and Networking Organizations

Community organizations often are frustrated with the lack of information received regarding patients cared for in the hospital. Developing linkages with other organizations—for example, social services agencies, long-term care facilities, nursing homes, and home health agencies—requires more than just a transfer agreement. Providing information on patients to other organizations through the assessment and care plan process and helping to make ongoing care accessible will ensure closer linkages with these organizations. Enhancing this relationship with community-based providers will bring in new patients and ensure that former patients will not be lost outside the hospital system.

Corporations

Corporate America pays billions of dollars each year for health care. By making direct contact with area employers not only for medical care services but for the whole variety of supportive services (as discussed in chapter 8), a hospital prepared to respond to corporate needs gains important allies and an important market share.

Be Proactive and Foster Innovation

Hospitals have come a long way in the 20th century, from religious and not-for-profit organizations helping to care for the ill and dying to modern businesses marketing diverse health care services to a variety of target audiences. Yet as we approach the turn of the century, much room still remains for original thinking within the broad spectrum of health care services.

In determining direction and managing operations, flexible administrations must take the leadership role in creating a top–down, bottom–up attitude that promotes continuity of care. The astute administrator of the 1990s and beyond will be *proactive*—that is, reward innovation, encourage risk taking, develop creative solutions to meeting patient needs, and compete effectively in this new health care environment. By capitalizing on trends, eliminating duplication and excess capacity, and responding to patient needs and demands, the conscientious hospital manager of the 1990s can help ensure success in this environment.

Quick response to change is essential. However, quick response does not negate the responsibility to conduct market research and feasibility studies for new products and services or to have the appropriate facilities and people in place. It does, however, require management and the board to take chances, to surge ahead of the competition. The most efficient and effective route to promoting change is to encourage everyone—patients, staff, physicians, the governing board, management, and the community—to participate.

Developing any new program within or outside the hospital requires a certain amount of risk. Although management tries to minimize risk, nothing is risk free. Therefore, it is important for senior management and governing board members to accept the possibility of failure but not be paralyzed by fear of embarking on a new venture.

Be Responsive to Your Community

The hospital's mission extends far beyond its walls to provide health care services to its surrounding community. As Bruce Vladeck, president of New York City's United Hospital Fund, said, "One thing the advocates of competition missed is that hospitals don't live in markets, they live in communities. . . . Over time, the most successful hospitals are those that provide the best service to their communities—and are recognized as such."[5]

Developing a community focus requires the hospital to become more involved with the world around it, guided by an administrator who is creative and flexible enough to respond to community needs. A close look at the community should reveal areas where the hospital can be of most help and where its efforts can be most rewarding in terms of securing a work force, bonding patients to the hospital, and opening up windows of opportunity for new business ventures. Opportunities may include involvement with socioeconomic development, for example, as in the Greater Southeast Center for the Aging, where involvement with socioeconomic development helped the community and the hospital. As part of the Greater Southeast Healthcare System, the center built 69 housing units for the elderly in their community. In fact, Greater Southeast has become the largest low-income housing developer in Washington, D.C.[6] Housing for the elderly was a normal extension of the services developed by the Greater Southeast Center for the Aging (see chapter 12). The center protected its essential health care services, provided another vehicle for referrals into the hospital, and provided a catalyst to bring community groups together to focus on the health and human services needs of the greater community.

Other hospitals have extended their mission into the community by providing training programs for care givers, setting up hypertension screening programs at churches and housing projects, and providing the management expertise and computer data base for a service credit program. *Service credit* is essentially a system where the elderly themselves provide basic services to each other such as companionship, homemaking, transportation, and so forth. These services are provided by volunteers who in turn accrue hours of service credit they may need in the future.

When a partnership between hospitals and communities is created, community leaders become hospital advocates, supporting the hospital in all sorts of political arenas (zoning, additional funds for indigent care, and elderly housing, for example).

Summary

Hospitals in the 1990s will need to focus market research and service efforts on the growing elderly market. A multiple management strategy will help health care institutions succeed in the future with this market. Hospitals will need to be quality- and service-conscious, maintain a strong reputation, keep their board, employees, and physicians informed, be proactive and innovative, and be responsive to community needs. Most important, hospitals must adopt a new definition of health care, one that transcends the traditional role of hospitals and focuses on continuity of care.

References

1. Peters, T. J. *Thriving on Chaos.* New York City: Harper & Row, 1987, p. 11.
2. Schorr, B. Senior backlash over Medicare stymies Congress. *Medical Business, South Florida Edition* 3(1):13, Jan. 2, 1990.
3. Brody, S. J., and Persily, N. A., editors. *Hospitals and the Aged: The New Old Market.* Rockville, MD: Aspen Publishers, 1984.
4. Peters, p. 120.
5. Johnson, J. Providers link health with human services. *Hospitals* 64(1):34, Jan. 5, 1990.
6. Johnson, pp. 35–37.

Chapter 2

The Growing Elderly Population and Health Care Utilization

Nancy Alfred Persily and Sonya R. Albury

Health care for the 1990s and beyond will be affected significantly by this nation's growing elderly population. For most of this century, the elderly population has grown more rapidly than any other age segment. The future indicates a similar trend between 1990 and well into the 21st century. This chapter lays the framework for eldercare services in tomorrow's market by demystifying the elderly population and determining their future impact on the health care system of tomorrow. The health status of the elderly and their health care utilization patterns will be explored, followed by an examination of how older adults view their own needs for the future. This book will use the terms *elderly* and *older adults* to refer to those age 65 or over.

An Aging Society

We live in an aging society. This trend has occurred because the number of young adults in the United States is shrinking while at the same time, the population of middle-age and elderly persons is rapidly increasing.[1]

Although the number of young adults age 18 to 24 years peaked in the early 1980s, this population is projected to decline by 12 percent during the 1990s.[2] During the same decade, the elderly population age 65 and over is projected to increase by 11 percent. The very old, those age 85 and over, will grow by 42 percent during the same period.[3] By the year 2011, the growth rate of the elderly population will dwarf the gains of the 1990s as the baby boomers start to hit age 65. For example, the 75 million baby boomers represent all Americans born between 1946 and 1964.[4] This powerful demographic tide will be followed by the baby bust, persons born between 1965 and 1976. Right now the baby boomers are between ages 26 and 44 years, and the baby-bust generation is 14 to 25 years of age.[5]

Although tomorrow's elderly population will certainly be larger than today's, it will not necessarily have the same characteristics. If tomorrow's elderly were the same as today's elderly, we would simply need to offer more and more of the same health care programs and services currently provided to the very old. This would create such a demand that no country could bear the financial burden.

Fortunately it does not seem likely that this will occur. The demographic, psychographic, and physical attributes of the elderly will not remain constant but will change with the times as shared attitudes and values carried by one generation are transformed by the next. Thus as Great Depression babies, baby boomers, and baby busters move through the life cycle, it is essential that planners for the future understand the attitudinal and behavioral traits as well as the improved physical health that characterize each generation. These individual improvements, coupled with economic and political changes, can create a whole new demographic profile.

There are sharp contrasts within the older adult market. Older adults represent a dynamic growing segment of the population with a diversity of interests, health statuses, and service needs. It is no more appropriate to lump together all persons age 65 to 85 than it would be to do the same for persons age 15 to 35. Because the older adult population includes the infirm nursing home resident as well as the active world traveler, it is difficult to articulate marketing messages that will reach all older persons clearly and effectively. The challenge, then, is to get to know tomorrow's older adult market: What are their health care needs, wants, and special interests? How can the health care industry respond to this growing population, and what will this new demography mean to health care providers of the future?

To understand where the elderly are headed, it is important to know the history of this population's emergence as a major patient market in the health care environment, their current economic status, patterns of longevity, and health status.

Population Size and Growth

At the turn of the century, only 4 percent of all Americans were age 65 or older. This percentage doubled by 1950, totaling over 12 million people, or 8.1 percent. By 1987 approximately 30 million older Americans were at least age 65, representing approximately 12 percent of the total population.[6]

In the next decade, growth of the over-65 population will slow, and then the pace will quicken again after the turn of the century as post-war baby boomers enter the ranks of older citizens. During the early part of the 21st century, the baby boomers will create a more dramatic increase in the numbers of elderly than experienced to date, with nearly one out of every five Americans reaching age 65 or older. By 2020, the elderly population (age 65 and older) will reach 52 million, and by 2030 the full impact of the graying of the baby boomers will be felt, when over 65 million persons will make up the elderly population. This climb from 13 percent of the total population in 2000 to nearly 22 percent by 2030 is charted in table 2-1.[7]

The unprecedented growth in the older population is demonstrated most dramatically among those age 85 and over (known as the *very old*). In 1950, more than a half million people in the United States were in this age group. By the turn of the century, however, the U.S. Census Bureau projects they will number nearly 5 million. Over a half century, the number of persons age 85 and over will have increased by a striking 700 percent.[8]

Despite their growing population size, very little is known about our oldest Americans. Until recently there were so few that no one paid them much attention. Persons age 85 and over currently represent 10 percent of the elderly population but will account for 13 percent by the end of the century. In fact, this group is expected to triple in size between 1980 and the year 2020, from 2.2 million to over 6.6 million.[9] The explosive growth of the very old is partly due to improved health care and better nutrition. With the advent of Medicare and Medicaid, there has been greater access to health care, and advanced medical technology has contributed and will continue to contribute to increased longevity.

Although the medical advances of today are significant, it is important to anticipate what the impact might be for tomorrow's health care delivery system. We already know that the very old are heavy users of health care. If current rates persist, the expected population growth among this group could strain the economy substantially. Efforts must be made to control the costs of delivering health care, and use of the health care system must change.[10] Avenues must be sought not only to increase life expectancy but also quality of life (or the "active" life span). Providers will need to develop high-touch *and* high-tech services to create a system that is market sensitive, effective, and of high quality.

Economic Status

Much has been said about the economic plight of the elderly and the need for long-term care services. The literature is replete with information on the economic woes of "spending down" one's assets and the burden imposed on limited resources by catastrophic illnesses. Most older adults in need of long-term care services (especially nursing home care) initially pay for this care with their own resources, which they often

Table 2-1. Actual and Projected Growth of the Older Population: 1900–2050 (in thousands)

Year	Total Population All Ages	55 to 64 years		65 to 74 years		75 to 84 years		85 years and older		65 years and older	
		Number	Percent	Number	Percent	Number	Percent	Number	Percent	Number	Percent
1900	76,303	4,009	5.3	2,189	2.9	772	1.0	123	0.2	3,084	4.0
1910	91,972	5,054	5.5	2,793	3.0	989	1.1	167	.2	3,950	4.3
1920	105,711	6,532	6.2	3,464	3.3	1,259	1.2	210	.2	4,933	4.7
1930	122,775	8,397	6.8	4,721	3.8	1,641	1.3	272	.2	6,634	5.4
1940	131,669	10,572	8.0	6,375	4.8	2,278	1.7	365	.3	9,019	6.8
1950	150,967	13,295	8.8	8,415	5.6	3,278	2.2	577	.4	12,270	8.1
1960	179,323	15,572	8.7	10,997	6.1	4,633	2.6	929	.5	16,560	9.2
1970	203,302	18,608	9.2	12,447	6.1	6,124	3.0	1,409	.7	19,980	9.8
1980	226,505	21,700	9.6	15,578	6.9	7,727	3.4	2,240	1.0	25,544	11.3
1990	250,410	21,364	8.5	18,373	7.3	9,933	3.9	3,254	1.3	31,559	12.6
2000	268,266	24,158	9.0	18,243	6.8	12,017	4.5	4,622	1.7	34,882	13.0
2010	282,575	35,430	12.5	21,039	7.4	12,208	4.3	6,115	2.2	39,362	13.9
2020	294,364	41,087	14.0	30,973	10.5	14,443	5.0	6,651	2.3	52,067	17.7
2030	300,629	34,947	11.6	35,988	12.0	21,487	7.1	8,129	2.7	65,604	21.8
2040	301,807	35,537	11.8	30,808	10.2	25,050	8.3	12,251	4.1	68,109	22.6
2050	299,849	37,004	12.3	31,591	10.5	21,655	7.2	15,287	5.1	68,532	22.9

Source: Projections are from Spencer, G. U.S. Bureau of the Census. *Projections of the Population of the United States, by Age, Sex, and Race: 1988 to 2080.* Current Population Reports Series P-25, No. 1018, Jan. 1989. 1900 to 1980 data tabulated from the Decennial Censuses of the Population, as reprinted in Special Committee on Aging. *Aging America: Trends and Projections,* (Washington, DC: U.S. Government Printing Office, 1989), p. 4.

deplete very quickly; that is, they "spend down" to the level of Medicaid eligibility. Concurrent with this phenomenon is a growing recognition of the elderly as a largely affluent consumer market to be targeted for new programs and services. This marketing strategy was coined by Estes (1979) more than a decade ago as "the aging enterprise," and there has been a plethora of activity to target this market with books, newsletters, and articles titled along the lines of "Selling to Seniors" and "The Mature Market Report."[11]

Marketing products to the elderly blossomed with the discovery that persons ages 55 and older control from one-third to one-half of the nation's discretionary income.[12] The elderly as a group have experienced significant gains in income, and some three-quarters own their own homes. Many also have impressive financial assets. For example, although they represent only 12 percent of the population, the elderly account for 40 percent of the total financial assets held by U.S. families.[13]

Given these disparate views of the economic status of the elderly, there is sure to be some confusion; yet both views are essentially valid. The truth is, the economic status of the elderly population varies substantially within its own ranks. There is a tremendous income variation within the elderly cohort, more than that experienced by any other age group. Average income statistics conceal the polarization of these groups, with many high-income elderly yet a large cluster of older adults just above the poverty level.[14]

To be sure, the elderly have made great economic gains over the past several years, particularly in relation to their younger age cohorts. One major influence has been the rise in Social Security benefits. Since 1970, benefits increased 46 percent in real terms, whereas the inflation-adjusted wages of the rest of the population decreased by 7 percent.[15] Consequently the gap in income between the elderly and nonelderly has been narrowed significantly. In fact, whereas the overall income of the nonelderly is higher, the elderly—having the highest discretionary income of any age group—are a little less likely to be poor than the rest of the adult population.[16]

At the other end of the spectrum, however, is a large concentration of persons age 65 and over who have incomes just above the poverty level.[17] According to U.S. census data, nearly 43 percent of the elderly live below 200 percent of the poverty line. The very old (persons age 85 and over) are more likely to fall in these low-income categories.[18] Because this is the fastest-growing population group in the country and is likely to create an enormous demand for long-term care, there is sure to be an impact on health care providers of the future. At the same time, it is important to consider that tomorrow's very old will not likely be the impoverished persons they are today. For example, more older women will receive Social Security benefits from both their husbands' and their own labor force participation. The typical 85-year-old of the future will likely be female and better educated than her predecessors. As a patient, she will have higher expectations regarding quality of care and convenience as well as assets to purchase health care services selectively.

For the next decade, the number of persons age 85 and over will remain relatively small in contrast to the younger elderly (age 55 to 74), although the former will continue to experience rapid growth. Over the next three decades, approximately three-quarters of the mature market will remain those between 55 and 75 years old, the group most likely to be well-off. In 1984, for example, approximately 63 percent of persons between age 55 and 64 had a net worth of $50,000 or higher; over 37 percent of this same group had a net worth of $100,000 or greater. Although these proportions declined with age, over half the elderly age 75 and over still had a net worth of $50,000 or greater during the same period.[19]

Longevity

The prominence of the large younger elderly market will diminish over time as the older age cohorts experience unprecedented growth. The large population of young elderly will increase by a modest 7 percent through the 1990s. In contrast, the population of persons age 75 to 84 is projected to grow by 21 percent, and the population of those 85 and over is expected to increase by 42 percent by 2000.[20] In fact, by the turn of the century, nearly half those over 65 will be over 75 years old.

The average life span of a baby born in 1987 is projected at 75 years, up from 47 years for a baby born at the turn of the century.[21] The increased longevity can be attributed to a number of factors. First, during the first half of this century, dramatic reductions occurred in deaths from infectious disease. Also, infant mortality was greatly reduced and childhood deaths decreased. Since then, more modest increases in life expectancy have been due primarily to decreased mortality among the middle-age and older population.[22]

These trends have led to a growing number of centenarians in our society today, with some surviving even into their eleventh decade. Census estimates show there were about 25,000 people age 100 years or older in 1986 and that by the turn of the century that number will quadruple. Even more dramatic, by the middle of the 21st century there will be one million Americans age 100 or older.[23] Although these changes point to a increasingly large population of the very old, does this mean there will be diametrically similar increases in illness and disease of the elderly? Is it possible that, as one demographer has predicted, we will need to build one new 100-bed nursing home every day for the next eight years just to keep up with the demand?[24] Alternatively, will the elderly live longer and be healthier than ever before? The health status of these much older adults and their younger cohorts will be the key to long-term care needs of the future.

Health Status

There has been much debate about how much care will be necessary for our burgeoning elderly population in the coming decades. According to R. A. Kane and R. L. Kane (1987), conflicting theories about whether there will be an increase or decrease in disability levels probably are accurate on both counts.[25] Current evidence indicates that the elderly today are healthier than prior generations. At the same time, more people are reaching old age with disabilities and functional limitations.[26]

With recent advances in preventive and curative medicine, many older adults are surviving diseases and conditions once considered fatal.[27] The elderly also generally have healthier life-styles than their younger counterparts, which contributes to their favorable health status.[28] Thus it is important to look at the general health status of the elderly as well as the disabled and functionally impaired elderly.

General Health Status of the Elderly

Not only are most elderly relatively healthy, but they perceive themselves to be in good to excellent health. Persons 65 and over are far less likely to exercise than their younger counterparts, but they are also less likely to be overweight or to drink or smoke. Furthermore, their health perceptions are positively correlated with income. For example, 25 percent of those with incomes over $35,000 rate their overall health as excellent in contrast to only 11 percent of those with low incomes (under $10,000).[29]

However, health and ability to function decline with advancing age. Over 80 percent of persons age 65 and over have at least one chronic condition, and the frequency of multiple conditions increases with age.[30] As of 1987, the most common chronic conditions among the elderly were arthritis, heart disease, hypertension, and hearing impairment. Other major debilitating conditions include orthopedic problems or deformities, cataracts, chronic sinusitis, diabetes, tinnitus, and visual impairment (figure 2-1).[31]

Heart disease is the leading cause of death among the elderly and the leading diagnosis for all short-term hospital stays. Whereas gains have been made in reducing the rate of death due to heart disease, it still remains a severe health problem. Heart disease, together with cancer and stroke, accounts for over 75 percent of all deaths among the elderly, 20 percent of doctor visits, and 40 percent of hospital days.[32]

The severity of a disease can differ widely from person to person. One person may be bedbound due to arthritis, whereas another may experience only occasional pain with limited loss of mobility. One way

Figure 2-1. The Top 10 Chronic Conditions for Persons 65 and Over: 1987

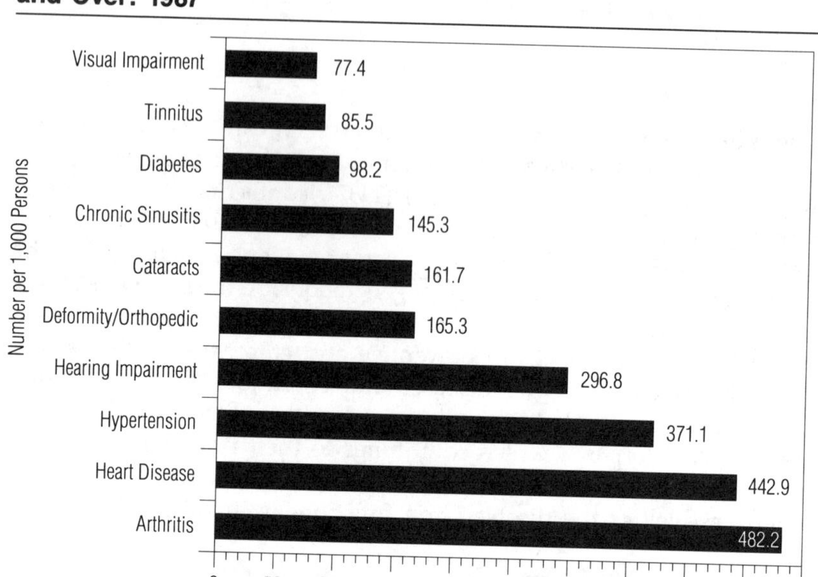

Source: National Center for Health Statistics, Health Interview Survey, 1987, as reprinted in *Aging America: Trends and Projections*, Special Committee on Aging (Washington, DC: U.S. Government Printing Office, 1989), p. 81.

of measuring severity is by examining the number of deficits or conditions that limit an elderly person's ability to function. Referred to as activities of daily living (ADLs), which cover personal care activities, and instrumental activities of daily living (IADLs), which cover home management tasks, these measures are useful in planning eldercare services. (These topics are covered in the section on the disabled elderly later in this chapter.) Women in particular are likely to have difficulties in performing these tasks. However, this may reflect the fact that more women live longer and that many older men do not routinely perform home management tasks, which would place them at lower risk of experiencing health-related difficulties with these activities.

One of the limitations of just examining ADLs is the lack of direct assessment of cognitive impairment. Some health providers include cognitive evaluations in their assessments to address this dimension. Any ADL deficits can be reflective of cognitive functioning but generally are not to be used as the only basis for determining cognitive impairment.[33]

Although various forms of dementia exist, the most widely recognized is Alzheimer's disease. Recent surveys indicate that this mental impairment is much more widespread than previously reported. Based on updated statistics from the National Institute on Aging (NIA), an estimated 4 million Americans are afflicted with Alzheimer's disease, and the number is expected to increase as the population ages. By the year 2040, the number of cases could reach between 12 and 14 million. Meanwhile, only 4 percent of those age 65 to 74 years have the disease, whereas nearly half of those age 85 or older are affected.[34]

Depression is another major health problem among the elderly. It is estimated that 15 percent of older persons living in the community suffer from symptoms of depression. The elderly often become depressed due to physical conditions that limit their ability to socialize or to live independently. Also, since older adults take more medications than other groups, they tend to suffer from more drug interactions often manifesting themselves through symptoms of depression. Finally, the elderly also experience significant losses (for example, loss of a spouse, loss of friends), which can lead to depression.[35]

At one time, the perception of health care professionals was that older people would not benefit from aggressive psychiatric care, so senility or depression among older adults was considered a normal part of the aging process and therefore not worthy of treatment. More recently, however, psychiatric care has been an acceptable mode of treatment for the elderly. Practitioners find that older adults can benefit from therapeutic interventions and that some conditions are reversible. It is also becoming clear that an older adult's physical health is integrally related to his or her mental health. As a result, more physicians realize that psychiatric consultation can have a positive effect on patient outcomes. In addition, the elderly are very responsive to drug therapy; and psychotropic drugs have been especially effective in the treatment of depression as well as other psychiatric disorders.

The Disabled and Functionally Impaired Elderly

According to the World Health Organization (WHO), *disability* can be defined as "any restriction or lack (resulting from an impairment) of ability to perform an activity in the manner considered normal for a human being."[36] This condition may be a result of disease, physical handicap, injury, or genetic defect.[37] Among the elderly, disabilities resulting from these impairments are related predominately to chronic conditions and other late-onset illnesses that limit them with respect to their ADLs.

The forecast for the future is that the elderly will continue to experience disabilities and illnesses for the same amount of time prior to death as the elderly do today. However, as the human life span is extended, onset of disabilities and illnesses will occur at a later age. Therefore, it would be inappropriate simply to calculate arithmetically the need for future nursing home beds by applying the present use rate to population projections. In fact, population projections of catastrophic growth among the disabled elderly do not take into account the changing nature of this population, such as innovations in service provision, future medical and technological advances, and later periods of onset of disability. These factors have contributed to the elderly being healthier and more physically fit than ever before. At the same time, the gross number of disabled has increased, creating greater demands on the health care system.

Many disabilities experienced by the elderly can be correlated with chronological age. For example, only a small proportion of 65- to 74-year-olds are disabled, whereas slightly more than half of the very old—age 85 and over—have at least one disability that limits their ADLs (figure 2-2).[38] For the most part, however, the elderly are functionally independent. In fact, over 75 percent fit this description, whereas only about 5 percent are severely disabled (those who have difficulty performing five or six activities of daily living).[39] The rest suffer limited disability, for example, general mobility problems and difficulty with some personal care activities.

The growing use of terms such as *activities of daily living* marks a shift from an exclusively acute-care orientation in health care to one that includes the prevalence of chronic illness and disability or changes in function, which limit but do not preclude independence. Insurance companies are also moving toward the use of ADL assessments to determine eligibility benefits for enrollees, following the lead of states that already utilize them for gauging benefit use. Activities of daily living,

Figure 2-2. Effects of Age on the Probability of Having an IADL or ADL Disability: 1984–1985

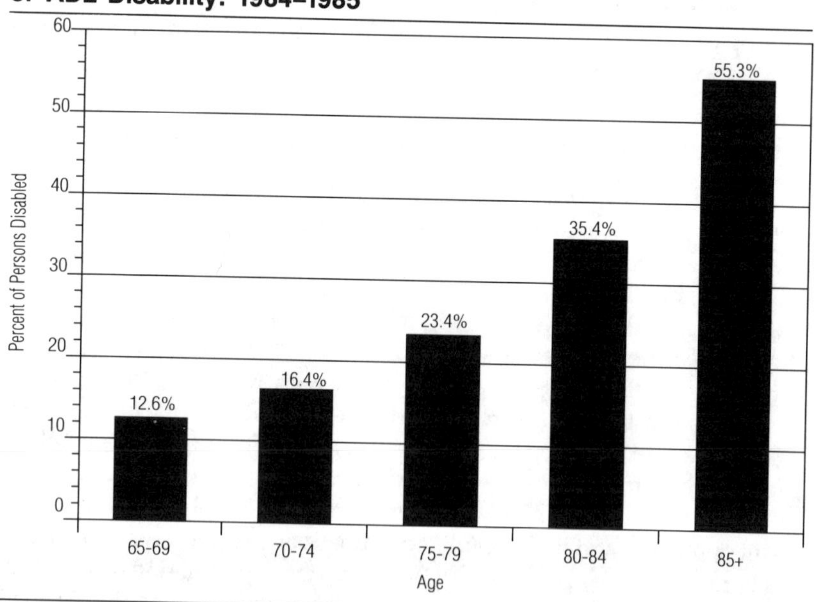

Source: National Long-Term Care Survey and National Nursing Home Survey adapted in Brody, S. J., and Pawlson, L. G., editors. *Geriatrics and Rehabilitation: Common Ground and Conflicts.* New York City: Springer Publishing Co., 1990, p. 25. Reprinted with permission.

therefore, are viewed as objective criteria with measurable components that can be applied consistently over time.[40]

The *activities of daily living* used by the federal national data gathering organizations include the following personal care activities: bathing, dressing, using the toilet, eating, transferring (getting into and out of bed or chairs), controlling continence, and regulating mobility. The term *instrumental activities of daily living* usually refers to home-management activities such as using the telephone, shopping, preparing food, housekeeping, doing laundry, using public transportation, taking medications, and managing finances.[41]

Disabilities involving multiple impairments (such as the inability to walk, eat, or dress) result from a number of diseases, often ones that follow an uncertain course. Some are long-term chronic conditions, whereas others can be intermittent over a long period of time. Although certain conditions may have resulted from childhood diseases and traumas, most age-related disabilities result from late onset of diseases or from recent trauma, such as falls or other accidents. A large portion of the elderly suffer from disabilities resulting from medical/surgical interventions that were effective but left them with residual impairments.[42]

The complexity of these disabling conditions makes long-term chronic illness difficult to treat. The chronically disabled population has multiple needs that cut across many health dimensions: medical, emotional, physical, functional, and social. Unfortunately, the acute-care system is largely calibrated by the severity of disease, not by the multiplicity of deficits, and thus is ill-suited to the need for continual care or continuity of care. Furthermore, because the disease itself often is the only focus of the acute-care system, the environmental, psychological, and long-term supportive care needs of the elderly remain largely unaddressed by this health system.

The essence of planning for eldercare health services, however, is the provision of continual care, not an attempt only to cure or treat the disease. The health care system must recognize the continued lifelong support needed to manage interactive chronic conditions among the elderly, throughout the varying stages of disease and illness. Providers of high-quality care to the chronically disabled must accept the limitations of the disabled and coordinate care with the realities of the physical and social environments in which they live. More care than cure may be required for complex problems. The goal of all health care should be to restore the individual's former level of functioning or maximize his or her remaining function, and to help the elderly continue to live the fullest lives possible.

Health Services Utilization

On average, elderly persons visit a physician eight times a year, in contrast to the general population, who visit physicians only five times annually.

Older adults are admitted to the hospital three times as often as the nonelderly, stay 50 percent longer, and use twice as many prescription drugs.[43]

General Health Care Consumption

Although the introduction of diagnosis-related groups (DRGs) was effective in mitigating the growth of health care costs—especially for hospital inpatient procedures—the United States has continued to experience rises in health care expenditures. Between 1977 and 1987, total personal health care expenditures tripled, from $150.3 billion to $447.0 billion. Some of this increase can be attributed to the growing number of persons age 65 and over, whose consumption of health care grew at an average annual rate of 13.6 percent, reaching $162.0 billion in 1987. Although the elderly represented only 12 percent of the population, they consumed 36 percent of all personal health care in 1987, up from 30 percent in 1977. The elderly population's impact on health care is even more evident when one considers that the elderly consume four times as much health care as the rest of the population.[44]

Hospital Usage

Hospital admissions for those over age 65 usually are for acute episodes of one or more chronic illnesses. In 1986, the most frequent diagnoses for these elderly were diseases of the circulatory system (31 percent), which include heart disease. Other major causes of hospitalization include digestive diseases (12 percent), respiratory diseases including pneumonia (11 percent), and neoplasms (10 percent). Although these were the primary diagnoses, the elderly have about 4 diagnoses per hospital discharge, whereas younger patients average only 2.5 diagnoses.[45]

It is not surprising, then, that the elderly account for a disproportionate share of hospital days. In 1986, persons 65 and over accounted for 31 percent of all hospital discharges and 42 percent of all short-stay days of care but represented only 12 percent of the population. For persons 75 and over, the rate of hospital utilization was even more dramatic. Although only 5 percent of the population was age 75 or older in 1986, this group accounted for 16 percent of hospital discharges and 23 percent of all hospital days.[46]

Coupled with this pattern of high utilization among the elderly, significant changes have occurred in health care utilization. Between 1975 and 1985, hospital admission rates, lengths of stay, and inpatient days declined for all ages. Most of the decrease in these rates was directly attributable to persons under age 65, a group that experienced a 14.6 percent decline in admissions alone. Lengths of stay decreased for the elderly, but their admission rates rose steadily from 1975 until 1983. Then with the advent of DRGs, admissions and lengths of stay declined for the older population as well as for their younger age cohorts.[47] By 1985, however, the decline in elderly admissions had steadied, whereas lengths of stay continued to fall. Admissions among persons age 65 and over are climbing once again, but lengths of stay continue to drop at a moderate pace.[48]

Physician Service Utilization

Physician service utilization also increases as people age. Those age 45 to 64 visit their physicians about 6 times a year, whereas persons 65 to 74 average 8 contacts and those 75 years or older see their physicians approximately 10 times each year. Among those age 75 and older, approximately 88 percent reported visiting their physician at least once during 1986, a number only slightly higher than the 83 percent of 65- to 74-year-olds who reported seeing their physician during the same period. Therefore, the likelihood of physician contact increases only slightly with age, but the frequency intensifies with age.[49]

The continued aging of America will create a greater demand on physician services. Estimates by the Administration on Aging project that for persons 65 and over, the demand for physician contact will increase by 21 percent between 1987 and 2000. For those persons age 75 and over, the demand will increase by over 50 percent. Between 1987 and 2030, the increase will more than double for all older persons.[50]

Nursing Home Stays

Another key component of eldercare is nursing home care. Whereas only 5 percent of the elderly are in a nursing home at any given time, each person reaching age 65 has a 36 to 63 percent chance of entering a nursing home sometime during his or her lifetime.[51]

Nursing home residents are disproportionately very old, female, and white. The vast majority (84 percent) are without a spouse, in contrast to 45 percent of those in the community. One out of three nursing home residents also have no children, compared with fewer than one in five of the noninstitutionalized elderly. These data suggest that among other social indicators, the absence of family members or informal supports can be the most decisive factor in the institutionalization of an older person.[52]

The utilization of nursing home care is changing, however. The 1985 National Nursing Home Survey indicates that a little over half of all nursing home residents stay in a nursing home for 90 days or less. These elderly often require a recuperative period to regain normal functioning following a period of hospitalization. They no longer require hospitalization, but are too ill to return home directly. Most of the residents (62 percent) do not remain in a facility beyond 179 days.[53] Although some die, many others return home after a short-term stay for convalescent or rehabilitative care.

Married individuals have a better chance of returning home. According to one study, a married person has a 1-in-3 chance of leaving a nursing home within 29 days, but for an unmarried individual the probability is 1 in 5, accentuating the importance of informal supports (table 2-2).[54] Based on these data, the implication for nursing homes is that many long-stay residents are unmarried individuals without adequate informal or formal support systems. Many are single women who must remain in a nursing home indefinitely or until adequate planning and provision of support services is initiated.

The Elderly as an Opportunity Market

The elderly are becoming the opportunity market of the future. Throughout the 1990s the number of persons age 50 and older will grow by 18.5 percent and by the end of the decade will number 76 million.[55] For the first time in American history, the elderly population exceeds the number of teenagers, and businesses compete feverishly to tap this older market by tailoring marketing messages to an older population and by developing eldercare products and services.

Table 2-2. Nursing Home Length of Stay Probabilities by Age of Entry and Marital Status (in percentages)

	Married			Unmarried		
Length of Stay (in days)	65 to 74	75 to 84	85-plus	65 to 74	75 to 84	85-plus
1 to 29	29	32	30	21	20	19
30 to 59	13	14	14	12	11	10
60 to 89	8	5	5	7	5	6
90 to 179	14	10	9	10	10	12
180 to 364	11	9	10	9	12	12
365 to 729	8	10	10	9	11	13
730 to 1,094	6	4	5	7	7	8
1,095 to 1,469	3	3	4	4	6	6
1,470 to 1,824	3	2	5	3	4	4
1,825 to 2,189	2	3	2	3	3	3
2,190 plus	4	7	6	15	10	9
Total	100	100	100	100	100	100

Source: Brookings Institution and Lewin/ICF calculations using data from the 1985 National Nursing Home Survey, as reprinted in Special Committee on Aging. *Aging America: Trends and Projections* (Washington, DC: U.S. Government Printing Office, 1989), p. 98.

Marketing Messages to the Elderly

Many companies, eager to cash in on this growing market, have aimed their products and marketing messages to the older population; but in their haste they developed new products without consulting their targets. However, they soon learned that in order to hit the bull's-eye, so to speak, they had to understand the needs and perceptions of older Americans.

A classic miscalculation on the part of one major company illustrates this type of marketing failure. A well-known maker of baby food, having observed that older adults were purchasing a great deal of conventional baby food, attempted to market a similar product to denture wearers. The new product bombed, however, because if older adults were to purchase "adult" baby food, it would be readily evident to cashiers that they were buying it not for their grandchildren but for themselves.[56] The conclusions to be drawn here are that the elderly do not want their dignity insulted or their noses rubbed in their age status. Most do not perceive themselves as old at all, and with their improved health and wealth, many feel much younger than their age. *Cognitive* age—the age a person feels—should be closely attended to by marketers. In fact, mature adults tend to view themselves as about 10 to 15 years younger than their actual age.

Makers of Affinity shampoo learned this lesson from results of their early advertisements. When first introduced, Affinity was marketed as a shampoo to ward off the effects of aging, which were *assumed* to be negative. Recognizing its mistake, Affinity altered its message to intimate that women can be attractive and alluring at any age. When a positive message of enhancing the beauty of aging was introduced, the market responded and Affinity sales took off.[57]

Another issue to consider when developing marketing messages to the elderly is the importance the older adult market places on life experiences rather than on possessions. Younger people, age 40 or under, tend to spend most of their discretionary dollars on possessions. During their middle years, ages 40 to 60, people generally spend money on catered experiences, for example, restaurants, art shows, sports events, or landscaping services. For persons ages 60 to 80, the emphasis shifts again as possessions and services provide less satisfaction and intangible life experiences become more important. This age group is more likely to spend discretionary income on products and services that enhance personal growth and development. Whatever the product or service, it should create opportunities beyond or in addition to its intrinsic value, such as social and learning opportunities, adding to life enjoyment, or enriching the lives of friends and family. These experiences may include playing a friendly game of cards, taking grandchildren on outings, attending lectures, enjoying a cruise, or touring the country overland.[58]

Conversely, negative advertising that focuses on age and mortality tends to create images that thwart the elderly's sense of well-being. For example, promoting a nursing home as a "rest home" is not nearly as effective as offering a short-term/rehabilitative nursing center. The first message suggests that the elderly want to do nothing further with their lives, whereas the other implies the possibility of regaining wholeness. This is particularly important in American society, where we *are* what we *do*. If a person does nothing in a nursing home, then the perception follows that a person *is* nothing. Because self-esteem is inextricably tied to productivity, the importance of leading a productive life becomes even more critical for retirees, who often find it difficult to contribute actively to their families and communities.

Psychologists recommend that human development continue throughout one's life. Given that the baby boomers are more likely than any prior generation to feel that learning is a lifelong activity, continued opportunities for human development should be afforded all elderly persons. Russian dissident Andrei Sakharov, for instance, proved by his lifestyle and unwavering commitment to his cause that people can be productive throughout the entire life cycle, contributing to society and leaving an ongoing legacy to others.

Desired Products and Services

If positive marketing messages are the key to reaching the elderly, then what are the service needs of the elderly? What "life experiences" can a health care provider offer?

One of the key responses to these questions is that the elderly prefer to live as independently as possible, and needs or preferences can vary among the different age groups. Although those aged 40 to 60 years may prefer to have someone else perform "mundane" tasks (such as laundry), the very old may seek to do these tasks themselves in order to feel "productive."

Because of these variances in age and perspective, a wide range of products and services is desired by today's elderly market. Key eldercare services to be considered include respite care, adult day care, home health services, homemaker services, personal care, and transportation. Even alternative housing options, such as adult congregate living facilities or alternate care facilities, should have as homelike an environment as possible. (These housing options will be described in chapter 3.)

Alternatives to nursing home care will continue to be developed as the elderly seek to remain in the community; yet at times, nursing home care will be inevitable as some elderly become too ill or too frail to be cared for at home. The nursing home experience, although sometimes necessary, does not always have to be a negative or even a long-term experience. With the emergence of new treatment alternatives, better assessment and case management, and improved postdischarge support services, the elderly patient can stay in a skilled nursing facility for a shorter period of time. As a result, short-term long-term care (characterized by a stay of 90 days or less) has become a viable alternative to long-term institutionalization, which usually lasts over 90 days and often for the rest of a person's lifetime.

All nursing homes provide nursing care, medical services, and personal care to persons unable to care for themselves due to illness or infirmity. Nursing homes may be licensed as skilled nursing facilities (SNFs), intermediate-care facilities (ICFs), or a combination of both. Skilled nursing facility beds can also be designated as extended-care facility (ECF) beds, which are certified by Medicare to provide a high level of restorative nursing care and rehabilitative services following hospitalization.

The temporarily needy and frail elderly may have transitory needs, which can be met through short-term institutional convalescent and rehabilitative care. The permanently frail and disabled elderly are not likely to be able to return home from a nursing home and are in need of continuous maintenance care within an institutional setting.

Most elderly will "age in place," meaning that even when they do move into retirement housing or personal care homes, the rule of thumb is that most relocate within 8 to 10 miles of their homes. Migration patterns indicate that long-distance changes usually are made for the purpose of living closer to children. Even retirees who move to the Sun Belt states frequently return to their home state or to their children when they become frail or lose a spouse.

Because they strongly want to remain independent for as long as possible, many elderly will remain in their own homes. Thus a large number will require some type of home care, which may include homemaker assistance, personal care, or transportation; heavy medical care usually is not required.

Special devices to enable the elderly to perform ADLs will continue to be in great demand. The manufacturing of durable medical equipment (DME), such as wheelchairs or home dialysis systems, and simple assistive devices, such as hospital beds, commodes, and walkers, will be a major growth industry in the decades to come.

Because the elderly are concerned with a product or service's ability to serve as an entrée to other experiences, they will be most interested in services that help them maintain dignity, enhance independence, and/or allow more life enjoyment. A short-term rehabilitation program, for example, can enable an elderly person to return home to family and friends. A senior housing complex can afford opportunities to participate in social activities and make new friends. An assistive device, such as a can opener for the handicapped, can allow a person to prepare his or her own meals and remain independent at home.

These same principles apply to hospitalization. The older adult market is most responsive to an environment that is sensitive to their special needs and life-styles. Hospitals frequently spend more on their marketing campaigns (more than $1 billion total in the United States in 1987) than on new program development or inservice training.[59] Hospitals often stop short of actually offering what the marketing messages say they will deliver. Glossy promotional and advertising campaigns are designed to capture the market, but the hospital must deliver on promises once elderly patients are admitted. Older patients can become frustrated when, despite the flashy promises, the system of care and service delivery remains virtually the same.

Hospitals must back up the services being extolled with sound programs that not only attract elderly patients but keep them and their families coming back for future treatment and service. This objective can be achieved by providing programs that truly help the elderly and their care givers through the acute-care process, such as an escort service, help in filing insurance forms, provision of care-giver education programs, and effective assessment and case-management services. The hospital should attempt to make the internal environment "user friendly," which can be done, for example, by making parking accessible to the older patient and providing transportation when necessary. Hospitals also should make sure that brochures are printed for easy reading and even look into providing telephones for the hearing-impaired.

All too often, hospitals lure certain market segments into the hospital, but once they are there, no appropriate accommodations are made for their stay. For instance (an extreme example), one hospital spent $125,000 on an advertising program for its senior membership plan. The advertising money was secured from the social services department budget when the social workers were laid off to free up hospital funds for advertising. Clearly, the hospital was able to bring older patients into the facility, but there was no mechanism in place to aid in planning for postdischarge services.

Looking Ahead

The profile of tomorrow's mature consumer is rapidly changing. Referred to by some as a moving target, the elderly population will be a challenging market to pursue in the coming decades.

As a whole, the elderly market will have many positive attributes. Particularly as the baby boomers come of age, older Americans will be more affluent and better educated. As a group they will have two or more incomes, multiple pensions, better retirement plans, and fewer relatives. They will be in better health and interested in maintaining healthy life-styles. Older consumers will want more information so that they can make informed decisions about their health care choices and alternative treatment settings to fit their varied life-styles.

No Depression era will shape the spending patterns of tomorrow's elderly population—as it did for today's retirees. This new generation of older persons will be used to a higher standard of living and probably will be more prone to spending their income and assets on luxury and convenience items.

Because older women will continue to outlive older men, products and services—including health care—tailored to their needs will capture their interest. Whereas past generations of elderly women lived on modest pensions (often from their husbands), older women of the future will be much more independent and financially secure. They will continue to serve as the gatekeepers of health care and will be much more aware of available alternatives.

Finally, the elderly are generally well-insured and will continue to have health insurance through Medicare. Many will continue to enjoy private insurance through their retirement benefit plans. Long-term care insurance will attract growing interest as consumer knowledge and acceptance increase, as more employers offer these benefits, and as more insurers enter the market with competitive and affordable plans.

Summary

The demographic profile of the elderly will change over the next decade and beyond. It cannot be said merely that increased population growth will require more of the same kinds of services now offered to an aging population. The diversity of the elderly population will challenge all of society to become more creative in health care delivery. The economic status of the elderly varies significantly and will continue to do so in the future. The percentage of elderly at or below the poverty level is decreasing and, on average, those over 65 have the highest level of discretionary disposable income of any age group. However, this does not preclude society from developing methods to protect the aging family from experiencing a variety of medical catastrophes, especially economic ones.[60]

Even though the majority of elderly are functionally independent, the disabled elderly population will continue to grow in terms of absolute numbers. Whatever the functional level or ability, the overall goal of older adults will be to remain as independent as possible. Chronic conditions leading to disabilities will foster the need for long-term care and greater continuity of care. To address this emerging need, the future health care provider will require an interdisciplinary team approach that manages both chronic and acute conditions through an integrated system of care.

References

1. Francese, P. Today's trends, tomorrow's markets. Presentation at "Demographic Outlook: Today's Trends, Tomorrow's Markets." Sent to subscribers of *American Demographics* (June 1, 1988), p. 2.
2. Francese, p. 2.
3. Buglass, K. The business of eldercare. *American Demographics* 11(9):32, Sept. 1989, and Special Committee on Aging, *Aging America: Trends and Projections.* Washington, DC: U.S. Government Printing Office, 1989, p. 4.
4. Longman, P. Justice between generations. *The Atlantic Monthly,* June 1985, p. 73.
5. Information provided pursuant to a conversation with Diane Cristo, research editor, *American Demographics,* Mar. 29, 1990.
6. Special Committee, p. 4.
7. Special Committee, p. 4.
8. Special Committee, p. 4.
9. Special Committee, p. 4.
10. Longino, C. F., Jr. A state by state look at the oldest Americans. *American Demographics* 8(11):39, Nov. 1986.
11. Minkler, M. Gold in gray: reflections on business' discovery of the elderly market. *The Gerontologist* 29(1):17, Feb. 1989.
12. Minkler, p. 18; Francese, p. 3.
13. Minkler, p. 18.
14. Special Committee, p. 25.
15. Minkler, p. 18.
16. Minkler, p. 18.
17. Special Committee, p. 25.
18. Minkler, p. 18.
19. Special Committee, pp. 4, 53.
20. Special Committee, p. 4.
21. Special Committee, p. 13.
22. Special Committee, p. 13.
23. Brody, S. J. Geriatrics and rehabilitation: common ground and conflicts. Presentation at the Conference on Rehabilitation and Geriatric Education: Perspectives and Potential, Dec. 4–7, 1988, p. 1.
24. Francese, p. 3.
25. Kane, R. A., and Kane, R. L. *Long-Term Care: Principles, Programs and Policies.* New York City: Springer Publishing Co., 1987, p. 366.
26. Brody, p. 4.
27. Kane and Kane, p. 366.

28. Special Committee, pp. 77–79.
29. Special Committee, p. 77.
30. Special Committee, p. 80.
31. Special Committee, p. 81.
32. Special Committee, p. 82.
33. McMorran, W. C. Activities of daily living trigger broader benefits. *Contemporary Longterm Care* 12(12):40, Oct. 1989.
34. Research on Alzheimer's disease holds hope for the future. *Alzheimer's and Related Diseases Association* 9(4):1, 7, Winter 1989; Fast facts. *Mature Market* 3(7):7, Aug./Sept. 1989.
35. Special Committee, p. 83.
36. Brody, p. 3.
37. Fox, D. M. Policy and epidemiology: financing health services for the chronically ill and disabled, 1930–1990. *Milbank Quarterly* 67 (supp. 2, part 2), 1989, p. 259.
38. Brody, pp. 7, 8.
39. Brody, p. 4.
40. McMorran, p. 40.
41. Brody, p. 3.
42. Brody, pp. 2, 8.
43. Special Committee, p. 91.
44. Waldo, D. R., and others. Health expenditures by age group, 1977 and 1987. *Medical Benefits* 6(18):2–3, Sept. 30, 1989.
45. Special Committee, pp. 93–94.
46. Special Committee, p. 93.
47. American Hospital Association. *Caring for the Elderly: New Directions for Hospitals.* Chicago: AHA, 1986, p. 91.
48. Special Committee, p. 91.
49. Special Committee, p. 95.
50. Special Committee, pp. 95–96.
51. Liang, J., and Jow-Ching Tu, E. Estimating lifetime risk of nursing home residency: a further note. *The Gerontologist* 26 (5):562, Oct. 1986; McConnel, C. E. A note on the lifetime risk of nursing home residence. *The Gerontologist* 24(2):196, Apr. 1984.
52. Special Committee, pp. 96–97.
53. National Center for Health Statistics. *The National Nursing Home Survey: 1985 Summary for the United States,* Series 13, No. 97. Hyattsville, MD: NCHS, Jan. 1989, p. 71.
54. Special Committee, p. 97.

55. Ostroff, J. An aging market. *American Demographics* 11(5):26, May 1989.
56. Wolfe, D. B. The ageless market. *American Demographics* 9(7):28, July 1987.
57. Wolfe, p. 28.
58. Wolfe, pp. 55–56.
59. Herzlinger, R. The failed health care revolution. *Fortune,* Dec. 19, 1988, p. 186.
60. Brody, S. J. Strategic planning: the catastrophic approach. *Gerontologist* 27(2):131, Apr. 1987.

Chapter 3

Health Care Service Delivery

Nancy Alfred Persily and Sonya R. Albury

Eldercare services or programs are becoming a familiar concept in the health care lexicon. In recognizing the elderly as a major consumer market, providers are tailoring new products and services to meet their needs. Along with these developments comes the need to change perceptions of health care service delivery and to restructure old health care models, which no longer fit the needs of a changing marketplace. This chapter highlights some of the trends spurring these changes along and their possible impact on future eldercare programming. In addition to changes in health care delivery systems and recognition of the elderly as a growing market, trends include the expansion of alternative treatment settings, hospital involvement in elderly housing needs, and the shortage of health care workers.

Driving Forces for Change in Delivery Systems

The general hospital of tomorrow cannot define itself as an acute-care institution whose primary purpose is to treat patients in acute phases of illness. Hospitals will not succeed unless they broaden their role in health care delivery and their view of patients. Hospitals must redefine themselves as health care centers that provide care at all phases of illness, and they must broaden service delivery to address the changing needs of patients at various stages of health and wellness. Current medical orientation, which is already changing, must focus on the long-term care needs of the growing elderly population. Coupled with this are the external changes of a more competitive environment and changing demographics that dictate the reshaping of the health care industry's future. Successful hospitals in the 1990s and beyond will focus on continuity of care and integration of services to better serve their markets and prosper in this new health care environment.

In fact, a number of hospitals have already sought new methods of care. Building on their existing acute-care services, they began looking at diversification opportunities that offer step-down and follow-up services in the home and in community settings. Despite being met with innumerable financial roadblocks, creative hospitals have found ways to move from an acute-care focus to a continuum-of-care focus. Such a transition can be a financially complex undertaking but one that opens many doors for the aggressive hospital.

Changing Patient Needs

Hospitals have evolved from primarily acute-care oriented facilities into centers with fuller health care delivery roles. This development has occurred mainly during the latter half of this century. Rarely are patients admitted to hospitals for the myriad of infectious diseases that were once the mainstay of most acute-care hospitals. Recent medical advances also have led to more patients being treated at home or in an ambulatory setting. No longer are patients hospitalized overnight for minor trauma or certain surgical procedures. As a result of hospitals losing much of their acute-care business, the question now is, Which patient markets are left?

With the exception of obstetrical patients, AIDS patients, and trauma patients (for example, those with injuries from automobile accidents or gunshots), the majority of patients now are admitted for acute flare-ups of chronic conditions (heart disease, cancer, arthritis, diabetes, for example). The elderly are the most likely to be admitted for these illnesses, and even hospitalization due to acute conditions (a broken hip or pneumonia) usually is caused by their frail condition and preexisting illnesses. With pneumonia, for instance, the elderly may not require hospitalization for the illness itself but because of the possible secondary complications that often occur. Other major conditions, such as chronic sinusitis, hypertension, and hearing loss, generally do not result in hospitalization. Although these conditions may cause considerable problems, often they can be treated on an ambulatory basis through coordinated and accessible outpatient medical support services.

Because the elderly prefer to live independently in the community, they often need help with day-to-day activities to maintain that independent life-style. Health care that helps them maintain independence and avoid institutionalization will fulfill a vital need. This is illustrated not only by the rise in outpatient care but in home health services utilization, adult day care, and the increasing demand for affordable housing alternatives with some assistance.[1] Thus hospitals must reassess their role as health care providers for these chronic care needs regardless of the treatment setting.

Changing Medical Orientation

For more than 250 years the philosophy of Rene Descartes has dominated medicine. This approach (the Cartesian model) tends to reduce complex medical problems into their smallest and simplest elements. By separating out the mind from the body, physicians have treated a variety of biological-based problems with successful results for a variety of illnesses. The Cartesian model has permeated medical teaching and practice as well as research. During the 19th century, for example, the doctrine of a specific etiology—cause and effect—emerged, leading to the effective treatment of several infectious diseases. Hence the approach became widely accepted among the medical community.[2]

The changing nature of health care for the elderly, however, runs against the Cartesian model. That is, the health care needs of the elderly are becoming increasingly more complex, and there is a growing consensus that favors treating the whole person and utilizing resources far beyond the acute-care medical model. Instead of focusing on human biology alone, health providers must develop teams of specialists from a variety of fields to address the array of short- and long-term needs of all patient population groups—especially the elderly and disabled.

Medical response has not always been in harmony with the changing health needs of the elderly, which challenge the way medical care is viewed. Societal attitudes, as well as entrenched philosophical approaches to medical treatment, often have obviated efforts to redefine the provision of care. In the area of rehabilitation, for example, it is not uncommon for physicians to think that this mode of treatment is a "contradiction in terms" if applied to the elderly. In the recent past, many physicians did not feel that older people could benefit from rehabilitation. In actual practice, however, many elderly can and do regain ability to function if appropriate rehabilitation is provided. Rehabilitation can further serve as a form of tertiary prevention to avert further deterioration.

A More Competitive Environment

The 1980s marked a series of shakedowns in the health care marketplace. Following skyrocketing costs for health care during the 1970s, in 1983, Congress passed the provision for the prospective payment system, which introduced the concept of diagnosis-related groups (DRGs). Diagnosis-related groups reimbursed hospitals prospectively based on a diagnostic group rather than on the actual cost of rendering care. Consequently, hospitals no longer benefited financially from longer patient stays. Faced with these new cost constraints, hospitals introduced many new strategies to remain solvent and in hopes of remaining competitive. Concurrently, ambulatory care and outpatient centers proliferated as technological advances reduced the need for inpatient care. Providers scrambled for patients as the health care system became less centralized and the patient census plummeted.

During this revolution in health care, entrepreneurs began to capitalize on new market opportunities. A variety of business ventures cropped up, providing such things as home health services, assisted living environments, and durable medical equipment. Backed by their faith in corporate organizational strategies, healthy competition, and a concern for the bottom line, entrepreneurs believed a more cost-efficient and user-friendly system of care would emerge.

The resultant health care environment has been a mixed bag of change. Hospital operations were streamlined, lengths of hospital stays were reduced, alternative treatment settings were introduced, and hospitals began to diversify their programs by linking up with long-term care facilities and other service delivery options.

During this same turbulent period, some hospitals began downsizing in order to remain competitive. Large health care corporations also began to look at what they did best and then sought to capitalize on that product or market. For example, National Medical Enterprises sold off some of its acute-care facilities while keeping its specialty hospitals to rebuild its image as a provider of high-quality specialty care. Other hospitals began to convert underutilized hospital beds for alternative programming such as hospital-based skilled nursing facilities, hotel/hospital services (for relatives and posthospital care), and adult day care programs.

Although downsizing and market adjustments are being implemented in some hospitals today, the majority are continuing to add new services to compete for new patients. As technological advances enable some traditional inpatient procedures to be performed on an outpatient basis, hospital administrators are forced to redirect their attention to same-day patient services. Others look toward expanding or adding services excluded from the DRG categories, mainly psychiatric, substance abuse, and rehabilitative care. Short-term long-term care, especially through hospital-based skilled nursing facilities, also is being examined to fill the gap between acute-care hospitalization and reentry to the community or longer-term institutionalization. These step-down services can help alleviate the pressure to discharge older persons and can provide additional revenue sources to the hospital. Congress's 1989 failure to pass the Catastrophic Coverage Act notwithstanding, the need for extended care among the elderly will continue to be an issue with hospital administrators.

Repositioning for tomorrow's competitive environment is not always based on the choices made by the provider, however. In most states, regulations require hospitals to go through the certificate-of-need (CON) process to add new services or to expand already-existing programs. Even though these laws have had many good results—such as ensuring accessibility to care and improving the quality of care—they also have cut down on competition among hospitals. These policies have prevented some hospitals from entering the market for regulated services if no "need" has been established. They also have prevented some hospitals from offering a full array of services and have given other providers a virtual franchise, thereby circumventing the desired overall containment of costs and reducing competition.

Another key concern to emerge in recent years is the impact of prospective payment on rural hospitals. In 1983, when Congress enacted the Medicare Prospective Payment System (PPS), an inherent bias existed toward larger and, more often than not, urban hospitals. The PPS program assumed that hospitals had the volume to balance losses on some cases against gains on others. This prescription for cost containment and financial viability placed rural hospitals at a distinct disadvantage. The low volume inherent in their facilities meant that one or two high-cost cases could spell disaster, especially because of the high percentage of Medicare patients treated in rural settings. The results have been dramatic. Since 1980, over 160 rural hospitals nationwide have closed their doors, and another 600 have been in danger of closing.[3]

In order to remain viable and compete for physicians and patients, rural hospitals more than ever are being forced to control their costs. One method for improving service delivery is to network with a regional facility or join a multisystem chain. Linking up with a tertiary care provider can help rural hospitals expedite appropriate referrals and engage in joint management and purchasing strategies, along with other resource-sharing arrangements. Other effective strategies that aid hospitals in managing length of stay and thus expedite discharge are:

- Linking up with nursing homes
- Designating swing beds
- Building or jointly developing older adult housing programs
- Providing home health services
- Instituting volunteer programs that provide older persons (and others) with telephone reassurance links, escort services, or companionship

Recognition of the Elderly as a Major Market

Nowhere has health care changed as radically as in the very nature of hospital patients themselves. Tomorrow's health care consumers will be older, more open to alternative health care settings, more likely to experience acute flare-ups of chronic conditions, and increasingly more selective in their health care choices. They will have higher expectations of both their physicians and their care providers. The market will be more consumer-driven, and patients will be subjected to a variety of marketing messages.

Hospitals are recognizing that persons age 65 and over represent an average of 42 percent—more than 80 percent at some facilities—of their total patient days. These patients use a disproportionate share of hospital services and will continue to consume the bulk of inpatient care. Many forward-thinking providers are recognizing the numerous opportunities that this elderly market affords.[4]

A primary advantage enjoyed by elderly patients is that they generally are well insured. In fact Medicare, a public insurance program, covers the majority of persons age 65 and over. Of all people covered by Medicare, 90.6 percent are over the age of 65. Of people over the age of 65, more than 98 percent are covered by Medicare.[5] In addition, many older persons also purchase private "Medigap" policies to pay that portion of charges not covered by Medicare. Together, these programs make the aged the most medically enfranchised group in the nation.

In contrast, many of those under age 65 are uninsured or underinsured. Much of this market is being captured by managed care programs—such as health maintenance organizations (HMOs) and preferred provider organizations (PPOs)—that market their products to businesses seeking the best value for their employees. Many hospitals contract with these third-party payers to compete for the younger employed patient market but rarely have direct access to them due to the additional administrative layer.

The elderly are an attractive market for a variety of other reasons as well. They place great value on their health, have a rising level of disposable income, and often give first priority to paying their health care bills. In fact, the elderly spend more on health care than any other consumer group. Even with Medicare, they pay for more out-of-pocket health costs than the nonelderly. These expenses also consume a higher share of their total budget, 9 to 15 percent in 1986, in contrast to only 4 percent for younger age cohorts.[6] In addition, although 42 percent of the elderly's out-of-pocket dollar went for nursing home care in 1984, just under one-third (31 percent) went for care other than physician and hospital services (figure 3-1), such as home health services, homemaker care, and day care.[7]

Elderly patients may fill otherwise empty beds at a reasonable reimbursement level, are more loyal to a particular institution than their younger counterparts, are reliable bill payers, and generate high levels of demand for privately paid services. They can provide opportunities for new service development and are an excellent referral network, often attracting other patients to the hospital.[8]

What this all means in terms of service development must be determined within each hospital, but the traditional acute-care model of health care delivery will not be sufficient to meet the needs of this growing market.

Figure 3-1. Where the Out-of-Pocket Health Care Dollar for the Elderly Goes: 1984

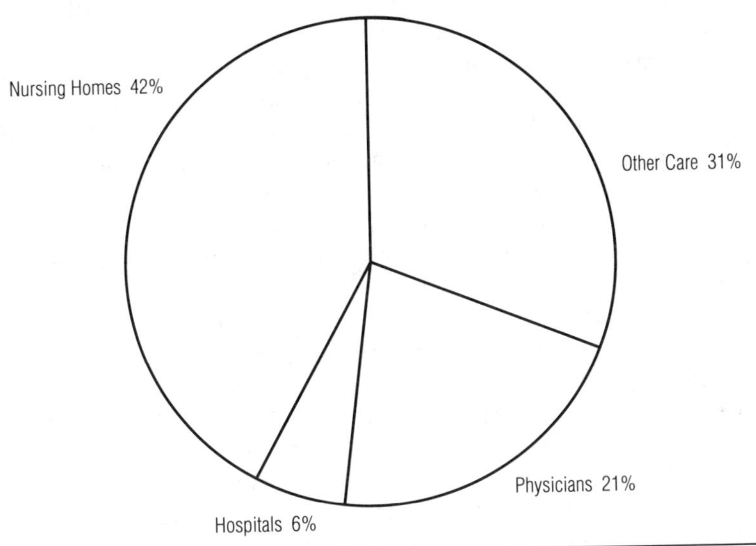

Source: Waldo, D. R., and Lazenby, H. C. Demographic characteristics and health care use and expenditures by the aged in the United States: 1977-1984. *Health Care Financing Review,* vol. 1, no. 1, Fall 1984. As cited by U.S. Senate Special Committee on Aging in *Aging in America: Trends and Projections,* 1987–88 edition, p. 130.

Expansion of Alternative Treatment Settings

Another trend in health care that has emerged in recent years has been the increase in alternative service delivery settings. A variety of treatment or care alternatives will be needed to meet consumer demand. These include, but are not limited to, ambulatory care, nursing home care, home health care, psychological services, and adult day care.

Ambulatory Care

Over the past decade, consumers have been directing more of their business to ambulatory outpatient centers. Whether called health care centers, ambulatory care centers, emergicenters, or surgicenters, these freestanding facilities have been established by hospitals, physicians, and some corporations. Not only is ambulatory care more convenient than hospitalization, it is often much less costly.

Most consumers prefer outpatient care, such as same-day surgery, rather than an overnight hospital stay. There are differences within age groups, but in every category the preference is for outpatient treatment. Over 85 percent of 25- to 44 year-olds prefer same-day surgery, in contrast to 73 percent of 55- to 64 year-olds and 65 percent of the over-65 population.[9]

One of the reasons for these lower preference levels among the elderly may relate to how much they know about outpatient services. Only 70 percent of those age 55 and older are aware of the outpatient service available at hospitals, compared to 80 percent of 18- to 54-year-old consumers. Coupled with the fact that the more educated consumer has a greater preference for same-day surgery, there is strong indication that as the affluent, well-educated baby boomers age, the demand for outpatient care will continue to rise. However, many elderly still will require hospitalization when a care giver is unavailable or incapable of providing postsurgery care at home.[10]

The introduction of ambulatory surgery has had a major impact on hospitals. Today 45 percent of all surgeries are conducted on an outpatient basis, up from 20 percent in 1983.[11] Although most of these surgeries are performed in hospitals, the number recorded in freestanding centers and in physicians' offices is on the rise.

Over time, the overhead of most hospitals may render them noncompetitive with other ambulatory care centers. Physicians recognize this opportunity to expand their office practice and capture a profitable ambulatory surgery and diagnostic service business.[12] Consumers are beginning to shop around for the "best" service, which they often see as being offered by the facility having the most amenities. Third-party payers also are negotiating for the lowest prices for health care; hospital-based services often lose out in this arena.

To be competitive in ambulatory care, hospitals must devise a variety of strategies that will attract patients on dimensions other than price. Hospitals need to become more "user friendly" by tailoring their outpatient programs to provide high-quality care and excellent customer service. In health care, the term *user friendly* means making the system of care more responsive to the needs of the patients whom the system serves.

In becoming service oriented, the hospital should become aware of prehospital, inpatient, and postdischarge needs of older patients. The patient relations staff or even volunteers can be helpful to patients by providing an escort service, which could help older patients get from one testing site to another or just to find their way around the hospital. To ensure continuity of care, the hospital also can develop integrated inpatient and outpatient tracking and recordkeeping systems, which can happen only in hospital-based programs, thus reducing or eliminating duplication of procedures. To make the outpatient programs more service oriented, the facility can provide pretreatment and aftercare information and care. For example, patients can be contacted prior to a scheduled test to inform them what the procedure will be like and how to prepare for it. The hospital also can provide immediate feedback to attending physicians and patients after diagnostic testing to ensure that appropriate follow-up care or treatment is rendered. After ambulatory surgery or other more involved procedures, home care, transportation, and other support services can be arranged for the patient through the social work or discharge planning department. These initiatives are designed for the elderly but also would apply in creating a user-friendly system for all patients—regardless of age.

In addition to the measures just outlined, a more specialized strategy employed by some hospitals is to develop tertiary clinics specializing in multidisciplinary diagnosis and treatment of special geriatric problems. For example, a variety of specialists from fields such as orthopedics, urology, rehabilitation, psychiatry, neurology, endocrinology, gynecology, and of course, geriatrics, can be involved. Some appropriate programs for the elderly include incontinence clinics, falls and immobility clinics, and memory disorder clinics. Hospitals have a unique opportunity to organize and promote these interdisciplinary programs, where some of these programs can generate their own revenue, and some will be "loss leaders" that will generate more inpatient business or increase income for other hospital-sponsored programs.

Outpatient services is an area where growth potential for hospitals is most promising. With pressure from third-party payers sure to mount, hospitals must continue to develop a solid base of effective alternatives to inpatient care. These include the following:

- Designing outpatient programs that bond the patient to the facility so that when inpatient care is needed, the patient will be more likely to select that hospital for acute-care services.
- Continuing to provide a strong core of inpatient care while also strengthening ambulatory programs. The hospital can then utilize both treatment settings as feeders from one care level to the next.
- Aligning their priorities with those of "buyers" and offering an affordable continuum of care to the entire family. This may mean developing more efficient and effective managerial skills and new clinical approaches, or it may mean developing joint relationships with physicians and other providers to deliver ambulatory care programs either at the hospital or at an alternative site.

Clearly, hospitals will be required to objectively evaluate the cost of delivering care and create a pricing structure that is both financially feasible and competitive in the marketplace.

Nursing Home Care

Nursing homes provide nursing care, medical services, and personal care services to persons unable to care for themselves due to illness or infirmity. Typical services include nursing care (both restorative and palliative care), preventive and health maintenance services, rehabilitation services, and ancillary and supportive social services.

Traditionally, the role of the nursing home has been to provide custodial care to the elderly. Residents often were those stricken with deteriorating conditions that required extended convalescent care and (most often) continued institutional care. Today's profile of nursing home residents, however, is much more diverse. Although still primarily an elderly group, many nursing home residents return home after a short-term stay. The common misperception that nursing home care is "the end of the road" is being dispelled.

The rise in short-term stays is due to a variety of factors. Most important have been the dramatic growth in the elderly market, improved technology, and prospective payment. The prospective payment system in particular has had a far-reaching impact. Since the introduction of diagnosis-related groups in 1983, hospitals have been forced to be more accountable from a financial standpoint as well as through professional review organization (PRO) pressure. As a result, nursing homes have had to keep patients who previously were sent to the hospital to die.

Another spin-off of these regulatory changes has been the quicker discharge of patients who no longer need acute hospital care.[13] These discharges, referred to as *sicker and quicker* discharges (although unverified by hospital evaluations), has had a ripple effect on health care in many communities. Caught unprepared, nursing homes, home health agencies, and social services providers have had to respond to these patients who are in need of short-term continuing medical care of a restorative or recuperative nature.

To be more responsive to the short-term/long-term care needs of these patients, innovative hospitals are taking a proactive stance in designing their own step-down programs, such as skilled nursing facilities, for example. Over half of all nursing home admissions originate from the hospital setting, making the hospital a primary source of referrals. Coupled with the incentive to discharge older patients in a timely manner because of DRGs, the stage clearly is being set to offer more diversified levels of care. It will be up to each provider to maximize these opportunities within the present regulatory environment in preparation for the future service delivery system.

Home Health Care

Home health care services took off in the 1980s. The increased utilization of home care can be attributed to the aging of the population, the shift from cost-based reimbursement to a prospective payment system, the expansion of HMOs, and an increase in high-tech home care services.

The country's burgeoning over-65 population accounts for approximately 80 percent of the recipients of home health care in America today.[14] Without home assistance, many of these elderly individuals would be at risk of institutionalization. The continuing care provided by home health agencies enables the elderly to remain at home and retain their autonomy and sense of dignity.

In addition to the increased demand for home care services among the elderly, sweeping changes have occurred in the reimbursement of health care services. Since the advent of prospective payment, the site of health care delivery has shifted from hospitals to the community. This pattern has opened the door to a wave of home health agencies—often with staff on site at the hospital—to assist in returning patients to their homes as quickly as possible. In addition, many hospitals established their own hospital-based home care agencies to protect their patient markets and keep them within the hospital system for subsequent admissions.

Health maintenance organizations have had an impact similar to that of DRGs. Arrangements with HMOs also offer incentives for hospitals to discharge patients earlier, thereby creating a greater demand for follow-up care in the home.

Regardless of whether or not hospitals are discharging patients prematurely, industry officials agree that home care patients are more acutely ill than they were a few years ago.[15] Home care patients now require a multiplicity of highly specialized services that must be given by qualified staff through a comprehensive, coordinated and continuous care program.

To meet these new challenges, a rapid development of high-tech home care products and services has been underway in health care. Many therapies previously performed in the institutional setting now are available in the home setting—for example, antibiotic therapy and hyperalimentation. Other advances include ventilator systems small enough to fit into a small suitcase, computers that monitor a patient's vital signs at home and transmit their information to a centralized monitoring station, and robotic devices that assist patients at home.

Along with these changes and medical advances, growth of home health care has been tempered by limitations in reimbursement. Medicare has strict guidelines on allowable charges and restrictions on length of treatment and the types of services offered. Therefore, many providers offer privately paid services, such as companions and nurses' aides, provide 24-hour care to supplement Medicare-covered home health services, and serve as a safety net in today's fragmented health care system.

Even with increased economic pressure, home care can be an effective and profitable service option for hospitals. As this area of health care delivery gains momentum, it will continue to evolve as an intrinsic part of the health care system.

Psychological Services

Geriatric psychiatry, or geropsychiatry, differs from general adult psychiatry in a variety of ways. Even though older adults may be troubled by the same disorders that plague younger persons, symptoms can manifest under altered conditions. Older adults often experience disorders related to the aging process, such as depression due to loss of functional ability, fear of death, chronic illness, or loss of a spouse. Iatrogenic diseases, those inadvertently introduced by physicians or their treatment, are prevalent among the elderly because of their more frequent exposure to medical interventions. Similarly, drug-induced disorders are a major concern, and coordinated intervention can help mitigate the effects of drugs through changing drug dosages and careful patient monitoring and education. The greater interplay of biomedical and social problems with the concurrent psychological disturbances in older patients demands a particular orientation and knowledge of intervention. Thus, the development of a separate and distinct geriatric psychiatry unit often is a preferred organizational structure. Physicians are able to manage patient care more effectively when they are grouped together and an array of services can be introduced in a specialized therapeutic milieu.[16]

The organization of geropsychiatric units has taken a variety of forms, but a common feature is a strong interdisciplinary diagnostic team. Patients are assessed for both medical and psychiatric conditions through in-depth diagnostic testing, with treatment often involving an array of therapeutic interventions. At South Shore Hospital in Miami Beach, Florida, for example, the frail elderly on the geropsychiatric unit participate in group therapy, communal dining, milieu therapy, drug therapy, socialization, recreational therapy, and occupational therapy. Physical therapy and speech therapy also are available.[17]

Geropsychiatric units have become increasingly popular due to their DRG-exempt status. Patients can be transferred from within the general acute hospital program or admitted from an external setting such as an outpatient mental health clinic, an assisted living environment, or a nursing home, with follow-up care being provided through transitional programs. Current options include day treatment programs, outpatient care and counseling along with discharge to housing programs or nursing homes where special mental health programs along with some medical monitoring are available to residents.

Adult Day Care

Adult day care programs have become popular settings for the provision of services to meet the health care and socialization needs of frail, moderately handicapped, and slightly confused elderly persons. Such programs also can serve as a form of respite care, making a tremendous difference in the lives of both care givers and older adults. Adult day care can provide the transition needed between 24-hour hospital or nursing home care and the community as well as aid in shortening hospital lengths of stay. Adult day care often helps in delaying or preventing premature institutionalization as well.

The patient mix in day care centers usually is composed of persons with dementia, the physically frail elderly, and older adults who need socialization or continued physical activity. Whereas many centers serve older persons with varying needs and disability levels, some specialization of adult day care programs has arisen during the past decade. These special-purpose centers service a single type of client—such as a mentally ill or Alzheimer's patient—who requires a variety of specialized services and an environment that is sensitive to their needs.

There are two basic models of day care: social day care and medical day care. *Medical day care* is designed with nursing services and a variety of therapeutic interventions, whereas *social day care* is oriented primarily toward socialization, counseling, and recreational activities. In recent years, social day care centers also have added more health-related services—especially in the areas of wellness and prevention.

Day care centers generally provide at minimum some social interaction, exercise, and a hot noontime meal.[18] Programs are located in various settings including senior centers, health centers, nursing homes, rehabilitation centers, mental health centers, hospitals, elderly housing complexes, churches, life care communities, and private homes. Weekend programs also are emerging; for example, the Weekend Day Care Program for Alzheimer's patients operated by Bon Secours Hospital/Villa Maria Nursing Center in North Miami, Florida. Day care centers located in hospitals often are referred to as *day hospitals* or *geriatric day programs,* which provide intensive medical, psychiatric nursing and/or rehabilitative services to individuals who do not require 24-hour nursing care but would need inpatient care if the day program were not available.

Whatever the setting, the elderly and their care givers are overwhelmingly pleased with the quality of services provided. According to a recent study, over 82 percent of the elderly and 92 percent of their care givers reported "the highest level of satisfaction" with their adult day care programs. Most were also pleased with the transportation provided, the amount of attention from staff, and the program hours.[19]

Day care, irrespective of the model, continues to be a financial bargain for the elderly and their care givers. The daily cost often is less than it would be if a home health nurse visited the patient for an hour—and day care lasts six to eight hours.

Nevertheless, proprietary day care is a relatively new phenomenon, and the cost-effectiveness of adult day care nationwide has yet to be determined. To society as a whole, day care may not be less costly than full-time care at home or in a nursing home. Yet, positive benefits experienced by the elderly and their care givers are believed to outweigh the disadvantages. Furthermore, when provided along with other supportive services to persons at high risk of institutionalization, real savings and long-term benefits can be realized. Hospital- and nursing home-based day care also provides an important feeder into the institution as well as a step-down resource for those recently discharged from acute inpatient care.

Hospital Involvement in Elderly Housing Needs

Housing for the elderly or the retired received substantial attention during the 1980s and will continue as a major concern during the next decade. Numerous living arrangements have been subjects of studies and pilot programs that examined the most effective and dignified approaches to maintaining older adults in a home setting.

The concept of home—whether a house, an apartment, or a mobile home—is central to American culture as the setting in which people live out their lives. A home also stands for familiar places and faces, a community, stores, personal possessions, and cherished memories. Because the qualities of home become more important as an individual ages, the elderly are prompted to remain in their homes even if a move is warranted for financial, health, or safety reasons.

Hospital staff workers are keenly aware of these feelings among the elderly; and patients are eager to return to their familiar surroundings, even if they fear being unable to manage for themselves. With the move toward prospective payment, hospital discharge workers have quickened the pace at which the elderly return home. Frequently, if appropriate in-home supports are not available, frail older adults can find themselves in dire situations that can lead to rehospitalization and/or institutionalization.

Concerned hospital administrators have taken a proactive role not only in working with other community providers to examine ways that enable the elderly to continue living in their own homes, but also in developing housing alternatives that allow the elderly to live as independently as possible. Some of these housing options, explored in the following sections, may be viewed as a continuum of programs (figure 3-2) ranging from those designed to enhance the quality of independent living (retirement communities and home equity conversions) to semi-independent living and sheltered arrangements (congregate housing and life care).

Shared Housing

The objective of shared housing is to match older adults with other persons or families who can share living expenses and offer companionship.

Figure 3-2. Alternative Living Arrangements and Institutional Care

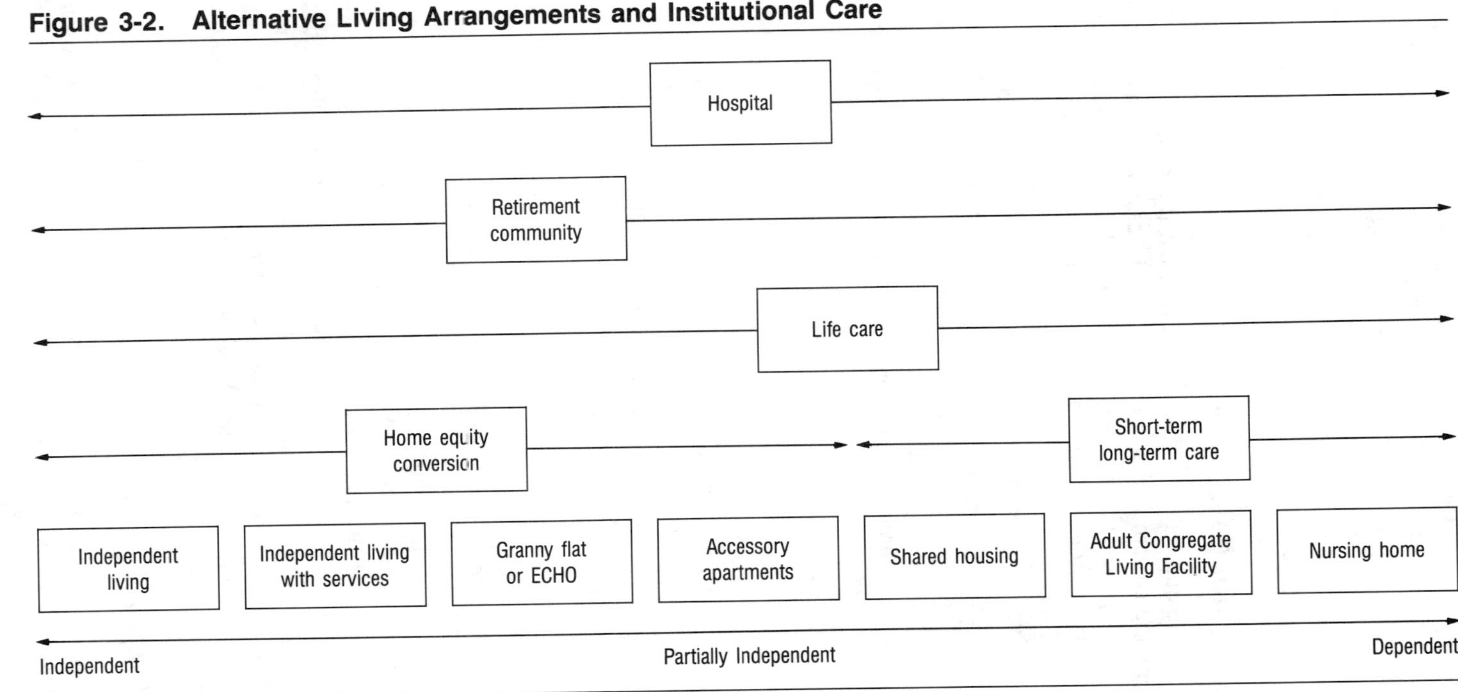

ECHO = elder cottage housing opportunity.

The elderly frequently suffer from loneliness and often have extra space in their homes that they can rent out. A boarder can reduce their isolation and also provide services such as cleaning, cooking, or transportation in exchange for reduced rent. Although it is often difficult to form successful or long-term matches, some programs are being met with modest success and seem to foster a positive community image.

Home Equity Conversions

About three-quarters of elderly persons own their own homes,[20] and some insurance companies are helping them "cash in" on a home equity conversion option. This option allows older adults to utilize the accumulated equity in their homes to serve as a source of discretionary income or pay for home repairs or health or social services. Usually the arrangement involves monthly payments to the older homeowner from the third-party investor who buys the home, and the homeowner is granted life tenancy in the house. Then the family who inherit the house may sell the house or keep it and pay off the bank loan. (For a further discussion on home equity conversion, see chapter 7 on financing eldercare programs.)

Retirement Communities

Although heavily concentrated in Sun Belt states such as Florida, Arizona, and Texas, retirement living communities are located throughout the country. These communities (or retirement villages) are self-contained complexes that provide a variety of services and amenities. Common features include recreational facilities, security, social activities, and sometimes preventive health services—for example, wellness or health screening programs.

Many developers believe that retirement communities need to be marketed more effectively, because few elderly actually have joined them. Other people who have studied the elderly consider this a very narrow market because they feel most older people prefer to "age in place." Whichever is the case, retirement communities continue to proliferate in a variety of configurations to appeal to the increasingly diverse tastes of the older adult market. Options include multiunit condominiums, mobile homes, town houses, single-family homes, or a combination of these choices. Century Villages in Florida and Sun City in Arizona are well-known retirement communities, as is Heritage Village in Connecticut. Many religious groups also have developed retirement communities throughout the country.

Continuing Care Retirement Communities

Continuing care retirement communities (CCRCs), or life care communities, offer a range of living arrangements from totally independent living units to skilled nursing care. Although CCRCs have existed for over 50 years, the concept gained recognition in the 1960s.[21]

Recent retirees are attracted to the concept of retaining their independence while also benefiting from financial security and guaranteed access to an array of services on a campuslike setting. Continuing care retirement communities are somewhat like long-term care insurance policies. For example, a group of approximately 300 to 500 individuals may affiliate and contribute to a self-insurance pool to purchase a full array of institutional and home-based services.[22] By contract, members are guaranteed access to appropriate long-term care services as needed, often with no additional copayments or out-of-pocket expenses. Most CCRCs guarantee lifetime residence, augmented by health care and various other supportive social services during the remainder of the resident's life.

Several variations of life care communities have evolved throughout the nation, and whatever their form, they represent an important alternative to institutional care. Continuing care retirement communities reduce isolation by providing opportunities for social interaction with peers, a variety of programs and activities as well as physical security, and a continuum of nursing care. All of these services and benefits are provided at the appropriate level according to the participants' needs as they age and need more care, thereby creating a healthy environment that reverses the alienation suffered by residents in institutional settings. These life care centers offer an opportunity for hospitals to provide a spectrum of medical care services to an aging community.

Assisted Living Facilities

The assisted living facilities market is another housing option referred to in some states as adult congregate living facilities (ACLFs) or alternate care facilities. These facilities may be separate and freestanding, or they may be one of the levels of care in a retirement community. These programs offer a variety of supportive services including meals, laundry, housekeeping services, recreational activities, and assistance with medication administration; some programs also offer transportation, personal care, and emergency response systems.

Hospitals, nursing homes, church groups, civic organizations, entrepreneurs, and a variety of other groups have entered the market of assisted living facilities. The Marriott Corporation is just one of many businesses engaging in diversification strategies to capitalize on the growing interest of aging consumers who seek alternatives to institutionalization.

Other Living Arrangements

Other living arrangements being explored have met with varying levels of success, and some have faltered because of zoning restrictions and financing difficulties. For example, accessory apartments call for private units installed in a single-family house—much like an attached rental unit. Each apartment generally houses only one elderly person and provides space for privacy while affording the security and companionship of living with relatives.

Elder cottage housing opportunity (ECHO) is a variation on this housing theme. Often referred to in Europe as "granny flats," these are separate units built on the property of an adult child's home but placed separately from the main house. The concept originated in Australia, where elderly persons rented low-cost mobile homes and placed them in their children's backyards. Both options—accessory apartments and ECHO units—require a care giver's or an adult child's participation, which can add to the complexity of program administration.

Shortage of Health Care Workers

The final trend to be addressed by this chapter is the health care worker shortage, one of the most dramatic personnel shortages in America's health care history. Patient care workers who provide personal care are in particularly short supply; these include registered nurses and nurses' aides. The shortage can be attributed to a variety of factors: the growth of the elderly population, alternative career options for health care workers, the development of new service alternatives, and recent advances in medical technology that heighten the demand for skilled patient care.

Hospital inpatients are also sicker than in the past, yet hospital stays generally are shorter. Patients who are less severely ill or who are discharged earlier are treated in ambulatory settings. Changes in technology also require health care workers with more advanced expertise, and patients often require more sophisticated care.[23]

These changes have made issues surrounding the quality of care of paramount concern, and nurses play an essential role in the delivery of high-quality patient care. One study confirmed what many people already believed, that the nursing shortage is putting an incredible strain on nursing care, and the continued delivery of high-quality patient care has emerged as a major concern to hospital CEOs.[24]

Coupled with these concerns have been the reductions and shortages of hospital staff in general, which can bog nurses down with responsibilities other than patient care and leave them with little time to monitor the quality of care delivered.[25] So far, the shortages have not yet forced hospitals to compromise quality of care, and high standards of performance are being maintained.[26]

Some hospitals seek to resolve the problem by providing extensive educational and training programs for employees. Whether for technical positions or those requiring sophisticated care, staff education is essential to upgrading skill levels. Some hospitals also offer tuition reimbursement, bonus incentive plans, career ladder opportunities, and salary incentives to attract *and* retain trained nursing personnel.

Hospitals are not the only health providers having difficulty in recruiting nursing personnel, however. Nursing homes and home health agencies also are competing for qualified staff to care for their patients, many of whom are elderly. What with new regulations at the state and federal levels, the requirement for more and more documentation of care provided and quality of care will lead to an increased need for professional nurses.

One of the principal changes at the federal level is the implementation of new regulations under the Omnibus Budget Reconciliation Act (OBRA) of 1987, which includes new R.N. staffing requirements for nursing homes, requires increased training and competency evaluations for nurses' aides, and sets guidelines for screening the mentally ill/mentally retarded and performing comprehensive medical assessments, among other provisions. With these nursing home regulations come concerns regarding adequate funding to comply with OBRA's stipulations. According to a recent survey, most administrators believe it will be difficult to meet the standards for nurses' aide training and competency evaluations as well as registered nurse staffing requirements and new inspection procedures. Implementation cost estimates range from under $5 to more than $15 per bed per day (figure 3-3).[27]

Home health agencies, on the other hand, are being confronted with new requirements for both Medicare and private home health providers. Florida, for example, has new regulations regarding case management and training requirements, two of which are that registered nurses must perform patient assessments every 60 days on an ongoing basis and that aides must have more training on an ongoing basis in order to keep their certification.

As hospitals move into the future, they will be competing with these other providers for scarce worker resources. It is essential, therefore, that hospitals know their strengths, use their personnel wisely, offer attractive incentives, and develop strategic plans for the recruitment and retention of high-quality personnel.

Summary

A myriad of trends has affected the way health care services are delivered today. Whether it be changes in patient illnesses, increased competition in the marketplace, the country's burgeoning older population, the introduction of new service alternatives, or the health care worker shortage, these trends all point to the redefinition of the hospital as it is known today.

Figure 3-3. Estimated Costs of Implementing OBRA 1987 per Bed per Day

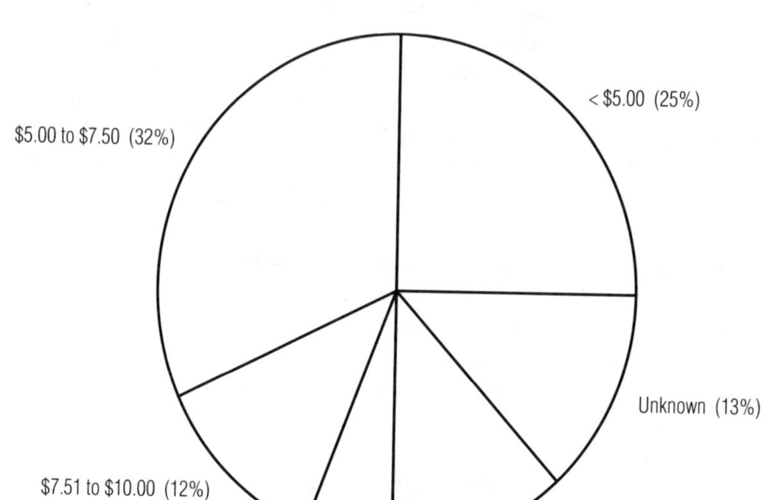

Source: Reprinted, with permission, from National Research Corporation, "Payment, rules are top strategic issues," *Modern Healthcare's Eldercare Business,* Jan. 15, 1990, p. 22.

Much needs to be done in the way of changing how society as a whole looks at health care and the role of hospitals. One way to have an impact on these perceptions is to offer educational programs for both the public and health professionals in geriatrics, rehabilitation, and other allied health fields. As changes in societal attitudes occur and the burgeoning elderly population becomes even stronger, there will be increased response through both public and private programs and legislation. Although the Catastrophic Coverage Act was revoked, Congress continues to seriously consider several bills that address continuity of eldercare. It is imperative that these issues remain on the nation's agenda for the future and that hospital administrators are positioned to act on new initiatives and opportunities for serving this population.

References

1. Spotts, H. E. Jr., and Schewe, C. D. Communication with the elderly consumer: the growing health care challenge. *Journal of Health Care Marketing* 9(3):36–44, Sept. 1989.

2. Brody, S. J. Geriatrics and rehabilitation: common ground and conflicts. Presentation at the Conference on Rehabilitation and Geriatric Education: Perspectives and Potential, Dec. 4–7, 1988, p. 1.

3. Slowly, perhaps inevitably, Congress faces rural aging. *Networks [National Council on the Aging, Inc., Washington, DC]*, 1(2):1, Dec. 15, 1989.

4. Special Committee on Aging. *Aging America: Trends and Projections*. Washington, DC: U.S. Government Printing Office, 1989, p. 93.

5. U.S. Census Estimates from a conversation with Mary Beth Vetter, U.S. Department of Commerce, Apr. 2, 1990; and U.S. Department of Health and Human Services, Health Care Financing Administration, Bureau of Data Management and Strategy, HCFA Pub. No. 03294, Sept. 1989.

6. Special Committee, pp. 58–59.

7. U.S. Senate Special Committee on Aging. *Aging America: Trends and Projections*. 1987–88 ed. Washington, DC: U.S. Government Printing Office, 1987, p. 130.

8. Spivack, S. A challenge to survival. In: S. J. Brody and N. A. Persily, editors. *Hospitals and the Aged: The New Old Market*. Rockville, MD: Aspen Publishers, 1984, pp. 9–10.

9. Jensen, J. Health care alternatives. *American Demographics* 8(3):38, Mar. 1986.

10. Jensen, p. 38.

11. Lutz, S. Ambulatory care keeps patients, hospitals on the move. *Modern Healthcare* 19(48):20, Dec. 1, 1989.

12. Spivack, p. 5.

13. Bowers, B., and Musser, K. Changing home health care marketplace in Wisconsin. *Home Health Services Quarterly* 8(4):7, Winter 1987–88.

14. Gilbert, S. Is America abandoning sick patients? *New York Times, The Good Health Magazine*, Apr. 29, 1990.

15. Coffey, R. M., Farly, D. E., Linel, K., and Wilson, R. *Secretary's Commission on Nursing: Support Studies and Background Information*. Vol. 11, Dec. 6, 1988, pp. 1–7.

16. Zubkoff, W. Telephone interview, Jan. 11, 1990. South Shore Hospital, Miami Beach, FL.

17. Zubkoff, Jan. 11, 1990.

18. Weissert, W. G., et al. Models of adult day care: findings from a national survey. *Gerontologist* 29(5):648, Oct. 1989.

19. Most day care recipients pleased with care. *Aging Action Alert*, No. 89-12. Washington, DC: Dec. 7, 1989, p. 73; Weissert, p. 647.

20. Minkler, M. Gold in gray: reflections on business' discovery of the elderly market. *Gerontologist* 29(1):18, Feb. 1989.

21. Winklevoss, H. E., and Powell, A. V. *Continuing Care Retirement Communities: An Empirical, Financial, and Legal Analysis*. Homewood, IL: Richard D. Irwin, 1984, p. 2.

22. Branch, L. G. Continuing care retirement communities: self-insuring for long term care. *Gerontologist* 27(1):4, Feb. 1987.

23. Department of Health and Human Services. *Secretary's Commission on Nursing.* Vol. I. Washington, DC: DHHS, Dec. 1988, p. 18.

24. Koska, M. T. RN shortage puts experience in forefront. *Hospitals* 63(9):22, May 5, 1989.

25. Koska, p. 22.

26. Lappa, K. Hiring standards: high quality still top priority. *Hospitals* Sept. 20, 1989, p. 89.

27. Jensen, J., and Sherman, J. F. Payment, rules are top strategic issues. *Modern Healthcare's Eldercare Business,* Jan. 15, 1990, pp. 22–24.

Chapter 4

Continuity of Care for the Elderly in Hospitals

Nancy Alfred Persily

The 1980s brought about a number of changes in the way hospitals conduct their business, moving them toward a whole new era of health care delivery. Hospitals are reexamining their roles in the service delivery system and developing numerous survival strategies for maintaining, repositioning, and introducing services in today's marketplace.

Prior to the 1980s, hospitals operated mostly in a noncompetitive, no-risk atmosphere, where market forces and reimbursement policies reinforced attitudes long held by administrators. Many administrators—driven by the urge to keep pace with technological advancements and services regardless of their cost-effectiveness—generally felt that their hospital's mission to serve the community justified unrestrained growth and expenditures. But as costs rose, so did hospital charges. The public and its legislators, forced to grope for measures that curbed skyrocketing expenses, struggled to contain costs to make health care affordable and accessible. Then in the early 1980s, new reimbursement constraints were introduced, pressuring hospitals to operate more efficiently while at the same time providing service that was consistent with their mission.

They started to shift their focus to a broader definition of health care, one that takes into account health or wellness as well as illness, and one that encompasses a consciousness of the need for continuity of care, even after patients have been discharged. Hospitals learned that their survival depends on their ability to reckon with these changes and respond to a variety of new market opportunities.

Marketplace Changes That Affect Eldercare

To understand the new challenges faced by hospitals and how they must be addressed, four major changes occurring in the health care marketplace are discussed in this section:

1. *Cost-based reimbursement has been replaced by other measures.* In the past, Medicare generally was a reliable—and fairly liberal—payment source, a cost-plus arrangement with few limits to reimbursement. Because most services were reimbursable, hospitals often developed new services and purchased expensive state-of-the-art equipment, based on what their internal groups judged the community to need. Hospitals operated in a noncompetitive atmosphere; the years 1966 to 1983 were an era of low-risk, no-challenge management. But revenues from both government and third-party payers decreased after 1983. As insurance companies began to redefine "allowable" charges, hospitals as well as consumers had to foot more of the bill. Diagnosis-related groups (DRGs) and other Medicare reimbursement limitations drastically altered the hospital's economic environment and forced providers to seek new methods for managing eldercare.
2. *Demand for inpatient care has declined for all but the elderly.* Today's Americans are healthier and taking better care of their families. Consumer awareness of options and costs has resulted in an increasing demand for health care (that is, preventive and maintenance services) in addition to acute and chronic medical care. Families seeking to provide for their older members have become sensitized to care-related costs.

   Meanwhile, the elderly are becoming the primary users of hospital inpatient services. In 1986, persons 65 and over represented 12 percent of the patient population but accounted for 31 percent of all discharges. They also stay in the hospital longer, representing 42 percent of all short-stay hospital days of care.[1]

   Younger persons, less likely to experience complications, benefit from new technological developments that make it possible to perform more outpatient procedures. These changes have led to an explosion of ambulatory services and centers operated by hospitals as well as a host of other competitors. Health insurers also have decreased the use of first-dollar coverage or deductibles, leading consumers to wait longer before going for care or to shop around for health care and, in many cases, choose outpatient services. As a result, the supply of hospital beds far exceeds the demand, forcing hospitals to compete with each other for the dwindling number of inpatients, many of whom are older adults.[2]

   At the same time, consumers—particularly older ones—are learning more about health care options and the cafeteria of benefits available to them because they are now under pressure to make the most of their own decreasing health care dollar.
3. *Other players have entered the medical market.* Competition in the health care market has increased as new players provide services formerly offered exclusively in the hospital setting. Insurance companies, physicians and physician groups, and corporations are building and

operating outpatient facilities, many of which are dedicated to a specific purpose (cataract surgery, mammography, diagnostic services, rehabilitation). These groups have an advantage over hospitals in that they are not subject to many of the regulatory restraints imposed on hospitals, such as certificates of need and rigorous auditing. The effect has been to attract patients away from the hospital setting, thus adversely affecting the traditional patient–hospital bond.

4. *Consumer health care choices have changed.* Health maintenance organizations and preferred provider organizations limit consumer ability to choose a hospital or physician. Large employers, seeing the costs of health care rise, use their size as leverage and in essence purchase health care in bulk, using financial incentives to influence employee choice. These new referral sources also are limiting the capacity of physicians to determine where they will admit their patients.

These major changes within the marketplace, particularly new cost-based reimbursement measures, have had a profound impact on health care for the elderly patient population. Based on DRG formulas, utilization review committees determined how long patient stays should be, and many physicians felt they had lost some power to make discharge decisions based on the individual medical needs of patients. Hospitals were accused of making "sicker and quicker" discharges because patients were being discharged without appropriate step-down arrangements. Thus posthospital care givers—most often family members—found themselves in the frustrating, many times heartbreaking, position of dealing with an elderly patient without respite or community support. Nursing home beds became scarce, and at times nursing home administrators had to deal with levels of illness and disability beyond their capacity.

At the same time, many hospitals did enter the eldercare market—either because neighboring hospitals had done so or because they saw a profitable service opportunity. Yet many did so without adequate research and planning. For example, senior membership programs sprouted up at hospitals across the country, but many were prepackaged carelessly and without follow-through. Most important, hospitals did not develop internal service-oriented systems for handling the continuity of care needs of older people once they developed external marketing programs. Hospitals also evaluated their efforts financially through a cost-center approach rather than through an evaluation of the total care package.

Overcoming Myths about the Eldercare Market

Demographic and sociological studies abound proving that, as the number and proportion of elderly persons increase dramatically during the next few decades, demand for health and social services for the elderly will be a critical factor affecting hospitals and other institutions.[3]

People are simply living longer; more are living into their 80s and 90s. Although better physical health contributes to this longer life span, longer life also brings with it more ill and disabled persons of extreme old age. To provide care for these older and chronically ill and disabled Americans, long-term care will increasingly become a planning issue for health care institutions, which must begin to consider a full spectrum of home, community, and institutional-based health care services for older adults.

To accurately and effectively gauge the elderly market in order to understand their needs, it is important to dispel some common myths.

Myth #1: The Elderly Can Be Treated as a Single Market

It would be a mistake to group this population segment into one market—those over age 65. Striking differences exist in terms of age, size, and growth rate; attempting to develop strategies for the group as a whole would be like creating a marketing plan for everyone under age 35.

Persons between ages 65 and 74, the *younger old,* make up the slowest growth sector and represent more than half the over-65 population.[4] This group is healthier and wealthier than other segments of the elderly market. They share the concerns of people about 10 years younger rather than the very different concerns of those age 75 to 84. Older adults in the 65- to 74-year-old group are active and generally are concerned about health and nutrition. They buy skin care products, vitamins and minerals, and medicines that ease pain and ease the performance of everyday activities. They exercise, usually by walking.

A more common image of the older adult fits better with the 75–84 age group, the *older old*. Health is more often an issue, mobility is more likely to be limited, and health care services and special care facilities are more in demand. This age group may be dependent on family members and concerned about their ability to pay for long-term care.

The *very old*—those over age 85—are more dependent than any other elderly group and require regular medical care and support services to perform everyday tasks. In addition, this group is likely to be surrounded by four or five generations within their families, which provides a broad spectrum of age groups likely to be involved in their health care decisions.

These demographic factors will create many business opportunities for hospitals. Certainly hospitals will continue their roles of providing acute and chronic care. But as technology improves the ability to treat the very ill, there remains the problem of what to do with an elderly patient who goes home once the illness is stabilized. As it ages, the population becomes more vulnerable; for example, 25 percent of older adults need some form of long-term care, either in an institution or in the community. Many are unable to live independently and need a variety of medical and support services.[5] Hospitals are in an ideal position to serve this elderly market because of their managerial expertise, sophisticated staff, data gathering experience, education and training programs, and broad experience in working with funding sources.

Myth #2: High-Tech Acute Care Can Solve the Problems of the Elderly

Twenty years of Medicare and its liberal reimbursement history have contributed to the myth that high-tech acute care solves most health problems. As mentioned previously, many of the elderly's problems realistically cannot be treated in an acute-care setting. Because elderly patients frequently experience acute flare-ups of a chronic disease, residual effects of a chronic condition lead to the need for a higher level of service or a continuum of care that includes preventive, therapeutic, rehabilitative, supportive, and maintenance care for the elderly and their families. This level of care, which takes place in both institutional and noninstitutional settings, can delay hospitalization, help improve the quality of life, and maximize functional capacity and self-care. The hospital acute-care experience is a small but important element in the cycle of chronic illness and disability.

The need for health care beyond acute hospitalization requires integration of services that extends the hospital further into the community. Outpatient facilities, long-term care facilities, senior housing developments, hospices, senior centers, and so on serve as physical sites for contact with the elderly. In addition, many opportunities exist for involvement and coordination with existing community services.

Myth #3: Finding a Niche and Exploiting It Is the Answer to Competition

Exploiting a niche or developing a particular program for the elderly may seem a simple solution, but it may not work in the long term. Often the niches hospitals choose duplicate services offered at other nearby hospitals. Sometimes these forays into the marketplace take place without real strategic planning, which can lead to fragmentation of services, a lack of continuity of care, and a decline in the quality of care provided. It is important for hospitals to diversify, but they must do so by integrating their own unique services and strengths. They must also examine the internal resources—staff, equipment, diagnostic resources—required to handle new programs and orient those resources to new services. In addition, in the scramble for market niches it is possible for a hospital to lose its ability to differentiate itself from competitors. Just adhering to the slogan "whoever gets there first, captures the market" without devoting time to planning and design often leads to failure.

Myth #4: Hospitals Must Diversify to Survive in Today's Marketplace

Because diversification alone does not guarantee survival in today's health care environment, hospitals must *integrate* their service delivery systems. *Diversification* occurs when a provider extends its business activities into various business lines that function independently. *Integration* is designed to build a continuum or network of care that complements and maximizes the effectiveness and profitability of the entire system. Although this system-building approach is a form of diversification, subsidiaries are vertically integrated to benefit the system as a whole rather than as individual components.[6] This concept was developed to strengthen the provider financially while enhancing its market attractiveness and efficacy in responding to community needs. When the hospital's role is evaluated within the greater social process and within its particular environment, an institution can take its rightful place as a leader in a health care system committed to a continuity of caring services—preventive, acute, transitory, and long-term.

Fortunately, in light of hard experience, hospital administrators and planners are rethinking their diversification strategies. Managers and administrators now know that time and resources spent on ill-conceived projects contribute little, if anything, to the bottom line. Unrealistic expectations, lack of clear objectives, and poor execution have forced hospitals to reorient themselves to new strategies.

Myth #5: The Older Person Is the Only Consumer

It is easy to view the older person as the only health care consumer, but this is not the case. Aging is a family affair, and adult children often make health care decisions for their aging parents. Consequently, they will perceive that the hospital that takes good care of their parents also will take good care of the rest of the family. Hospitals that focus on the family (from youth through old age) as part of their mission will create a long-lasting bond.

Planning for Organizational Change

Before practical decisions can be made about the long-term direction a hospital might take, its current and future development must be analyzed. Additionally, research must be conducted to gauge more accurately where the hospital is positioned currently in relation to where it wants to be in the future.

In their campaign to move hospitals toward continuity of care in an orderly and successful manner, many hospital planners already employ departments and staff dedicated to patient assessment and discharge planning. However, without a global mission statement that brings every internal group into the process, it is easy to revert to creating quick fixes (that is, niches) without the benefit of strategic planning and proper follow-through. In creating a mission statement that focuses on meaningful continuity of health care, the hospital and all its internal groups can move away from the concept of acute care or high-tech care toward reevaluation of the hospital's fundamental mission to fulfill changing patient needs.

Administrators, trustees, physicians, nurses, and staff can and should be involved in planning any strategy that focuses on changing existing systems to meet the long-term care needs of the elderly. Hospital leadership must provide a proactive atmosphere in which myths and barriers are overcome and the new definition for continuity of care permeates the process. Again, the hospital's new mission should turn on its role as a health care center, not just as an acute-care facility.

The first step in achieving facilitywide commitment to continuity of care is to reeducate and reorient internal groups so that resistance to change and fear of risk taking are eliminated. In other words, a foundation must be laid that brings administrators, hospital board members, physicians, nurses, and all staff through the process of redefining the mission and then planning to fulfill it. The next step is to involve the various groups that can help plan and implement an integrated program of eldercare services.

Providing Education in Eldercare

An umbrella campaign should be launched to educate and motivate the entire hospital to take an interest in the eldercare market. Such a program would bring together all levels—from the governing board to hourly workers. For example, a program goal could be to broaden staff awareness regarding special care needs of the elderly. Of particular importance is getting staff to understand that the needs of the elderly change, not necessarily due to age but to changing functional ability. Participants should learn skills that help them develop sensitivity to special aging-related problems. These include multiplicity of diseases, chronic disability, and social problems unique to older adults who are without family or other immediate care givers. These types of educational exercises have been introduced at a variety of institutions, including South Shore Hospital and Medical Center, Miami Beach; Greater Southeast Community Hospital, Washington, D.C.; and The Mount Sinai Medical Center, New York City.

In developing such a "think elderly" program, employees across many levels within the hospital can be involved in planning various components in a *quality circle* arrangement, which brings multidisciplinary groups together to work on resolving specific problem areas. For instance:

- Plant and equipment personnel can provide input on ease of access into the hospital.
- Volunteers may offer an elderly escort program.
- The department responsible for signage can ensure that signs throughout the hospital are in large letters.
- Parking can be evaluated to determine whether specific areas should be reserved for the elderly or if valet parking should be instituted. (Consideration should be given to the fact that some elderly people have a fear of parking garages and may need special access, escort service, or a parking area that is closer to the hospital.)
- The hospital sometimes can tie its goals in with existing transportation systems, for which older adults may be willing to pay.

Hospital staff would benefit from exposure to special needs and demands of the elderly population. These include major considerations such as care management; less comprehensive needs such as assistance due to lack of mobility; and sensitivity to hearing impairment. Training courses can teach basic skills in customer relations, serving to remind employees that a hospital environment can intimidate an elderly patient who already may suffer functional loss, confusion, or impairment. There should be a focus on patients' psychological and social well-being as well as their physical status. Discharge planning and case management studies can serve as a basis for a task force assessing those needs.

Working with Internal and External Audiences in the Change Process

Whether initiated from administrators or the governing body of the hospital, the commitment to eldercare must remain strong at the very top echelons. In determining direction and managing hospital operations, administration must take the leadership role in creating a top–down attitude that embraces the "geriatric imperative" for continuity of care. In addition, administrators must create allies among all staff levels by involving them in the proactive planning process. These groups include the governing board, medical staff, volunteers, the elderly, and the community.

The Governing Board

If the governing board is to participate in the process of examining a new mission proposal, administrators must proceed on the premise that such involvement is mission related as well as economics related. Economics is forcing these hospital players into more active roles.[7] Certainly the traditional detachment between management and the governing body must be replaced by active partnership roles.

As members of the community and as business leaders within that community, board members can bring to the educational process a mission orientation that has wide-reaching social benefits. Board members also serve as important advocates to the business community and may have prior care-giver experience, for example, as a nurse or physician, which can be particularly beneficial to this process. Discussing the status of the elderly in the community, their own experiences in care giving and those of their peers, local and national demographic trends, limitations in existing social services, and available alternatives will give board members food for thought as they begin their own internal processes of reorientation.

Hospital administrators should consider bringing in a consultant to conduct this planning and training phase involving governing board members. A consultant can provide information about activities at other sites, analyze data more objectively, and give additional insight into a hospital's strengths and weaknesses. The outside consultant also can help develop a geriatrics planning committee among board members to gather data, plan programs, develop consensus, and fuel momentum. Such consultants should not be promotion-oriented only, but should enhance internal organizational aspects of the planning process. Committee discussions can take place in a variety of venues, such as retreats or a series of educational sessions with medical staff, to provide information on local aging issues. Educational institutions or area agencies that work with the elderly might provide faculty for such sessions. Position papers and conferences should echo a central theme of older persons' needs in the community. Circulation of appropriate literature can prepare members for discussions.

In essence, the governing board should be encouraged to consider two questions: How can existing hospital services meet the needs of the elderly in the community? How can the hospital respond as a community facility to the social and medical problems of older adults in the community?

The Medical Staff

Physician advocacy of an eldercare program can add significant power and prestige to the planning process. As mentioned earlier, physicians, especially those who treat a large number of elderly patients, already experience frustration over the lack of posthospitalization follow-through for their patients, as well as a perceived lack of control over their decision-making powers due to DRG regulations on lengths of stays.

Additionally, eldercare problems can be alleviated by introducing special skill training among medical staff (physicians are more motivated to treat older adults if they understand their needs). Moreover, when hospitals provide the necessary case-management services and counseling to adult children and other family members, the physician is more likely to want to be involved, knowing that the total burden for these services will not rest on his or her shoulders.

An ad hoc geriatrics planning committee, composed of administrative staff, physicians, board members, nurses, and social workers, can explore ways to bring physicians into the "think elderly" program. Those physicians known to treat and admit large numbers of elderly and those in certain specialties—cardiology, urology, rheumatology, neurology, ophthalmology, for example—are ideal to serve on such a committee. The committee can develop standards of geriatric care and serve in an advisory capacity for other hospital programs as well. For example, members can lead educational programs for staff and the governing body. Seminars within specialty groups can educate physicians about the needs of the elderly and how physicians might take advantage of opportunities to increase their practice base.

Continuing education programs for physicians, particularly for primary care physicians—can increase sensitivity to the need for geriatric medicine, as well as offer a convenient way for physicians to comply with continuing education requirements. These programs, when opened to physicians outside the hospital sphere, broaden the image of the hospital as an eldercare provider. If expanded to nursing homes and other health care facilities, these programs can create a network of feeder patterns into the hospital. When conducted by selected physicians within the institution, they become a means by which medical staff can market the hospital.

Depending on the competition among physicians and the hospital structure, size, and its orientation, each geriatric program will develop differently. The hospital might appoint a chief of geriatric medicine, create a department of geriatric medicine, develop inpatient and/or outpatient geriatric assessment units, or develop its own unique structure. Physicians generally prefer to admit patients to a hospital-based service or one the hospital is affiliated with, because they have less fear of patient loss. Whatever the choices, through careful and thoughtful planning the hospital will arrive at solutions best suited to its needs.

Volunteers

Volunteers are valuable human resources who can assist the hospital in meeting its eldercare goals. An important feature of volunteerism is that it provides additional personalized attention that communicates caring and kindness. Because many volunteers tend to be older, they offer a special viewpoint with regard to the needs of older people. Within the hospital, they can be involved in escorting, transporting, and providing information to patients and their families, even serving as counselors to help with health insurance forms.

Special training programs in the care of elderly patients should be developed for volunteers. The content of these programs, developed by the hospital, will give volunteers an understanding of the continuum of care and their role as part of the patient care team. This care-giver training will assist them in providing care within the hospital setting and elsewhere, for example, when caring for their own parents, older siblings, or spouses.

Volunteers can be taught to assist older patients in the community with processing their paperwork. It is no wonder that for the hospitalized elderly (three times the number of younger inpatients), hospital paperwork can be the most traumatic part of their hospital stay.[8] Confronted with admission forms, insurance papers and consent forms, an elderly patient easily can become overwhelmed.

The hospital with a patient advocate or volunteer who can help patients wade through the paper maze can help alleviate stress associated with this process. This service can be integrated with a senior membership program that offers a variety of services, thus making hospitalization less overwhelming and more personalized for the elderly patient and acknowledging the volunteer as an integral member of the hospital team.

Volunteers can teach self-care and even be sent out to senior centers, churches, and housing developments to help take blood pressures or provide information and referral assistance. This has been particularly successful at Greater Southeast Community Hospital, which runs hypertension screening programs through a volunteer network composed of 25 churches. Within the hospital setting, volunteers can provide a "guidance system" for elderly patients, who many times are fearful of finding their way around alone.

Because volunteers may be considered "hospital authorities" within their own circle of friends, they can serve as hospital spokespersons. Entire senior groups have been known to join hospital-based membership programs or an HMO based on a volunteer's informal promotion.

The Elderly

Elderly involvement with the hospital can have far-reaching benefits. As noted earlier, if the hospital provides excellent care for a grandparent or parent and is involved with that patient even after hospitalization, then the perception will follow that the hospital also provides excellent care for the nonelderly family members.

Hospital-sponsored self-help groups and wellness activities can bring families into the hospital. Volunteers, especially older volunteers, not only provide tremendous resources for relief and patient relations, they also receive the benefits of meaningful activity. In addition, inviting elderly community members, such as business retirees, to serve on governing boards and advisory committees is an ideal way to show the hospital's commitment to serving the needs of older adults while taking advantage of their unique life experiences.

The Community

A "think elderly" program also can involve the community. For example, local chapters of the American Association of Retired Persons (AARP) or Area Agencies on Aging often lack input from hospital people; nor do hospitals attempt to benefit from the vast community knowledge these organizations have—much less their political clout. For example, such groups can:

- Provide much of the information and resources necessary for a comprehensive program
- Lead seminars and lectures geared toward selected groups
- Serve as conduits through which the hospital's intentions are publicized to the community
- Provide access to social services agencies, corporations, and other interest groups active in the area
- Provide zoning and lobbying assistance

Hospital staff members can contribute to these voluntary organizations by serving in an advisory capacity or as active volunteers.

Summary

Considering the demographic evolution our society will undergo in the next few decades and society's response to new needs, hospitals must begin planning to ensure their own survival as well as to take advantage of new opportunities. At the same time, hospital management must resist the urge to rush into creating services without careful thought and planning. A commitment to continuity of care necessitates serious evaluation of a hospital's current mission and thoughtful regard to redirecting the hospital's role in society.

Health care needs of the elderly will continue to grow and diversify, so that it will become impossible for a hospital to provide all necessary services. At the same time, no other community institution serves more elderly than the hospital, and therefore none is in a better position both to capitalize on the elderly market and to provide leadership for improving quality of life for older persons.

To plan and deliver effective and successful continuity of care, hospitals must interact and create partnerships with both internal and external audiences. Cooperative relationships with internal groups and external agencies can ensure that continuity of care is delivered in an integrated, coordinated manner.

References

1. Special Committee on Aging. *Aging America: Trends and Projections* Washington, DC: U.S. Government Printing Office, 1989, p. 93.
2. Spivack, S. A challenge to survival. In: S. J. Brody and N. A. Persily, editors. *Hospitals and the Aged: The New Old Market.* Rockville, MD: Aspen Publishers, 1984, pp. 4–9.
3. Greenwald, M. Bad news for the baby boom. *American Demographics* 2(2):34, Feb. 1989.
4. Special Committee, p. 4.
5. *Exploding the Myths: Caregiving in America,* a study by the Subcommittee on Human Services of the Select Committee on Aging, House of Representatives, Jan. 1987, p. 9.
6. Graham, J. Diversified hospitals review plans after some bumpy rides. *Modern Healthcare* 17(17):30–40, Aug. 14, 1987.
7. Signer, C. A. Economics forces hospital "players" to assume new, complementary roles. *Modern Healthcare* 15(25):60, Dec. 6, 1985.
8. Special Committee, p. 91.

Chapter 5

Service Options in Eldercare

Nancy Alfred Persily

No one hospital can develop all the different health care services available to the eldercare market. Alternative services will differ depending on each hospital's environment, location, internal structure, and market base. Research that examines the hospital's internal strengths and weaknesses as well as external threats and opportunities will be vital when determining the specific services to be considered. This chapter addresses specific questions about marketing strategies and service options for the elderly, including:

- How do hospital planners determine which services are most appropriate to develop on-site, off-site, or in cooperation with other agencies and groups?
- What services should be offered to the elderly?
- How should service options be structured and what marketing approach implemented?
- What services will generate revenues?
- How can a system be created that will serve the hospital's mission?

Opportunities in the Eldercare Market

As noted previously, opportunities abound in today's marketplace. The U.S. elderly population is increasing, and the creative health care manager will study demographic trends and conditions carefully to explore a variety of service ideas and options. Each offering should be examined to determine its "fit" within the hospital's existing structure, mission, and service environment. Many options will require some reorganization, whereas others may be as simple as strengthening, expanding, or marketing existing services. Because several of the desired service components may already exist within the community, it may be viable for hospitals to consider networking with other groups to provide them. Community resources can be mobilized to develop a cohesive network among providers that deliver eldercare services. Such a network, when coordinated by a hospital, can lead to a stronger market image and increased patient referrals, as well as foster hospital bonding with community organizations.

To be responsive to today's marketplace, hospital administrators must reexamine the hospital's structure and its mission. As discussed in preceding chapters, the United States is no longer "a nation of the young." Therefore, insurers and health care providers must redesign the health care financing and delivery system to meet the needs of older adults who suffer from various chronic conditions. By matching products and services with the preferences and needs of the community, hospitals can begin to address effectively the requirements of the elderly population.

The gap between America's existing medical system and the evolving needs of an aging population has stimulated new ways of thinking about health care. Multiple gaps exist within and between these two system components, resulting in fragmented and overlapping services without a single access point. New outcome measurements must be developed that are geared to the level of *function* as opposed to the level of *illness.* An effective eldercare services system will integrate medical, health, social, and support services to meet the diversity of older persons' needs. This eldercare system will merge with the disparate acute-care, long-term care, and social services systems that currently exist.

The hospital is strategically positioned to serve as the central coordinator for eldercare services because it cares for older people during the time when they need services the most and because it has a cadre of personnel who are available to provide not only medical care services but also information, referral, and in some instances, even case-management services. Entry into the system can be facilitated through the hospital or affiliated providers connected through a variety of formal and informal relationships. The effectiveness of this network is measured in terms of efficient utilization of resources—how older patients are served in the least restrictive environment in accordance with their needs. By moving patients into the least intensive level of care, resources can be used more appropriately and costs minimized across all care settings.

Market Research

The first step in determining which market strategies and service options to consider is to perform some preliminary market research. This step includes gathering internal, external, and qualitative data.

Internal Data

Planning a new hospital program begins most appropriately with the gathering of internal data. Management information systems can provide a wealth of demographic information on inpatients and outpatients. The ages of the inpatient and outpatient populations are the most important data elements, and data should be segmented generally in 10-year increments to determine trends and examine current and future Medicare demands.

Similarly, correlating the sex of inpatients or outpatients with their ages can give the hospital valuable information on which to base service decisions. (For example, in 1987 there were three women for every two men over age 65.)[1] Older men also tend to marry younger women, which means that more elderly women live alone, and more aging men may have care givers to coordinate and render necessary services.[2] If this is true, there is a need for services directed particularly at elderly women, many of whom live alone and some who have no care givers. These services include transportation and community support programs, such as homemakers, emergency response systems, day care, and even guardianship programs.

Patient origin studies reveal where patients live and provide valuable information for determining the composition of primary, secondary, and tertiary service areas. From this information, the need for transportation services and even satellite facilities can be suggested. Other internal data to be gathered include type and volume of diagnosis related groups (DRGs) by age and admitting physician and modes of entry of patients (that is, number that enter through the emergency room).

Diagnostic Groups

What services draw elderly patients to the hospital? Does the hospital have a reputation for treating a particular illness? Several factors determine why a patient or family chooses a hospital: reputation of the service offered, the physician practicing there, location, presence of other competitive facilities, and personal preference based on experience.

If certain elderly population groups (by age, for instance) come to the hospital for specific health problems, such as pulmonary or cardiac problems, that information can be used by the hospital to promote the service to other interested patient, physician, or community groups.

It is of vital importance that information on patient groups correlate with that of referring physicians. Physicians who admit a majority of elderly patients should have their data broken down by specialty, department, office location, admissions by diagnosis, and total hospital revenue generated. Those who admit significant numbers of elderly persons can render valuable information about the patients' needs and the physicians' desires. If a physician perceives that the hospital is interested in elderly patients, referral patterns can become more positive.

Length of stay data can indicate severity of illness, and comparing length of stay data to usage by age groups can provide important information for establishing optimum patient mix. When correlated by type of service (such as intensive care and rehabilitation), length of stay data also can be an important factor in determining the success or failure of discharge planning and the availability or need for aftercare services. Changes in Medicare reimbursement formulas make it necessary for hospitals to track such information for financial survival as well as for the patient's well-being.

Modes of Entry

It is useful to discover modes of entry by patients, whether through the emergency department, outpatient clinic, private physician referral, skilled nursing facility (SNF), or health maintenance organization (HMO).

Open 24 hours a day, 7 days a week, the emergency department is the site for a significant proportion of elderly admissions to the hospital. Emergency room data can provide information about type and severity of cases, patient origin, type of medical or social problem, and the number of readmissions. Admissions through the outpatient department can provide information about services used, frequency of admitting diagnoses, method of payment, and overall referral patterns. Reviewing utilization of services (for example, radiology, pathology, or rehabilitation) can determine what the split is on inpatient and outpatient usage, the financial implications of promoting more outpatient care, and the profitability of various services. Referral patterns should indicate which physicians use outpatient services, and the next step would be to determine why.

An analysis of inpatient admissions and outpatient services provided to HMO patients can advise administration as to the profitability of the arrangement with the HMO, because this will shed light on whether or not managed care groups just use the hospital for the inpatient stay or for continuing care as well.

Skilled nursing facility referrals should be analyzed for appropriateness, length of stay, admitting diagnosis, and ease of return following discharge. Ongoing analysis of these admissions can ensure legitimate use of inpatient acute beds. It can also track appropriateness of admissions by nursing homes and can flag quality of care issues, for example, if certain nursing homes consistently send the hospitals patients with decubiti (bed sores).

In addition, length of stay data in general can provide important information on the need for hospice care, rehabilitation, home care, and convalescent care. When hospitals have "length of stay problems," they are often related to the lack of appropriate services in the community or lack of services for the medically indigent. It is important for a hospital to sort out these problems to determine what may be best in terms of their future financial health.

External Data

A number of commercial sources can provide information about the community. For example, banks and utility companies carry out their own marketing research; real estate and taxation information is available to the public; and sociology, economics, and geography departments at local academic institutions continually examine the surrounding community for purposes of training. Many of these resources are readily available to local hospitals. A hospital could even work with a teaching facility by volunteering to be a research project site.

More sophisticated demographic and trend analysis data on the elderly are available from many sources. For example, government and hospital publications publish national, state, and regional demographic trend analyses; health services distribution; and hospital delivery patterns. Census data also are available from the U.S. Census Bureau, the National Center for Health Statistics, state and local regional planning agencies, agencies on aging, health systems agencies, hospital cost containment boards, and local health departments.

Data on the number of individuals on nursing home waiting lists can suggest ways hospitals might serve patients in line for those beds and indicate what the demand is for alternative long-term services.

Congregate care facilities—those offering protective environments with services that include meals, housekeeping, nursing, transportation, and social activities—should be inventoried regarding the number of such facilities in the community, the average age of residents, affiliations with medical institutions, and ownership of the facilities. Condominiums and other residential developments heavily occupied by older adults can provide opportunities for emergency in-home medical services, home care, screenings, clinics, emergency response systems, oxygen therapy, and durable medical equipment (DME).

A thorough analysis of competitors and their programs for older adults is of particular importance and also a source for new ideas, but that does not necessarily mean their programs should be replicated. An inventory of comparable providers—institutions with similar organizational structures and similar markets—should be developed and closely examined.

Qualitative Data

Whereas the research activities discussed so far involve the gathering of *quantitative* information, there also exists a need to determine what is unique about the hospital's product and services in relation to the area's elderly and their families. *Qualitative* research seeks to uncover perceptions that exist in the minds of patients, physicians, and the community at large; what their expectations are; and what their experiences have been. Qualitative data also offer valuable information on perceptions, preferences, and attitudes toward services being planned by the hospital.

These perceptions are important because community leaders, providers, and physicians play a crucial role in influencing health care choices made by the elderly. Physicians, for example, often serve as referral gatekeepers in that a new program or service must be marketed to them as well as to the patient to ensure that in their eyes it is acceptable, accessible, and appropriate for their patients. Because today's competitive atmosphere also calls for consumers to choose from a pool of similar services, a hospital must understand consumer preference and demand.

Several tools facilitate qualitative research, including questionnaires, telephone interviews, personal interviews, focus groups, and Delphi processes. For example, a Delphi study might involve polling key community leaders to determine their perceptions regarding the need for institutional or community services. Focus groups can garner information needed to determine community perceptions of facilities and long-term services. *Focus groups* are specially constructed discussion groups that can provide in-depth information from respondents on any matter of interest. The focus group enables older people, for instance, to report in their own words those things that are most important to them regarding community facilities and services. The well-run focus group will provide insights to the hospital that are easily translated into strategic plans and/or questionnaires for in-depth probing with other individuals, if necessary.

Data from qualitative questionnaires tell how the hospital and its services are perceived by patients, donors, and physicians. For instance, in terms of quality, service adequacy, and staff concern, what are their attitudes toward the hospital and the care provided?

This basic qualitative and quantitative market research will provide the administrative staff with the necessary data to educate the governing board, medical staff, and other internal groups so they have the appropriate tools to create a strategic initiative toward a hospitalwide program of eldercare.

Marketing New Services

When planning any new service, keep in mind the four elements of marketing:

1. Product
2. Price
3. Place
4. Promotion

Product refers to the service being offered; *price* denotes anything given up by the consumer (inconvenience, change in behavior patterns, out-of-pocket money); *place* includes location, access, availability, referral mechanism, and hours of operation; and *promotion* involves advertising, public relations, and community education.

These precepts serve as important marketing guidelines during the design, delivery, and promotion of a new product or service. Each new service or product line should be evaluated continually in terms of how it is to be packaged, priced, and promoted and where the service or product will be marketed and delivered. The development of hospital service initiatives, however, must go beyond the four marketing elements. The hospital must determine how the new service will fit within the existing organization, how it will be managed, where the operating funds will come from, and the role of existing staff in program implementation. These components should be examined for each service option to determine its true success potential, especially in terms of how the new service relates to the entire hospital system.

Financial Viability of New Services

Competition for new services can be fierce, and the financial ramifications of adding new services for the elderly will concern many people within the hospital. However, when evaluating these ramifications, planners must research the effect of a new program or service on the entire hospital system and not simply develop the most profitable service that might benefit only one department. Planners should develop a methodology to learn how patients are referred to the hospital and how the hospital can reach those patients, and then maximize referrals throughout the system by creating complementary programs. Rather than evaluating profit or loss by cost center, this type of patient tracking can determine how new spin-offs affect the total system. If the services are well planned and well integrated into the total delivery system, health care can be provided in a high-quality, cost-effective, and efficient manner.

One study indicates that hospital service expansion efforts continue to be successful, and a number of the top-ranking options relate to the eldercare market: freestanding outpatient diagnosis, inpatient rehabilitation, home health, nursing facilities, and retirement housing, for example. Top-ranking ones had a success rate of 54 percent or more, of which many were money makers (figure 5-1). For retirement housing projects, more than 34 percent were breaking even, and over 25 percent were making money. For skilled nursing facilities, the success rate was even higher: 34 percent broke even, and 34 percent made a profit. The result? Through the development of integrated health care delivery, hospitals can serve the elderly and still realize a profit that benefits the entire system.[3]

Figure 5-1. Hospital Service Expansion Strategies Ranked by Success in Generating a Profit or Breaking Even

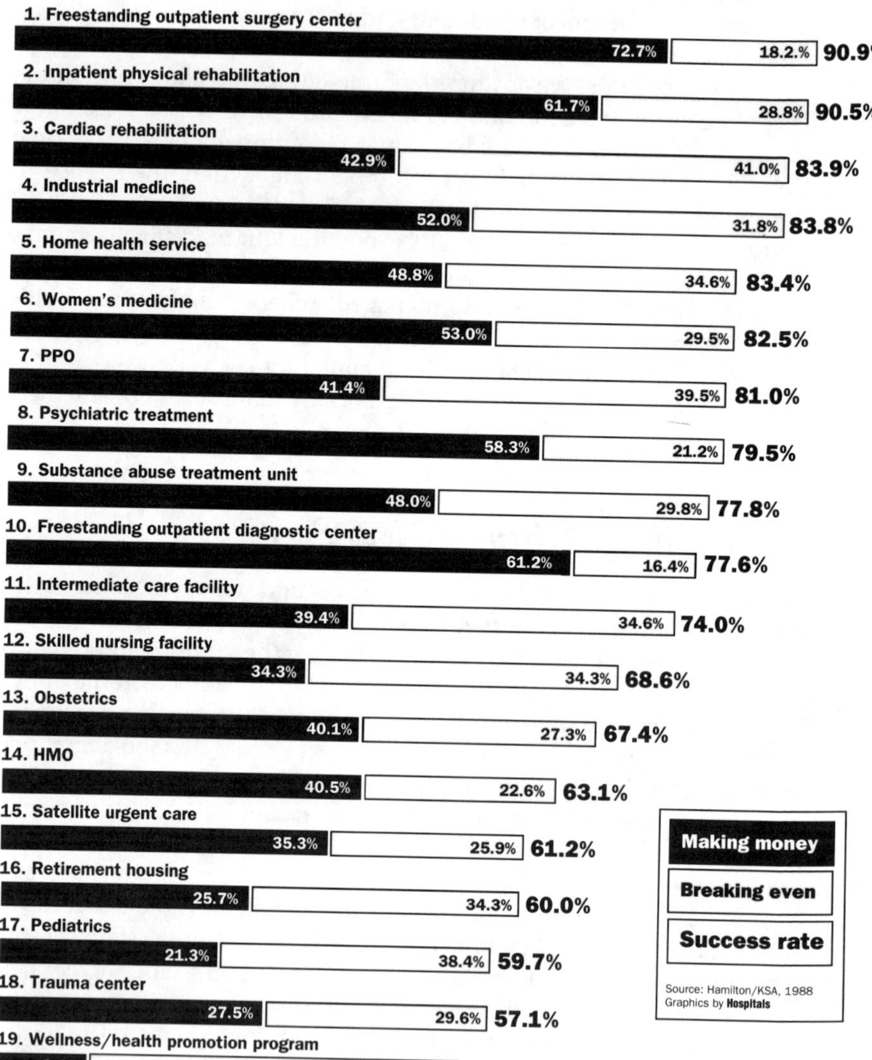

Source: Hamilton/KSA, 1989. Adapted, with permission, from Sabatino, F. Survey: managed care led '89 diversification improvements. *Hospitals* 64(1):56–59, Jan. 5, 1990.

Note: Numbers to the right of the bars indicate success rates.

Selecting Market Segments for New Services

The diversity within the eldercare market was highlighted in previous chapters. Once the market segments have been identified—for example, the younger old (65–74 years), the older old (75–84 years), and the very old (85 and over)—the appropriate service development must be determined. The hospital must decide which market it wants to target and what services it will provide. A number of factors will influence the decision, including the following:

- The hospital's mission
- Available and profitable markets
- Profit potential
- Existing provider resources
- Strengths and weaknesses of the facility
- Physician and community services
- Competition
- Other current and anticipated market conditions

Hospitals might consider pursuing several emerging markets. For example, the younger old market, which tends to be healthier and more active than its older counterparts, is composed of older adults who remain viable through diet, exercise, education, and staying abreast of the latest health information. Preventive, diagnostic, and wellness programs are some services that would appeal to this market, along with inpatient and outpatient psychiatric services and a long-term care insurance program.

The mildly disabled elderly is another market that could be targeted. This group experiences limitations in activities of daily living (ADL), but may function on their own or with modest assistance. Appropriate services include helping with paperwork, financial planning, assisted living programs/residential housing, home health care, short-term rehabilitative care, and transportation.

The frail elderly often are severely disabled and require intensive services as well as long-term institutional care. Other options may include comprehensive in-home services as well as infusion therapy, DME, and nursing home and hospice care.

Another emerging market is that of care givers to the elderly, an informal support system that provides a variety of eldercare services. Children, spouses, and siblings are the most prevalent care givers, with distant relatives, friends, and neighbors playing smaller roles. Services for this group could include case management, respite care, care-giver education, and training as well as care-giver support groups. Services for the frail elderly—adult day care, home health, homemaker, shopping and chore services—also could be marketed directly to the care givers. These services could alleviate the burden of care for individuals who are experiencing multiple demands and responsibilities.

The impact of these care demands has been particularly acute for women who, although previously available to provide home care, may now be in the work force. As primary users of health care facilities and heads of families, women tend to decide where the health care dollar is to be spent. Finally, because they generally live longer than their spouses, women often are the primary caretakers for ailing husbands.[4]

In determining which market to pursue and what services to offer or coordinate, health care managers can draw from the findings derived from internal and external assessments conducted during the planning process stage.

Researching Service Options

A number of market opportunities will emerge from the initial research performed on the internal and external environments. These findings need to be evaluated in terms of the hospital's current programs, resources, and priorities. Once a menu of options has surfaced, the institution can research the marketability of those services and then determine which ones it can provide (both managerially and financially), which are fiscally sound, and how they should be promoted in the marketplace.

To measure product marketability, hospitals will need to conduct more focused research to examine consumer feelings, preferences, and reactions to proposed service options. The most common and widely used techniques are survey research, personal interviews, and focus-group interviews.

The primary objective of this research is to learn how to package, design, and market services during the planning stages of program development. Although some services may be necessary or appropriate for the elderly market, they may not be well received due to a number of reasons: cultural or religious concerns, regional or public opinions, fear, or preferences of some elderly to perform the service themselves. Moreover, although a service may be needed, consumers might balk at the price set to offset the costs. From the hospital's perspective, if the service is incapable of generating adequate benefits to the entire system, then the product cannot be considered financially sound.

This phase of planning also is critical in ascertaining how the service or product should be promoted to the public. Because the elderly often consider their cognizant age to be 10 to 15 years younger than their actual age, promotional campaigns that portray them as poor, helpless, and frail will tend to offend rather than attract. The elderly prefer being portrayed as dignified, intelligent, and still having something to offer. The best strategy for promoting services to older adults is to refrain from depicting them as too old or treating age in a negative light.

Site Location for New Services

Eldercare services can be located on-site or off-site – depending on the program and target market. For example, if the hospital is located in an urban area and has a large low-income patient base, a satellite service site in a suburban area may attract a larger private pay or Medicare market – particularly effective if the satellite program is located near a retirement community. Conversely, if the hospital has attractive grounds that are underutilized, and is located in a suburban area, an extended-care unit or nursing home could be located on campus rather than off-site.

Organizational Options for Eldercare Programs

Organizational options that should be considered for eldercare program development include hospital-owned and sponsored services, joint ventures, formal cooperative relationships, and networking strategies.

Hospital-Owned and Sponsored Services

Hospital-sponsored programs span educational programs to rehabilitative day hospitals and skilled nursing facilities.

One problem confronting eldercare program development is that the programs must compete with specialized programs designed for other markets, and large capital outlays are required to initiate services. Many of these specialized services may be money makers, so they easily capture the administration's attention. The deciding factor, however, should be how the service will benefit the entire system in achieving its goals, with particular emphasis on effecting continuity of care for patients throughout their illness and through convalescence.

A variety of options provide greater continuity of care – educational, discharge planning, and case-management programs; programs for geriatric units or for geriatric rehabilitation; or programs for hospital-owned day hospitals, home health care, and skilled nursing facilities. (Case-management programs are discussed in depth in chapter 6.)

Educational Programs

According to a 1986 American Hospital Association survey, the most frequently offered hospital-based services to the elderly were patient education and information programs.[5] Educational programs for the elderly are certainly the most likely to dovetail with existing hospital programs. These can be provided by hospital staff or coordinated with community agency programs. Key topics may include informational programs on money management, long-term care insurance, medications, different diseases, self-care, exercise, and safety.

Educational programs also can be designed for specific eldercare groups or special events. For example, care-giver classes can serve as both educational programs and support groups, offering needed skill training and support to care givers while a loved one is in the hospital. Senior citizen clubs provide activities and opportunities for socialization. Outside or in-house experts can be used for one-time sessions or a series of classes.

In-house experts are valuable because they are knowledgeable about the specific health care problems affecting the hospital and its community. In addition, staff physicians can heighten hospital visibility by conducting seminars that are open to the entire community. The educational programs help market the hospital and can be tied in to other local or regional activities, for example, Older Americans Month.

Program location is important. Health promotion programs for the elderly can be offered at the hospital or at local retirement communities, nursing homes, condominiums, community schools, churches, or senior centers. Some hospitals provide transportation for the elderly to the classes at the hospital or have vans that bring services to them.

Many older adults often are lonely due to loss of their loved ones; many have moved upon retirement, leaving friends and family. As a result, educational programs that offer opportunities for social interaction can attract the older adult market. A major need among older adults is companionship, and educational activities can afford opportunities not only to enhance their own self-care abilities but to meet others who share similar interests and concerns. The primary benefit to the hospital is increased awareness in the community as an institution that cares for older adults. This translates into bonding of entire families with the total hospital/health care organization and can lead to more patients and increased private pay as well as Medicare sources.

Discharge Planning

Discharge planning is a routine hospital process, and under prospective reimbursement effective and efficient discharge planning has become a fiscal necessity for hospitals. Third-party payers increasingly have a role in when and how patients are discharged and what services they will use following discharge. Hospitals are forming closer bonds with nursing homes and home health care agencies to ensure continuity of care so that patients can be discharged on a timely basis. Standard flagging should be in place in every facility for discharging "at-risk" patients in order to identify special needs. By averting unnecessary rushing at the end of the patient's stay, inappropriate placements (such as premature institutionalization) can be avoided. At-risk patients commonly include people over age 85, who are most likely to have loss of function; those over age 75 who live alone; disoriented patients; and those with multiple needs. Other candidates for discharge planning include patients in certain diagnostic categories (such as oncological, neurological, or psychiatric) or those who have repeat hospitalizations. If discharge planning begins upon admission and effective assessment tools are utilized, a timely discharge can be facilitated.

Discharge planning is an essential part of the case-management process, discussed in depth in chapter 6.

Geriatric Units

Geriatric units are developed specifically to provide medical services to elderly patients who suffer from a variety of medical conditions. Geriatric units within hospitals have met with resounding success in some select environments, whereas others have had only modest success. The main questions to ask when considering the development of a geriatric unit are: What are the expected payoffs, and what are the potential risks or drawbacks? Answers to these two questions will provide helpful insights into the program's success potential.

Veterans Administration (VA) hospitals are successful program sites for geriatric units. Elderly patients treated in VA geriatric evaluation units are often less likely to eventually need nursing home care than patients treated in the traditional VA system, where there is no multidisciplinary assessment of the patient. Under a multidisciplinary team approach, VA patients regain functioning through the diagnosis and treatment of conditions that otherwise may be overlooked. Those conditions, which are often not the primary diagnosis, may include balance problems, problems with sight and hearing, forgetfulness, and so on. These conditions can exacerbate medical conditions (when patients forget to take medications) or can lead to more traumatic medical problems like falling and breaking a hip. A likely reason for the success of VA geriatric units is the cadre of VA hospital–based physicians who have access to a variety of training programs at the facility. Also, competition among physicians for patients is not a major factor because the physicians are all on staff at the hospital and do not get reimbursed on a per-patient basis.[6]

Montefiore Medical Center in New York City has a successful geriatric unit, where the inpatient service program uses a multidisciplinary team approach. The team includes physicians and nurses, rehabilitation specialists, social workers, a psychologist, a pharmacist, a dietitian, and a lawyer who advises on patients' rights and competency matters; all are skilled in geriatric care.

Initial costs for such evaluation units are high. However, costs can be recouped due to a decreased need for acute-care hospitalization and post-hospital nursing home care. The length of stay can be managed by a cooperative staff and a responsive information system. It is generally believed that for a carefully selected subgroup of elderly persons, a comprehensive geriatric evaluation and follow-up program can yield impressive benefits to the institution without increasing the ultimate cost of health care.

Geriatric units, however, can be perceived as a threat to physicians outside the unit who view the program as fostering competition for patients. A patient may be "lost" if admitted to a special unit for treatment by a physician specially trained in geriatric care. Yet dedicated geriatric units can be viewed as an adjunct to the overall medical treatment provided by all physicians. When this type of assessment is done within the hospital setting and as part of the medical process, it gets physicians involved in the "think elderly" atmosphere.

An outpatient geriatric unit can allay these physician concerns by providing a mechanism through which a patient can be assessed by a geriatric specialty team and then referred back to the primary physician. This approach is used in many teaching hospitals that incorporate geriatric assessment programs. In these environments, geriatric physicians, fellows, social workers, and nurse specialists along with other professionals assess the patient to develop a comprehensive plan of care, involving both medical and social monitoring. The plan is discussed with significant others and then the patient is referred back to the primary physician for ongoing care.

Another eldercare service option is to develop a specialized clinic for the treatment of a specific problem or disease. Rather than focusing on the entire medical field, the clinic addresses a particular medical condition. Examples may include incontinence, falls and burns, back injury, or memory disorder clinics; a multidisciplinary team of specialists from a variety of fields participates. An incontinence clinic, for instance, encompasses the disciplines of urology, neurology, internal medicine, psychiatry, gynecology, nursing, and social services. Patients and their families often self-refer to the clinic; referrals are generated from a number of outside sources, such as other hospitals and physicians.

Geriatric Rehabilitation

Rehabilitation services can constitute preventive care for older persons. Once an elderly patient's ability and potential for rehabilitation are recognized, he or she receives services that will help prevent a serious disability. Educational programs with nurses, physicians, care givers, and patients can be effective toward heightening awareness of the rehabilitation potential of the elderly population. Rehabilitation care also can serve as an effective tool to promote the hospital as a caring and progressive provider of eldercare services to the community. Considerable growth has occurred in recent years in the rehabilitation field, where programs include medical rehabilitation units, rehabilitation hospitals, hospital inpatient rehabilitation units, outpatient facilities and services, physical therapy centers, and comprehensive outpatient rehabilitation facilities (CORFs). Although these programs are not specifically geared only to geriatric patients, they do comprise a large share of the total patient population.

Growth in the rehabilitation service arena has been spurred by changes in the reimbursement system. Unlike other hospital-based care, reimbursement for rehabilitative care is exempt from the prospective payment system. As a result, it has emerged in recent years as an attractive source of revenue for the hospital while freeing up other beds for short-stay patients. The need for rehabilitative care has also increased due to elderly population growth and advances in medical technology, which allow people to survive conditions once considered fatal.

Hospitals that already have rehabilitation programs know the difficulties of effective management and marketing of these services. Stiff competition requires planners to create innovative services, programs, and facilities to capture and maintain market share. Many hospitals advertise their rehabilitation programs through promotional campaigns and media exposure. However, because of the complexity and diversity of services, rehabilitation programs require a total marketing effort that targets physicians, case managers, major employers, and discharge planners. A shotgun promotional approach directed solely at potential patients will not be as effective as a broader and more focused approach that seeks to attract patients through key access points.

Rehabilitation services can be well worth the effort. As indicated in an 1989 study by *Hospitals* magazine, inpatient physical rehabilitation was generating a profit in 61.7 percent of the hospitals surveyed. Another 28.8 percent were breaking even, indicating a strikingly high success rate of 90.5 percent, second only to freestanding outpatient diagnostic services (90.9 percent).[7] Most important, however, rehabilitation beds can generate revenue by reducing lengths of stay of older adults, thus freeing up acute-care beds for other patients, and reduce discharge problems by increasing levels of function for the patient and level of involvement by family members. In terms of continuity of care, rehabilitation programs keep the patients in the system, monitor their progress, and often achieve the goal of increased independence.

Hospital Day Care

Often the elderly may need day care services, and these can be provided in the hospital setting. It should be noted that day care itself is not reimbursable by Medicare, although rehabilitation-oriented therapies—such as physical and occupational therapies—are. Receiving therapy in a day-hospital setting keeps patients within a hospital's circle of care without continued hospitalization. For patients who do not need 24-hour care, day care programs can provide needed services such as speech, physical, and occupational therapy training in the activities of daily living as well as recreational outings and social activities.

Home Health Care

Home care is a vital component of health care and continuity of care for the elderly. Home health care provides nursing services, therapy, and other health-related services to patients in their own home; benefits families who need medical assistance in the ongoing care of their loved ones; and ensures physician access to follow-up and recuperative care. Home health care also extends hospital services beyond the acute-care setting.

The field of home health care has enormous growth potential, and the range of medical products and services has increased dramatically. Home health care also tends to be less expensive than institutional care, especially when just out-of-pocket expenses are examined as opposed to informal care-giving costs. Because of tightened reimbursement regulations and confusion over what constitutes covered care, many hospitals are also developing agencies that offer home health services over and above those covered by Medicare, thus carrying continuity of care even further.

The services generally offered by home health agencies include skilled nursing personal care (such as bathing, shaving, oral hygiene); physician referral; physical, speech, and occupational therapy; and other related services. Innovative providers are expanding to offer counseling services, homemaker/companion services, emergency response systems, transportation, shopping assistance, and home-delivered meals.

Home health care usually is administered by a separate department in the hospital, through a subsidiary agency, or through a joint venture with physicians and/or other private entrepreneurial groups. (Joint venture strategies will be covered later in this chapter.)

Skilled Nursing Facilities

Skilled nursing facilities (SNFs) can serve the temporarily needy and frail elderly who have transitory needs that might follow an acute-care hospital discharge. These step-down services, although now recognized as part of the acute-illness episode, do not require the same level of acute care. Skilled nursing facilities can be developed on-site by a hospital or through linkages with continuing care services.

Hospital-based SNFs can be a way for hospitals to extend their services beyond hospitalization, especially those hospitals that, due to empty beds, have available medical and support services, staff, and space. Through creative use of space and innovative programming that builds on existing products and resources, these programs can also be developed off-site. This depends on the hospital resources and existing market conditions—for example, competition and the needs in the community. In addition, Medicare pays a higher rate to beneficiaries treated in hospital-based SNFs than to those who go to freestanding nursing homes.

Forsyth Memorial Hospital in Winston-Salem, North Carolina, experienced a 30 percent decline in one year in the number of days patients spent waiting for nursing home placements. This happened when the holding company that owns the hospital built a 151-bed nursing home on campus. Hospital officials note that it is easier now for hospitals to discharge patients who are difficult to place, such as ventilator-dependent patients, tracheotomy patients, and those with decubital ulcers.[8]

Joint Ventures

Joint ventures are legal relationships formed through the combined resources of two separate organizations in which the whole is often greater than the sum of its parts. Through their combined action, companies can reap the benefits of expanded client base and revenues without assuming the full financial risks or burdens of a new venture. These joint activities often provide infusions of capital and enable businesses to compete in a more efficient and productive manner through shared resources and expertise, resulting in increased effectiveness in service or product delivery.

In the health care setting, joint venture strategies enable hospitals to enter the home health care market without going it alone. They may acquire existing agencies or contract with outside management companies that have expertise in home health care. Collectively these efforts have created a situation in which, as early as 1986, nearly 55 percent of all community hospitals either owned and operated a home health agency (33.3 percent) or had access through a formal contract (21.6 percent).[9] Some benefits associated with joint venture arrangements are more striking than others, yet the less-obvious ones also are significant. For example, obvious benefits to a hospital joint venture include the reduction of risk experienced by a single sponsor, control over costs, and control over quality of care. In addition, as hospitals redefine and extend their mission, they increase their spheres of influence over a wider market base; that is, existing markets are expanded and protected through the assurance of high-quality care. New funding sources can be freed up to provide step-down care and community-based services to expedite discharge planning and enable the hospital to operate more efficiently. Patient–physician relationships can be enhanced, which can lead to greater loyalty and stronger ties to the hospital.

Prospective partners for hospitals in joint ventures include the following:

- Other hospitals
- Physicians and physician groups
- Long-term care facilities
- Home health agencies
- Private for-profit corporations
- Insurance companies
- HMOs
- Real estate developers

The most common joint ventures are physician–hospital relationships. The benefits for physicians include a hedge against shrinking market share and greater support systems. Hospitals benefit because not only can physicians provide expertise to staff ventures, but also an infusion of capital and loyalty in terms of a referral base. Physicians who focus on eldercare typically joint venture with home health programs, durable medical equipment firms, nursing homes, and assisted living centers. A spin-off advantage occurs when physicians discharge to facilities where they have a financial interest and commitment.

Note, however, that stricter Medicare fraud and abuse laws impose on physicians and other health care providers new federal and state regulations covering Medicare reimbursement, referral arrangements, and profit-sharing agreements.

Nursing Homes

Mutually beneficial partnerships can be formed between hospitals and developers of long-term care facilities, or nursing homes. Hospitals gain access to long-term care beds and the expertise of long-term care providers in designing cost-effective programs. By joint venturing with a nursing home, hospitals can free beds up for other patients as acute-care lengths of stays are reduced. Nursing homes benefit from a steady influx of patient/residents and assurance that a resident's condition has not deteriorated as a result of a drawn-out and costly hospital search for an appropriate placement.

Hospitals can influence the quality of patient care in the nursing home by conducting training seminars (for staff and community) on topics such as Alzheimer's disease or diabetes, for example. The nursing home may not have the resources to hire staff with the clinical expertise in these specialized fields. Thus unnecessary and preventable rehospitalizations can be avoided. Similarly, nursing home staff can contribute to the hospital's knowledge base through education of hospital personnel on the complexities of caring for long-term patients with chronic disabilities.

Long-Term Housing/Assisted Living

Some hospitals might consider joint venturing with a developer to build long-term housing on hospital property with the hospital providing medical care for residents. Such agreements also can be made with a group of physicians, national corporations (such as the Marriott Corporation or Brimm), or a local entrepreneurial group. The hospital neither owns nor has a financial commitment to the facility but receives a patient population from it. The long-term care facility benefits because the hospital cares for its residents and makes referrals to it. They also benefit by enhancing the facility's credibility by being associated with a high-quality medical center.

Other Joint Venture Service Options

Hospitals can develop joint ventures with other hospitals. Jointly sponsored programs may include options such as home health services, long-term care facilities, and preferred provider organizations (PPOs). These collaborative activities can prevent duplication of services while realizing greater economies of scale and capitalizing on program diversification across more than one setting. This is especially appealing in a large geographic area or within a health system's network.

Hospitals located in very close proximity to one another may not find it feasible to form joint ventures because of overlapping service areas, which creates a competitive environment. However, more widely dispersed institutions can reap several benefits from joint arrangements without infringing on service boundaries. This may be especially appealing for rural hospitals that link up with larger urban facilities to provide mutually needed services or marketing programs.

In some communities, however, it is possible for hospitals in close proximity to develop joint venture arrangements. For example, the Five-Hospital Homebound Elderly Program was formed in Chicago to provide community-based long-term care to frail elderly persons at risk of institutionalization. The program had five voluntary short-term community teaching hospitals—Augustana, Columbus, Grant, Illinois Masonic, and St. Joseph—averaging 500 beds per institution. Originally designed to offer ambulatory medical and social services to older adults ineligible for Medicare-reimbursed home care, the program later was incorporated and expanded to offer more intensive skilled nursing care through its designation as a Medicare-certified home health agency. The vertical integration resulted in several benefits to the participating hospitals. They gained flexibility during the discharge planning process, showed a reduction in the incidence of unnecessarily lengthy hospital stays, enhanced their public image, and improved continuity of care by involving hospital-affiliated physicians in the program.

SeniorCare, a senior membership program developed by leading nonprofit hospitals on Florida's west coast, is a joint venture arrangement that spans four distinct communities. Participating institutions include Morton Plant (Clearwater), St. Anthony's (St. Petersburg), Sarasota Memorial (Sarasota), St. Joseph's (Tampa), and University Community (Tampa). The program offers a variety of health and educational services: expedited hospital admission, Medicare/insurance claims education, health education, physician referral service, Lifeline (emergency response system), and a newsletter. Each hospital offers specific programs and services for senior adults that address the special needs in its community.

The program protects market share for each institution while also developing a strategy for generating an expanded patient referral base and enhancing their image as leaders in health care for older adults.

An alternative for a specialty or small community hospital would be to joint venture with a large tertiary hospital. Large teaching hospitals also can benefit from formal linkages with smaller institutions to capture new patient markets. Jackson Memorial Hospital (the primary teaching hospital of the University of Miami) and the Veterans Administration Medical Center located in Miami both have developed joint ventures with South Shore Hospital and Medical Center to reach the sizable aged population on Miami Beach for both primary and tertiary care. Florida's first Clinical Geriatric Fellowship was established at South Shore under the joint sponsorship of the University of Miami School of Medicine and the Miami Veterans Administration Hospital. The Geriatric Assessment and Planning Program was established in collaboration with these institutions as well. The VA also established an Adult Day Health Care Program at South Shore Hospital. Other cooperative initiatives and programs developed at South Shore include a Lifeline program, a pain center, and various educational programs. (See the case studies in Part Two for a further explanation of these and other related programs.)

Joint venture relationships can also be developed with members of industry, home health care agencies, durable medical equipment suppliers, and pharmaceutical companies. New England Medical Center in Boston teamed with Caremark, Inc., a national chain of home health agencies, to provide home health care. The hospital also plans to joint venture with another hospital and a nursing home owner to operate a 224-bed nursing home.

Any number of creative joint venture relationships is possible; however, state licensing laws can impede hospitals from directly investing in new businesses. Holding companies set up to make such investments or provide capital pools for investment can provide mechanisms for such ventures within established legal parameters.

Some limitations and risks are involved in joint ventures, but it also is true that with increased risk comes increased reward. The risk assumed can be substantially reduced by conducting the necessary preliminary market research and trend analysis, coupled with good judgment. This approach will take hospitals far in launching new businesses with a good chance for survival.

Formal Cooperative Relationships

Hospitals need not be limited to conventional joint ventures that involve large capital outlays. Continuity of patient care also can be fostered through a variety of cooperative relationships that can take the form of contractual agreements for specific services. According to one American Hospital

Association survey, the most frequently provided hospital services offered through contractual arrangements were home health services, skilled nursing facilities, homemaker services, intermediate care, and hospital care.[10] These arrangements also include joint management of nursing homes and reserving nursing home beds for a specific hospital's discharges.

A hospital contracting with a nursing home to reserve beds ensures that long-term care placements are readily available for discharged patients. With this type of contract, a hospital pays a monthly fee to the nursing home to reserve a specific number of beds, regardless of whether or not the beds are used. In determining whether to enter into such an agreement, hospitals need to decide whether the contractual expense is offset by the cost of holding Medicare patients in acute-care beds until there is a nursing home bed available. Note that Health Care Financing Administration (HCFA) rules only allow the hospital to reserve the space, not to pay the nursing home to provide care on behalf of the hospital.[11]

Good Samaritan Health Services in Portland, Oregon, has been actively involved in contractual agreements with 12 nursing homes throughout the state. The hospital provides nutritional consultation, laboratory services, nursing education consultation, medical directorship, and utilization review to nursing homes.[12] In such a relationship, the hospital creates an atmosphere of goodwill and generates an active referral base of elderly patients from these facilities.

The hospital also brings a wide array of strengths to a contractual arrangement; for example, strong management capabilities, high-tech medical equipment, a large physical plant, and expertise in a variety of health care specialties and treatment modalities. Building on these strengths requires ingenuity and creativity. Presenting them to other providers can be initiated on a very small scale to "break the ice" and lay the foundation for future relationships through the establishment of trust. Joint purchasing agreements and other administrative arrangements that save both groups money or lead to more efficient management can be the first steps in developing an ongoing or fuller contractual relationship.

Carrying this idea further, cooperative agreements can be based on something as simple as a common patient transfer agreement between a hospital and a nursing home. These agreements can be amended to include other service agreements such as utilizing the chief of geriatrics at the hospital as the medical director at the nursing home.

An option adopted by Mount Sinai School of Medicine of the City University of New York has been to endow a chair at an affiliated nursing home. This enables the Mount Sinai Medical Center, a major teaching hospital, to assign a faculty member to the nursing home for the majority of his (in this case, Dr. Leslie Libow) academic commitment. Medical students, residents, and geriatric fellows rotate through the nursing home. This is a win-win situation for the medical school, the hospital, the nursing home, and the patients. The staff benefits by being involved with a variety of educational and training programs, which may include didactic as well as clinical instruction.

Institutions that perform geriatric patient assessments can provide these completed assessments to participating nursing homes in order to facilitate their care plan development and as an overture for establishing or maintaining good relations.

The Greater Southeast Community Hospital in Washington, D.C., developed a unique educational project for nurses employed in long-term care settings. The program was designed to help nurses refine their physical assessment and other related skills. Using a rotation schedule of nine nurses per month, the program can reach approximately 90 nurses per year. Thus the hospital is able to have an impact on the delivery of high-quality nursing care to long-term patients in the community as well as foster bonding between participating nursing homes and the hospital.

Another option would be to provide nursing and related health care services directly to a retirement or assisted living facility. Sunrise Retirement Homes, located in Arlington, Virginia, offers a "Specialized Care Program" of this type. This program was developed in response to families who wanted to hire an additional short-term nursing aide or nursing assistant help for a resident when necessary. Hospitals are in an excellent position to offer these services, which may range from more intensive nursing to special dietary and nutritional consultations and other forms of assistance as needed. These services will generate additional revenue for the hospital, make use of greater economies of scale in a hospital setting, and enable residents to remain in their chosen environment.

The benefits of cooperative relationships are diverse. They serve as a strategic approach for hospitals seeking to expand their service and referral base without investing the resources required to develop a new program or become a full partner in a joint venture. Yet many of the same benefits can be realized, such as facilitating patient discharge, enhancing continuity of care, developing a broader referral base, and having greater control over the quality of health care in the community.

Networking Strategies

The development of informal relationships with other providers and agencies in the community often lays the very foundation upon which future agreements are built. Networking serves as a beneficial way of tying into existing programs without a significant initial investment of resources. A broad base of influence can be accomplished easily at minimal cost. Networking also provides opportunities for the hospital to determine which providers it may want to associate with on a more formal basis and will keep the hospital in touch with the most current activities and opportunities as they occur in the community.

An increasing number of hospitals have joined together with other agencies, for example, social services agencies, home health agencies, long-term care facilities, senior housing, day care centers, and voluntary organizations. No one hospital and no one agency can be all things to all people, but by establishing working relationships in the community, resources and personnel can be used most effectively. A hospital does not have to own a service to take advantage of its benefits.

Both the University of California at Los Angeles (UCLA) and South Shore Hospital in Miami Beach provide models of community networking to provide continuity of care for the elderly. In seeking an agency that would help it extend its base of operations beyond the academic setting into the community, UCLA ultimately formed its partnership with Jewish Family Service (JFS), which had an existing site for the delivery of social services to the elderly population. After research established the need for medical services in the same locale, UCLA and JFS developed a health services agency that bonds academia and the community (see chapter 22).

Similarly, South Shore Hospital joined forces with the University of Miami in an effort to match the long-term care needs of the elderly in the South Miami Beach community with available community services. South Shore saw itself as a natural geriatric laboratory for the development of elderly programs and gained important linkages with the community. The hospital set up a long-term care advisory committee composed of representatives from nursing homes, senior housing programs, county social services agencies, and voluntary groups. All of these relationships resulted in referrals in all directions, between the hospital and the community-based agencies and the long-term care institutions.

Summary

The first step in exploring service options is market research, which includes gathering internal, external, and qualitative data. Service options also must be developed using the four elements of marketing—product, price, place, promotion—and evaluated based on financial viability.

It is important to remember that area elderly may be made up of several market segments by age, health status, and sex. Many alternatives for elderly programming exist for the hospital that has made a conscious and thoughtful commitment to expanding its services to enhance greater continuity of care. Examples of creativity and entrepreneurship abound in the organizational structure of these programs and in the way hospitals have joined together with other service entities to provide them. Programs may be hospital-owned and sponsored or provided through joint ventures or other formal cooperative relationships. Networking provides informal opportunities for exploring service options and assessing potential partners.

A hospital truly cannot be all things to all people, and it benefits the hospital and society in general to form bonds to provide the vast array of services that will be needed to manage the social and physical needs of our communities in the future.

References

1. Special Committee on Aging. *Aging America: Trends and Projections.* Washington, DC: U.S. Government Printing Office, 1989, p. 10.
2. Special Committee on Aging, p. 107.
3. Sabatino, F. Survey: managed care led '89 diversification improvements. *Hospitals* 64(1):56–59, Jan. 5, 1990.
4. Special Committee on Aging, p. 107.
5. American Hospital Association. *Emerging Trends in Aging and Long-Term Care Services.* Chicago: Hospital Research and Educational Trust, 1986, pp. 4–5.
6. Veterans Administration. *Caring for the Older Veteran.* Washington, DC: U.S. Government Printing Office, 1984, pp. 65–68.
7. Sabatino, p. 57.
8. Hospitals seeing benefits in offering long-term care. *Modern Healthcare* 19(12):40–43, Mar. 24, 1989.
9. American Hospital Association, p. 5.
10. American Hospital Association, pp. 3–5.
11. Hospitals reserving nursing home beds. *Modern Healthcare* 15(9):68, Apr. 26, 1985.
12. Newald, J. Hospitals and nursing homes: tying the knot. *Hospitals* 60(10):91–92, May 20, 1986.

Chapter 6

Case-Management Initiatives in Eldercare

Carolee A. DeVito, Nancy Alfred Persily, William Zubkoff, and Sonya R. Albury

Many hospitals are targeting the growing elderly population as their primary patient market for the future. The focus on the elderly market will surely intensify well into the next decade.

Relationships among medical specialties and health care organizations are becoming absolutely necessary to facilitate the continuity of long-term care and to avoid fragmentation of services for the elderly. Coordination among providers in complex health care systems is necessary, and appropriate medical treatment of multiple chronic conditions in frail older persons must include a plan for continuity of care. It will be particularly important for hospitals to encourage and foster ongoing care coordination among providers and to develop case-management initiatives to help bond older patients to the hospital and to develop accurate data on care needed and the care delivered.

Effective geriatric assessment and case management is the most essential service to offer in order to ensure effective eldercare programming. It should serve as the linchpin around which all services for the elderly are coordinated and monitored, during and following hospitalization.

This chapter will discuss in detail how the hospital participates in the case-management process. As the major provider in the community, the hospital will initiate many case-management services (such as intake, assessment, care planning—acute and postacute—and arranging for service delivery), for it is here in the acute-care setting that many older adults enter the long-term care service system. By initiating case-management services, the hospital ensures that integrated assessment and care planning is provided in the hospital and then sets the stage for ongoing case management to be provided in the community (including monitoring and reevaluation of service needs).

This chapter also will describe the essential dimensions of case management and care coordination and the rationale for initiating these services in the acute-care setting. Furthermore, it will describe typical models of case management as well as hospital planning and implementation techniques.

Definition of Case Management

The term *case management* as used here encompasses monitoring and coordination of services for the patient, and in some cases for the family, from initial intake or admission to the discontinuation of care. It draws on the skills of a team of professionals, which may include the attending physician, nurses, social workers, mental health therapists, clinical pharmacists, and physical and occupational therapists, as well as other relevant health care providers who work in concert to develop and implement the most appropriate plan of care for the patient.

Key features of case management include:

- Assumption of responsibility for mobilizing medical, social, and health services to ensure continuity of care
- Comprehensive and systematic assessment and planning with involvement of multidisciplinary personnel
- Assumption of responsibility to provide or coordinate the multiple services needed by the the patient and family over time[1]

Uses of Case Management in Eldercare

The case-management process can be used to establish quality controls, identify "at risk" patients, develop tracking systems, serve as a feeder for new or existing services, and measure program effectiveness. Many key components (staff, skills, and other resources) already are in place in the hospital, as this process is really a streamlining of typical hospital procedures, leading to a more efficient and continuous approach to the needs of elderly patients.

Astute hospital administrators recognize that for patients with illnesses that require high-cost treatment or complex medical care, case management also can help monitor and control patient flow so that appropriate services are rendered in an efficient and caring manner.

All too often, long-term care and acute care are provided to the elderly literally at the same time. The elderly—in particular the very old—often have more than one disabling chronic condition, and the second condition (such as hypertension, arthritis, diabetes) does not disappear when they have an acute episode. Therefore, any caring process has to take into consideration all their conditions, not just the illness that precipitated the admission to the hospital.

As Drs. Rosalie and Robert Kane have said, "Effective care of the frail elderly requires a long-range perspective."[2] Appropriate assessment of an elderly patient upon admission, coupled with other components of a case-management initiative, can have potential long-range effects on their future status and abilities to function following discharge. The patient's future use of medical and social services and the total cost of care (to the patient and to providers and insurers) may all be guided by careful case management. This is because case management can reduce duplicate efforts in providing care and promote the efficient coordination of resources. These facts together with the current prospective payment system, which puts even greater pressure on hospitals to discharge patients earlier, make the provision of case-management services even more important for elderly and disabled populations. With a good case-management system in place to coordinate care, rehospitalization or institutionalization may be prevented or postponed.

However, appropriate assessment and case management during the hospital stay often is not enough. Equally important is the provision of continuous care for older patients being transferred from the hospital into the community or to another institution. Continuous case management to the point where elderly patients no longer need continued services ensures that patients are not discharged without appropriate follow-up.

When an elderly person is hospitalized, the institution has a responsibility as well as an opportunity. Even though providing for acute care may be the reason for admission, the management of ongoing care is the true challenge.

Although the particular circumstances surrounding a hospitalization may be a *new* acute problem, admission is more likely to represent an exacerbation of chronic problems or an acute problem due to preexisting conditions. Many of these patients needing longer-term care come to the acute-care hospital with a history of relationships with a variety of medical, health, and personal care providers, none of whom may have provided the case management necessary to develop resources needed before, during, and after an acute episode.

A case-management initiative can truly help the patient by decreasing length of stay, reducing recidivism, and helping the older person remain as independent as possible. At the same time, it can bond that person more closely to the hospital and its affiliated providers, giving the hospital the opportunity to "do well by doing good."

Patient–hospital bonding through case management can result in the following benefits: control of specialty service referrals, control of physician referrals, control of long-term care service referrals, and tracking of providers who bring patients to the hospital.

Controlling Specialty Service Referrals

Case management is a vital mechanism in identifying target populations for adjunct programs for the elderly such as rehabilitation services, which target high-risk groups. To the extent that the hospital controls meaningful information, it can control referrals. For instance, the hospital could provide referrals to specialized rehabilitation programs (at a hospital-based or hospital-owned rehabilitation center or skilled nursing facility [SNF]), or to other programs within the system such as a fall-prevention clinic operated at the hospital or by a group of community physicians affiliated with the institution. This control of specialty referrals increases continuity and helps ensure high-quality service while at the same time controlling utilization.

Controlling Physician Referrals

An effective case-management program can provide referrals for a cadre of specialty and primary care physicians affiliated with the institution who have particular expertise in caring for older patients. Case managers can identify a primary source of general medical care and coordinate ongoing medical services as well. Ongoing case management also ensures continuity of record keeping and often reduces the necessity for repeated diagnostic testing, which occurs when referral mechanisms break down.

Although patients hospitalized for recurring medical problems may be likely to return to ongoing community-based care, those hospitalized for surgical problems or relatively new acute problems may need significant coordination of care to effect a smooth transition from the hospital to another institution (for example, a specialty hospital or nursing home) or back to their own home. With the elderly patient who is hospitalized for a hip fracture, for example, inpatient care may be dominated by surgical and orthopedic physicians but may also include a cardiology and/or neurological consultant. Whichever disciplines are involved, there will be a need for continuity of medical care and management of physician referrals during the posthospital phase of treatment. Similarly, coordination is important for the newly diagnosed diabetic patient, who has a variety of health care needs and most likely would not get appropriate ongoing care unless a case-management program were incorporated throughout the hospital system. Too often, individuals with newly diagnosed diseases as well as indigents get lost in the shuffle and are not monitored adequately subsequent to discharge. By assessing the patient at time of admission, monitoring his or her stay, and preparing for effective postdischarge case management, the patient will be assured of more appropriate treatment and effective ongoing care.

Controlling Long-Term Care Service Referrals

To maintain market share, hospitals take many steps to keep patients within their health care system.

A good case management system can provide significant control regarding the future care of older patients. For example, patients discharged from acute-care institutions to SNFs, intermediate care facilities, or even other levels of institutional care, routinely may be "lost" to the original provider—to the disadvantage of both the patient and the institution. Mechanisms to link the hospital with community-based providers by tracking patient care and/or providing for their ongoing care can lead to improved patient case management and to a higher likelihood that the sponsoring hospital will be the site of the next rehospitalization. Most important, mutual trust develops whereby long-term care facilities and other community providers begin to rely on the hospital's case-management program and its personnel to provide them with good information about the patient upon discharge. The facility in the community has a contact who knows the patient well and can share additional information that may prove helpful in the patient's continuing care. This mutual reliance can result in a symbiotic referral relationship, where the long-term care facility recognizes the hospital as the site for continuing ambulatory and inpatient care.

Tracking Providers Who Bring Patients to the Hospital

A good case-management program, coupled with an effective information system, can help the hospital track and assess its relationships with other providers. A tracking system is the only way to document the financial benefits of relationships with other providers (see chapter 7, which covers financial issues). For example, patient rehospitalization rates can be identified for selected physicians. Similarly, summaries of transfers and readmissions to housing and nursing facilities following hospitalization can be provided to document the mutual benefits accruing to these organizations. Ultimately, sophisticated tracking systems can be utilized as quality assurance monitors to assess success and failures of referrals to nursing homes, senior housing facilities, and community agencies. For instance, if the hospital discovers that an inordinate number of patients from one nursing home have repeated admissions for medical problems such as decubiti (severe bedsores), then the hospital may decide to forgo referral to that facility or attempt to educate the personnel there on preventing such a medical condition.

Dimensions of Case Management

In developing a case-management initiative, it is essential to understand its key components. This section describes the case-management function, its basic models and organizational settings, and then identifies who performs case management in the hospital setting.

The Case-Management Function

The care coordination process has been described in a variety of ways and with multiple terms. The traditional and most common is the term *case management,* which is utilized in this chapter for uniformity and clarity. However, many other terms have been widely applied. The National Council on the Aging, for example, now uses the term *care management* in its standards because it conveys that the process is the management of care rather than the "case" or the "person."[3] Other terms, such as *case coordination, service coordination,* or *service management* also are used to describe the process.

Regardless of terminology, the essential purpose of the case-management process is to make the system of community-based care work more effectively. Case managers seek to ensure that individuals receive assistance that is responsive to their needs in the most affordable, appropriate, and effective manner.[4]

Although more specific definitions of eldercare case management vary considerably, most contain seven fundamental functions that serve as key components of the process:

1. Intake/screening
2. Geriatric assessment
3. Care planning
4. Arranging for services
5. Ongoing monitoring
6. Reassessment
7. Discharge

Intake/Screening

Screening at initial intake or admission allows the hospital to identify patients who are at particular risk and will require extensive monitoring. Risk factors for the elderly include a variety of medical, psychosocial, and environmental characteristics. Patient characteristics that can be utilized as screening criteria include age, diagnostic condition, ability to perform activities of daily living (ADLs), marital status, mental status, social support, and economic status.[5]

The most important guideline in screening potential patients for case management is to keep the process simple. Four or five key questions can help elicit the information needed to determine which patients may be appropriate for a comprehensive assessment. A sample of key questions are:

- Does this patient live alone?
- How many times has this patient been admitted this year?
- Is the patient confused?
- Does this patient have more than one disabling condition?

Geriatric Assessment

In the hospital setting, comprehensive geriatric assessments help facilitate the discharge planning process. These "in-house" assessments afford staff the time to arrange services needed both within the hospital setting and upon discharge. Family involvement can be initiated earlier to ensure that family members are fully aware of alternative treatment and discharge plans. Adequate preparations for discharge can be made with the family's participation and assistance.

Comprehensive geriatric assessment includes an evaluation of the patient's mental and health status, family and social support systems, finances, functional level, and environment. The assessment process systematically gathers information for identifying major needs on each dimension. To be effective, the assessment must be carried out in a manner analogous and complementary to the diagnostic workups prepared by physicians, which precede medical treatment decisions. Collectively, this information base serves as the foundation for linking social services needs with medical treatments and services during the hospital stay and following discharge.[6]

Care Planning

Upon completion of the geriatric assessment, an individualized care plan is developed. Specific treatment goals and objectives are established based on the initial assessment and in coordination with the patient, family, physician, and other participants on the care-planning team. This step includes designating type and intensity of services deemed necessary to meet identified patient needs. These services may be provided by family and friends, directly by the hospital staff, and/or by the formal system of community-based agencies and professionals.[7]

Arranging for Services

Once care plans have been developed, case managers are responsible for facilitating implementation, which involves locating and arranging for the patient's access to the agreed-on package of services. The case manager arranges for the provision of services as prescribed in the care plan, maximizing familial resources and financial payment sources.

Ongoing Monitoring and Reassessment

Ongoing monitoring of care is essential to ensure that services both in and out of the hospital are delivered as planned and care plans are modified as necessary.

Periodic follow-up and evaluation of the patient's needs is the final and often-forgotten step of the case-management process. It consists of supervising the reliability, quality, and appropriateness of the services provided. This ongoing patient tracking allows the case manager to reassess the elderly person's condition and help avert unnecessary rehospitalizations. It often involves communicating with family members to determine whether or not they are still physically and/or psychologically able to continue care-giving responsibilities.

Discharge

Discharge, or termination, occurs when the hospital's involvement with the patient or care giver is completed. Although referred to interchangeably here, the hospital may want to distinguish between discharge and termination. The term *discharge* can refer to the process that ends the hospital's involvement with the patient, except for case management, because the relationship between the patient and the case manager can and should continue following discharge. *Termination,* on the other hand, actually occurs when the case manager is no longer involved. Despite the finality these terms denote, they are used for the purposes of record keeping and staff function only. Potential reasons for termination often include improvement in the patient's condition so that case management is no longer needed, relocation of the patient, or death of the patient.

When possible, the hospital should seek to continue a "relationship" with the patient and/or the family at some level, perhaps through preventive education programs, support groups, or ongoing communications, so that the hospital remains the facility of choice for possible future hospitalizations.

Case-Management Models

There are two basic case-management models. One is the *broker model,* in which the case manager performs an assessment and develops a plan of care. The case manager then arranges for services by coordinating with providers of care and helping the patient access funding. Under the *consolidation model,* services and financing are all in one program. The case manager performs a comprehensive assessment, controls the type of services offered, and has the authority to purchase care on behalf of the patient.[8] Many variations on these models have emerged, with some providers offering a limited number of services directly and others indirectly by coordinating efforts with other community-based organizations. (Examples of these models and their distinctive applications are provided in the case studies in Part Two of this book.) Programs evolving from these models range from basic case-management programs to information and referral, hospital-based SNFs, and social health maintenance organizations (SHMOs).

In the hospital-specific setting, four distinct models have emerged. These models were identified through a study of 24 hospitals, which participated in the Robert Wood Johnson Foundation's *Hospital Initiatives in Long-Term Care* program. The models reflect the changes that have occurred as growing health care competition prompts many hospitals to look beyond the "four walls" of inpatient care to serve older adults.[9] The four descriptive models include medical management, aftercare case management, nursing home diversion, and community care coordination. A brief discussion of each model demonstrates how a case-management initiative can function within the context of a total project.

Medical Management

The medical management model provides assessment and ongoing medical care service planning and coordination to chronically ill patients. The goals are oriented toward reducing acute flare-ups of chronic conditions through coordinated medical management on an ongoing basis. Focus is placed on arranging needed medical care or health care appointments, following up on self-care strategies, and scheduling service delivery.[10]

Aftercare Case Management

Aftercare case management programs are designed to enhance and extend the discharge planning process beyond the acute-care setting. Short-term care plans and service arrangements are made after performing a comprehensive assessment. Care and patient status usually is monitored for up to three months in the community following discharge. Older adults who require long-term care monitoring and coordination are referred to community-based programs for continued case management.[11]

Nursing Home Diversion

Nursing home diversion focuses on providing alternatives to institutional placement subsequent to discharge. Many involve Medicaid waivers, which allow the hospital to offer case management and related services as long as the patient remains Medicaid eligible in the community. The beneficiaries would otherwise require nursing home placement without the delivery of community care services.[12]

Community Care Coordination

Community care coordination providers are similar to nursing home diversion programs; however, they generally do not have financial control over service provision. These programs serve a wider patient population because they are not confined by strict eligibility criteria and can encompass a diverse mixture of medical conditions and functional impairments. They often are linked to geriatric outpatient clinics and other existing community case management programs.[13]

Organizational Settings for Case Management

Clearly the process of case management does not occur in isolation but is part of the total community care system that includes an array of services, providers, and community resources. Each hospital has a unique set of circumstances. Every community is different, with a special combination of existing services, agencies, institutions, and resources. The type and amount of funds available also will be a key factor in determining the most appropriate setting and case-management model (or models) in each community.

Common organizational settings include hospitals, senior centers, area agencies on aging, family service agencies, public agencies, HMOs, and experimental "social" HMOs. Insurance companies, home health agencies, and agencies specifically designed for case management are becoming more prevalent. In addition, social workers, nurses, and other health care professionals are setting up private case-management practices.[14]

Whatever the setting, it is important for hospitals to be knowledgeable of their local area and local case management resources. Effective coordination with existing providers is crucial in order to share information, create meaningful care plans, maximize resources, and ensure closer bonding.

Responsibility for Case Management

Case management is a function that encompasses a broad range of disciplines. Physicians, nurses, social workers, and therapists, among other specialists, may be involved. In eldercare, a family medicine specialist, a geriatrician, an orthopedist, or a psychiatrist may be the appropriate physician to participate on the multidisciplinary case-management team. This enables the team to assess the individual's entire spectrum of needs and develop a care plan that treats the whole person, not just the medical condition.

Generally the case manager is a social worker or nurse who has responsibility for coordinating the care of an individual patient. The case manager should have both inpatient and community experience in identifying long-term services for the elderly. He or she should have training and/or several years' experience working with at least multidisciplinary (if not interdisciplinary) approaches to care as well as experience in problem-oriented assessment and care planning. Generally, minimum education requirements may be master's-level credentials.

The case manager must have responsibility and influence to implement the likely daily program tasks and avoid known interdepartmental or interdisciplinary rivalries, building on strengths and leaving out "turf" issues.

Roles performed by the case manager include:

- *Service coordinator.* Identifying and coordinating service delivery.
- *Patient advocate.* Ensuring that the patient and/or care giver receives appropriate high-quality services in a timely manner. Case managers also may seek to change or expand existing service programs to meet needs or intervene in order to make the current system more responsive.
- *Counselor.* Providing assistance to individuals and their families in recognizing and addressing their problems and needs. The case manager educates the family regarding the availability of services and how to access them. He or she encourages them to assume responsibility for care to the greatest extent possible, thereby fostering independence of the elderly person.
- *Gatekeeper.* Containing costs by ensuring that clients receive only appropriate care and are able to justify the expenditure of funds.[15]

Depending on the specific program, one or more of the above roles may take on greater emphasis, but all are crucial in assisting older adults and their care givers in gaining access to needed care and services. From the hospital's perspective, the case manager also serves an important role by ensuring that the hospital's resources are efficiently utilized to orchestrate the smooth coordination of care within and outside its walls.

Planning for a Case-Management Initiative

Planning a case-management initiative requires developing a planning staff, conducting an environmental analysis, and performing the necessary development steps. The planning of a case-management initiative should proceed with attention to certain goals:

- Provide details for a proposed program that is "doable" at the proposed site. That is, the program implementation should be achievable in the proposed time frame and with the likely resource allocation (cash, capital, staff) available.

- Provide details for a proposed program that is consistent with the overall goals of the organization. In fact, if program implementation will require important changes in the organization's goals or mission, these changes should be recognized as a prerequisite to program implementation. A separate and deliberate effort may be necessary to achieve a new mission statement that is accepted by all key players. It is unlikely that a new case-management initiative and a handful of program proponents can affect longstanding expectations of the hospital's management (especially if the program planning implementation staff are outsiders or newcomers). Important achievable organizational change comes best from within as an attempt to meet well-accepted hospital goals.
- Provide details for a proposed program that is likely to yield outcomes desired by the hospital management. The hospital administration should have full knowledge and understanding of the expected program effects on patient care, including the components of care, any likely changes in patient mix, change in recidivism, and/or the impact on patient referral sources. Expected program effects on organizational growth should also be presented to hospital management. Any effects on organizational status, such as the likelihood of academic affiliations or the ability to attract public and private grant dollars, should be part of any discussion with hospital leadership. The program's chances for success are increased greatly if hospital management "buys into" the program and gives visible support.

Developing a Planning Staff

The planning staff must have the skills, authority, resources, and support to gather and use meaningful information. Although the necessary expertise can be found in outside consultants in the health/hospital industry, newcomers or outsiders to the hospital may encounter difficulty in meaningful planning and implementation if full cooperation by inside staff is not secured first. Significant change requires identifying leaders and "change agents" within the hospital and empowering them to carry out all planning/implementation steps with any consultants as guides and advisers.

The individuals within the hospital who are proponents of the development of a case-management initiative can have important input and a catalyzing effect for the development of a program planning staff. However, both the planning and implementation phases are likely to fail unless an appropriate array of expertise is represented on the staff and unless this staff is given specific time frames and enough time in which to conduct the planning effort. Although the members and numbers of the hospital staff may vary from hospital to hospital, they should represent experience and knowledge in acute and long-term care. The members of the planning staff should represent the following areas within the hospital:

- Administration (inpatient as well as ambulatory services)
- Finance
- Nursing
- Social work
- General medical care
- Rehabilitation
- Education/training
- Data processing/information systems
- Clerical support
- Utilization review/quality assurance

The planning staff must have designated leadership with specified reporting responsibilities to middle and upper management. The selection of the chairperson/leader of the planning staff and that individual's discipline/affiliation can have a significant effect on the program. Senior management must consider the implications and inherent power to effect change represented by all committee members, especially the committee chair.

Conducting an Environmental Analysis

To devise the best case-management initiative for a given hospital, the institution must first examine its external and internal environment.

A review of the hospital's external environment includes identifying the existing strengths and limitations in community care, recognizing potential new markets, and identifying opportunities for problem solving. A review of the internal environment includes a review of the patient mix, admissions, and referral patterns.

It is important to be cognizant of the limitations as well as the capabilities of the existing system of health care within the community. The inability of existing care providers to offer continuity of care for the elderly is often readily evident. A lack of patient-centered/need-driven care planning is often attributable to the large number of providers available and the lack of communication among them. Case management can open up the lines of communication and solve many patient needs.

Some providers, such as home health agencies, are perceived (particularly by physicians) as offering case management when in actuality most traditional agencies do not offer this service. This wrong perception can leave older adults without continuity of care or a comprehensive plan of care and necessary service arrangements—an unmet need that provides an opportunity for the hospital.

The hospital should conduct a thorough institutional assessment prior to the implementation of a case-management program for the elderly. Although current information may be available in some settings, this phase should be another exhaustive, carefully designed effort to gather and/or synthesize information describing virtually all environmental and organizational issues related to identifying and meeting patient needs.

Environmental factors are often difficult to change, at least in the short run. An in-depth understanding of external factors such as competitors, funding sources, and actual and potential markets helps to define the case-management program's focus, potential, and limitations. This is also true for internal environmental factors such as staff qualifications, organizational hierarchies and lines of authority, and physical plant capabilities and restrictions. On the other hand, certain organizational attributes may be quite alterable.

With an understanding of environmental issues in hand, the program planners must specify the extent of change that their new program implies and the potential mechanisms needed to create meaningful change within the organization. If the new case-management program builds on existing staff capabilities and existing procedures, then program implementation may be relatively easy. However, if the new case-management program requires significant reallocation of resources and new staffing or procedures or fails to attract meaningful support at any level, then implementation will be more difficult.

The institutional assessment provides an opportunity to identify and accommodate difficulties in program implementation, as well as an information-gathering function and a negotiating forum in which to plan a program that will be as close as possible to the ideal and can really work in that setting. Additionally, likely leadership figures, other change agents, and facilitators can be identified.

The initial assessment phase also must be used to identify the staff and management roles for the implementation phase. The implementation staff may or may not completely overlap in membership with the planning staff. However, just as outside consultants in isolation may be restricted in planning, an implementation staff that has had no hand in program planning can resist changes in responsibility and authority. Even if planners argue that the case-management initiative will reduce or streamline hospital efforts (paperwork, staffing requirements, and so forth) in the long run, implementation itself—or any change for that matter—requires extra effort and a staff committed to the program design and specific procedures.

Performing the Necessary Development Steps

Although the exact process may vary somewhat, a number of steps can be described for developing a case-management initiative at any hospital. Those steps include:

1. Conducting a review of patient needs
2. Integrating different perspectives and developing a statement of need
3. Conducting an inventory and assessment of community services
4. Providing an interim assessment
5. Identifying possible changes in staffing or responsibilities
6. Identifying core staff needed
7. Modifying and testing training, procedures, and forms

Conducting a Review of Patient Needs

Patient needs should be reviewed by accessing available information from primary care staff, nursing, social services organizations, community providers, and other key informants.

This step helps set the limits of the case-management program. At its inception, any case-management program can be defined as a broad attempt to match patient needs with services. The planning staff as a group must invest sufficient time to conceptualize their model more adequately. They must specify their definition and the expected boundaries for "patient needs" and "services." At this stage, a variety of questions must be answered:

- At what points in the care continuum will the program apply? That is, will the program be designed to have an impact on inpatient care (thereby requiring the staff to define sets of inpatient care needs and inpatient care services), discharge planning, and/or aftercare?
- Will the program target all elderly patients or a subset of them, such as all elderly patients with certain levels of functioning, certain diagnoses, in certain inpatient units, and so forth?
- Will the program include the provision of care, or will it direct the care given by others through mandating requirements, protocols, or making recommendations?
- Will the program request the cooperation/collaboration of other providers including community-based attending physicians, other institutions, and/or family members?
- How can differences in assessment of patient needs (between disciplines, for example) be reconciled in this setting?
- How can differences in care plans (services) necessary to meet needs be reconciled in this setting?

The planning staff members must then gather specific information from each discipline they represent. They should obtain demographic, medical, psychosocial, and functional information on patients who will be targeted by the program. Information also should be gathered regarding patient care needs and type, timing, and amount of service necessary to meet those needs. A description should be provided from each discipline's perspective of the patients who are served and those who would most likely benefit and be targeted for the new program. In general, the physician member of the team can gather information from the medical staff, the nurse can gather information from nursing staff, and so on. This process can include record review, informal conversations, or even formal meetings and focus groups with peers. Depending on the detail desired and the amount of time allocated to the project, this effort is likely to take one to three months.

Integrating Different Perspectives and Developing a Statement of Need

In order to integrate different perspectives and develop a statement of need, the planning staff must examine intraorganizational structures, lines of authority, information flow, information systems, staff resources, training strategies, and documents/forms relevant to long-term care assessment, planning, and linkage of patients to services. This step may require an additional two to three months. Because it constitutes the most tedious efforts, support staff (data collectors, for example) can be very useful to keep the progress timely.

A useful strategy to accomplish this step is to review all relevant written documents from charters, mission statements, five-year plans, and so on, as well as organizational charts, policies and procedures, flowcharts, forms, and associated training/education materials. Additionally, periodic and annual reports of relevant departments and special studies and quality assurance programs often provide valuable insight regarding the process of care in the institution. The full committee or a designated subcommittee of two to three individuals can synthesize this information for presentation to the staff.

Conducting an Inventory and Assessment of Community Services

It is important to identify and assess each service provider in the community. The extent of this effort depends on the general nature of the case-management initiative. A program that focuses on discharge planning will need a fairly comprehensive listing of service availability and accessibility, including the history of associations between provider agencies and the hospital. Case-management programs that will include aftercare must obtain more detailed information about community providers (social services agencies, long-term care facilities, senior housing, and so forth) and long-term accessibility to services, staffing, paperwork, and so forth.

Providing an Interim Assessment

At this point, a description or interim assessment of what is needed by patients and of the current systems (under the direct control of the hospital) available to meet those needs can provide a powerful interim report to administration. Generally, a commitment from administration, including a commitment of resources, will be needed at this time.

A presentation to senior administration, followed by a series of meetings with middle management, is a likely mechanism for this step. A preliminary proposal including a time line should be the result of this exercise.

Identifying Possible Changes in Staffing or Responsibilities

Possible changes in staffing or responsibilities must be identified. This step requires the various disciplines to negotiate actual program components, such as identifying changes in responsibility (for existing and/or new personnel), and identifying changes in procedures and documentation. A series of two or three half-day sessions could provide sufficient time for these efforts.

Identifying Core Staff Needed

The planning staff should agree on the initial core staff for the case-management initiative. If recruiting is necessary, it should occur at this time. All subsequent planning and implementation will benefit from including the individuals who will have program responsibility. Providing necessary resources to hire staff and/or redefine current responsibilities is a management commitment in the program, and it must be initiated in a timely fashion.

The specific department(s) in which case management is housed depends on the organizational structure and size of the hospital. Typically, discharge planning departments offer leadership and core staff to provide this service. The planning staff should carefully assess the implications of the departmental structure in the program's daily functioning. For instance, a new and separate entity of discharge planning may have difficulty participating meaningfully in any inpatient care decisions and therefore may have to be evaluated for long-term potential. Strong support must be available from administration; medical staff; and departments of nursing, social services, rehabilitation, and data processing to make any department the successful recipient of this responsibility.

Modifying and Testing Training, Procedures, and Forms

Usually it is necessary to modify various systems already in place in the hospital to fully integrate a case-management initiative. This includes modifying training, some hospital procedures, and forms used, a step that can take several months depending on the extent of change dictated by the program design. Without good direction and leadership as well as the cooperation of the hospital (for example, medical records committee, data processing), project plans often are bogged down at this point. The extent of revisions and the extent and type of pilot testing should be agreed on well in advance of these activities. Specific questions such as the following must be asked:

- Will we duplicate the current assessment/planning process to pilot test?
- Will we test on one unit or all?
- Will we have only a few providers or many providers?

The expectations and necessary refinement of procedures and forms also should be discussed with administration with a clear end point in view for program development. In general, the results of the pilot testing and revised procedures and of forms and training materials can form the basis of another interim report to administration. Regular interim reports indicate that the development phase is moving forward and can identify any snags and solutions.

Program Implementation

Because a case-management program must interface with many departments and services, at the inception of the program special attention should be placed on eliciting the full support and active participation of key members of the administrative and medical staff. This is essential to the success of any institutionwide geriatric program. As noted in chapter 4, overcoming resistance on the part of the medical staff and administration and promoting their cooperation and support are the key elements in the process of developing geriatric initiatives.

Three factors are critical to program implementation: staff training, program initiation, and evaluation.

Staff Training

Orientation and training are essential to making any assessment and planning process an integral part of "usual and customary" care. This ensures that everyone affected by and involved in the process recognizes the need for a case-management initiative and understands the steps involved in assessment. Initial orientation and training, periodic retraining, and routine training for new staff members (or individuals who change roles) are necessary for all shifts and all involved disciplines. Training materials, specific written procedures, and ongoing information must be adapted and directed at various groups in the system according to status and roles:

- *Hospitalwide.* Orientation in the case-management process should be conducted for foundation/board members, medical staff, nursing staff, ancillary departments, and community providers.
- *By group.* Special effort should be made to bring together professional groups in their usual forums (for example, medical staff meetings) to explain the case-management initiative. Presentations are best made by a peer group member of the planning staff along with top administration to ensure credibility. Presentations should be brief and to the point. Materials should be provided if they are of specific use to the group (for example, telephone numbers or beeper access information for the new staff). A clear explanation of how the case-management initiative may affect them and/or their patients should be offered, and any concomitant changes in process or paperwork should be explained. Further, a target date to report back on the program's progress and a mechanism for everyone to share ideas and problems should be provided.
- *By department.* Specific orientation to all departments across all shifts affected by the program (such as admitting, medical records, transportation services, and so forth), and mechanisms for periodic retraining/reinforcement as well as training of new employees should be initiated. Specific training is needed for all departmental personnel on all shifts responsible for contributing to the geriatric assessment and case-management process or who will be utilizing the information produced. Mechanisms for periodic retraining/reinforcement should be addressed, as well as training of new employees.

This training must be very detailed. Written learning objectives and educational strategies must be developed for each discipline having specific responsibility in the case-management initiative. This includes those who will provide information and those who will use the information and/or refer to the service. The case-management training materials should reflect the standard of all other hospital materials, including audiovisual aids and handouts, as necessary.

The best forum for training would be group meetings such as routine in-service sessions; but, depending on the nature of the case-management initiative, special sessions may be needed. In general, all sessions should include training staff who have participated in program development and who are known authority figures to the specific discipline.

Program Initiation

After basic training, the case-management program can begin. Regardless of the extent and intensity of training, any program that requires new processes and forms can be disruptive. One strategy to facilitate implementation is to begin the program (where possible) with duplicate staff.

With specified time limitations the planning staff can participate in actual program implementation as a technical resource pool to the core case-management staff. They can convene daily or weekly for a predefined period of time to provide feedback to administration, incorporate ideas from the core case-management staff, and thereby refine the program to enhance its chances of successful implementation. Specifically, this period of time can be used to train core staff extensively with regard to case-management process implementation. It can also be used to teach staff training techniques to implement the program throughout the site.

Evaluation

Evaluation should take two forms: *formative evaluation,* that is, constant feedback during initial phases that is used to tailor the case-management program; and *summative evaluation,* to determine the value and success of the program.

Summative evaluation, which must be planned in conjunction with program goals, should take place every three months during the first year of the program and every six months thereafter. Every expectation of administration should be played with a time frame and set of information needed to evaluate the efforts (for example, recidivism for certain patient types before and after the program).

The successful program will schedule periodic reporting and readjustments based on these outcomes. The most meaningful programs will schedule reevaluation of need and service availability (environmental and organizational assessment) in conjunction with changing hospital goals.

Summary

This discussion of case management for the elderly demonstrates that the process is much more than traditional discharge planning.

Continuous monitoring and evaluation of older patients over the long term has not generally been recognized as the hospital's role. However, the process of effective geriatric assessment and care planning can impact on the short-term and long-term care of older adults.

Case management, as discussed in this chapter, strengthens, integrates, and can streamline the usual care processes within an institution. The difficulty in simultaneously maximizing safety, function, and independent living requires sophisticated planning as well as total commitment and endorsement of top administration. The dimensions of case management include different case-management models and organizational settings, and different personnel may perform the case-management initiative. Planning a case-management initiative requires developing a planning staff, conducting an environmental analysis, and performing the necessary development steps. The benefits of a case-management initiative are great, both from the hospital's perspective of rendering high-quality care and generating a future market for services, as well as from the patient's and family's perspective of ensuring greater independence and peace of mind.

References

1. Brody, S. J. DRGs: the second revolution in health care for the elderly. *Journal of the American Geriatric Society* 32(9):676–79, Sept. 1984.
2. Kane, R. A., and Kane, R. L. *Long-Term Care: Principles, Programs, and Policies.* New York City: Springer Publishing Co., 1987, p. 280.
3. National Council on the Aging. *Care Management Standards, Guidelines for Practice.* Washington, DC: NCOA, 1988.
4. National Council on the Aging, p. 1.
5. Kane and Kane, p. 31.
6. Jette, A. M., and Zielstorff, R. D. *Comprehensive Functional Assessment.* 1989.
7. Jette and Zielstorff.
8. Quinn, J. Case management: the key to integrating long-term care services. *Perspectives on Aging* 15(5):7, Sept./Oct. 1986.
9. MacAdam, M., Capitman, J., Yee, D., Prottas, J., Leutz, W., and Westwater. Case management for frail elders: the Robert Wood Johnson Foundation's program for hospital initiatives in long-term care. *Gerontologist* 29(6):737, 1989.
10. MacAdam and others, p. 739.
11. MacAdam and others, p. 739.
12. MacAdam and others, p. 739.
13. MacAdam and others, p. 739.
14. National Council on the Aging, p. 1.
15. National Council on the Aging, p. 7.

Chapter 7

Financing for Eldercare Health Services

Jay Wolfson and Peter J. Levin

This chapter will review reimbursement and financing issues that are central to providing health services to older adults. It also will examine the financial realities hospitals will face in developing appropriate service capabilities. The following questions will be addressed:

- Which reimbursement and financing mechanisms are currently in place to pay for health services to the aging?
- How can hospitals determine which aging services they should develop?
- How can these new ventures be financed?

The first question is concerned with how hospitals get paid for various services (issues of reimbursement). The second and third speak to strategic financial management, planning, and product development.

As the older adult population grows and becomes a powerful economic force in the health care marketplace, an expanded scope of services and programs will be required to meet their health and social welfare needs. In preparing to address the financial challenges attendant to providing these services, hospitals and other providers must ask these questions:

- Who will pay?
- Which products are profitable, and which generate other profitable services?
- What can hospitals do to maximize existing reimbursement provisions?

The scope of eldercare services, although broad, fits on a continuum of care, which has at its core information and referral and primary care services and includes products ranging from acute and chronic inpatient care, skilled nursing facilities (SNFs), respite care, hospice, and death management services (figure 7-1). Within this panoply providers may also consider organ transplant centers, prosthesis programs, and other special services for private pay patients.

The discussion begins by summarizing some of the challenges affecting hospitals. The analysis then turns to a review of current sources of funding for eldercare programs and services and continues with a review of financing and reimbursement alternatives for eldercare services, such as home equity conversions and reverse mortgages, as well as effective reimbursement management and utilization review. The evaluation of appropriate, vertically integrated products for the elderly is discussed. In this context two techniques are stressed: product line management and the ability to link services financially; and basic decision-analysis techniques, which employ present value and other option strategies. Finally we look at the role hospitals play in their communities and some factors they must consider to prosper in the marketplace.

Changes in Health Care

This section will briefly list some of the challenges faced by hospitals today and then will describe how the health care environment changed during the past 20 years.

Challenges in the 1990s

In the United States the $200 billion hospital industry is struggling to survive changes in reimbursement patterns and problems in obtaining and retaining personnel. The financial crises consist of changing levels of profitability, cash flow, vastly modified capital needs, a shift to outpatient services, and a dramatically increased level of control by both government and the private sector over what they will pay.[1-4] Personnel problems in health care include increased costs associated with obtaining and retaining nurses and ancillary staff and the frequently cited issue of nursing and other staff shortages.[5-8]

Background

Between the 1960s and the 1980s, the nation's health care system was reshaped—indeed, transformed. It evolved from a medical care delivery system comprising physicians and hospitals into a complex, *health* services industry affected by capital and technology. Within this new industry insurance companies, federal and state governments, and employers became increasingly involved in financing, monitoring, regulating, and containing costs.[9]

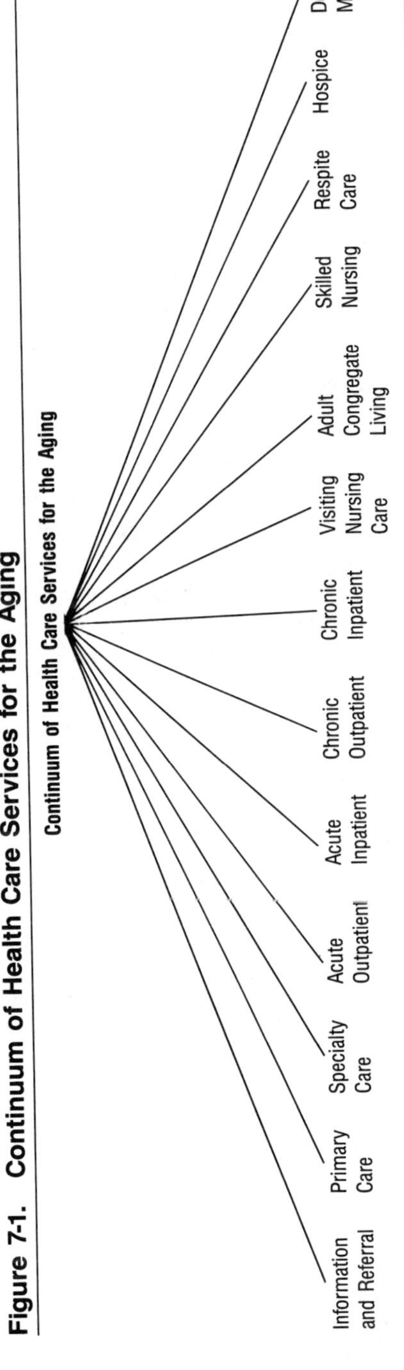

Figure 7-1. Continuum of Health Care Services for the Aging

For almost 20 years, beginning in the late 1960s, the health care system experienced a substantial infusion of government money and attention, sparking growth and change. In a 1959 article, Shain and Roemer noted that hospital beds, once built, would get filled by virtue of the relationship between physicians and hospitals;[10] "Roemer's law" seemed to reflect the reality of the market. In the 1970s, however, the advent of massive public and private insurance revenues in the marketplace added a corollary to Roemer's law: If it gets paid for, it is done; if it is not reimbursed, it is less likely to be done.

Changing reimbursement policies and different utilization patterns have changed the way hospitals do business.[11] The reimbursement climate that propelled the hospital industry through the 1970s virtually crumbled in the mid-1980s. This was in part a result of changes from prospective payment under the Tax Equity and Fiscal Responsibility Act of 1983 (TEFRA).

During the early 1980s, the increases in national health care costs captured the attention of both federal and state governments because of the high demands placed on public funds from Medicare and Medicaid.[12] (See table 7-1.) At the same time, the private sector became sensitized to the fact that it was paying more each year for employee health benefits.[13]

The growing awareness and concern of the public and private sector led to formal efforts to control health costs. Most of these efforts focused on stricter reimbursement management, such as obtaining second opinions for surgery, preadmission authorization and testing, better coordination of benefits, and the growth of managed health care programs in the forms of HMOs and PPOs.

Insurers began to respond to client demands by adopting more data-oriented (utilization and cost data) reimbursement systems. Claims management and processing moved into the age of computers. Third-party payers enlisted the active participation of health professionals to oversee "utilization management"—clinically based review of claims (bills) for medical care and the development of standards (protocols). At the same time, changes in Medicare and among private insurers began to encourage the provision of health care services outside the traditional

Table 7-1. National Health Care Expenditures (in billions)

	1970	1975	1980	1985
Total	75.0	132.7	248.1	419.0
Private	47.2	76.4	142.9	244.0
Public	27.8	56.3	105.2	175.0
Federal	17.7	37.0	71.0	123.0
State	10.0	19.3	34.2	52.0

Source: Health Care Financing Administration, 1989.

hospital inpatient setting. This resulted in some procedures being shifted more toward ambulatory care—and increased attention on the control of hospital-based costs and services.[14]

Between 1984 and 1988, following the introduction of prospective payment and the effects of TEFRA, major for-profit hospital corporations began to divest themselves of a considerable number of facilities. Previously, hospitals had acquired other institutions to obtain tax breaks and spur long-term financial growth. By 1986 the tax rules had changed, reducing substantially the attractiveness of various joint venture and capital investment strategies. Besides, many of the "buyable" profitable hospitals had been bought and the chains—most notably, Hospital Corporation of America (HCA), National Medical Enterprises (NME), and American Medical International (AMI)—began to divest themselves of hospitals that were not performing well.

These same forces affected the long-term care industry. Beverly Enterprises and ARA Corporation (Philadelphia, Penn.), two of the nation's largest skilled care providers, experienced a series of major financial blows, resulting in efforts to sell facilities, attempted employee buyouts (Beverly), and massive financial losses.

One of the most troublesome problems to affect health care institutions recently is the relative shortage of working capital. The monitoring of cash flow on a weekly, if not daily, basis has focused inordinate management attention on daily operational issues. New lines of short- and intermediate-term credit have been established to help hospitals and others pay their bills and/or satisfy the terms of their bond covenants. In many instances, funded depreciation has become a source of operating capital for hospitals.

The health care industry continues to change and can be adversely affected by reimbursement issues. However, as the population continues to age, the reimbursement issues for the eldercare market must be evaluated in terms of future success and growth.

Reimbursement Programs for Eldercare Health Services

Reimbursement programs for services for the elderly include Medicare, Medicaid, and private supplemental insurance. First the major federal funding sources for eldercare products and services will be examined. Then the historical background of two federal programs that helped spur growth in the health care industry—Medicare and Medicaid—will be presented, along with a discussion of each current major payer source. After reviewing these reimbursement programs in relation to services for the elderly, this chapter finally will summarize other financing alternatives for eldercare services.

Federal Funding Sources and Eldercare

Seven major federal program/funding sources can be correlated with a range of health and social services needs of the aging population. See table 7-2 for funding source links with services.[15]

Whereas Medicare, Medicaid, private supplemental insurance, and out-of-pocket money pay for a substantial amount of elderly health care, significant limitations or entire gaps in coverage do exist. As noted earlier in this book, limitations in Medicare remain, especially after the 1989 Congressional repeal of the Medicare Catastrophic Coverage Act. Until this is revisited, Medicare will continue to place imposing limitations on the use of skilled nursing care, hospice services, and home care. Furthermore, without major changes Medicare essentially will not reimburse respite services for care givers or expand its prescription drug coverage. Nor does Medicare pay for intermediate-type care provided in adult congregate living facilities (ACLFs).

Some states have sought to expand their Medicaid (health services for the medically indigent) provisions to allow middle-income older adults ease in becoming eligible for Medicaid without "spending down" all of their liquid assets. Other state lawmakers have expanded Medicaid, or they have considered special programs to create pharmaceutical insurance–type programs for Medicare beneficiaries at very low cost.

Specific eldercare services that hospitals must now consider in terms of reimbursement include those on both sides of the continuum of hospital care – acute care and chronic care. The range of reimbursable and nonreimbursable services includes:

- Information and referral
- Primary care (perhaps satellite-based)
- Case-management services for the chronically ill
- Home care services
- Congregate living and life care facilities
- Skilled nursing care
- Hospice centers
- Death management services
- Respite services for care givers
- Other services for care givers, family members, and the very old

Hospitals must now critically assess these and other health care product lines to determine which, if any, they should provide by establishing networks with other providers and which ones they might own or manage.

For hospitals, the financial advantages of these services will vary, and each hospital will differ with respect to the scope of services and programs it can offer. Later in this chapter, some basic guidelines are presented, to be used in assessing and evaluating the prospect of creating, acquiring, or affiliating with such service alternatives.

Table 7-2. Major Programs to Fund Community Services for the Elderly

	Funding Source						
Services Funded	**Medicaid**	**Medicare**	**Social Services (Social Security)**	**Supplemental Security Income**	**Administration on Aging**	**Veterans Administration**	**Housing and Urban Development**
Medical services	X	X			X	X	
Home nursing	X	X					
Home/health aide	X	X	X		X	X	
Homemaker			X		X		
Personal care	X		X			X	
Chore/home repair			X		X		
Home delivered meals			X		X		
Shopping assistance			X		X		
Transportation			X		X		
Adult day care			X				
Housing assistance							X
Congregate housing			X	X		X	X
Adult foster care			X	X			
Respite care			X				
Congregate meals			X		X		
Day hospital services	X						
Social/recreation					X		
Legal and Financial			X		X		
Mental Health		X	X				
Information and referral			X		X	X	X

Source: U.S. General Accounting Office, 1979.

Incentives for Growth: Early Medicare and Medicaid

Following the introduction of Medicare (health insurance for the elderly and permanently disabled) and Medicaid (health benefits for the medically indigent), there was a sudden infusion of federal and state revenue into the health care system. Prior to 1966, zero percent of hospital revenues came from Medicare. By the end of 1966, 19.1 million people were enrolled in the new federal program, and $891 million in benefit payments was made to hospitals under Medicare Part A.[16] (See table 7-3.) In 1970, only four years into Medicare, national health expenditures (all health services and supplies) totaled $75 billion (table 7-1), of which Medicare Part A contributed $5.1 billion, or 14.6 percent.[17] By 1980, national health care expenditures had risen to $248 billion, and Medicare Part A payments had increased to $25 billion, or about 11 percent.[18] During the first ten years of Medicare, Part A payments to hospitals totaled $48.8 billion.[19]

Under Medicaid, the combined state-federal–funded program, sizable sums were spent on the indigent elderly and on Aid to Families with Dependent Children (AFDC). From the onset the benefit payouts were larger than those for AFDC recipients—despite the fact that the number of elderly who were Medicaid eligible was much smaller than the number who were AFDC eligible (see table 7-4).

Table 7-3. Medicare Part A Enrollees and Payouts: 1966–1976

Year	Number Enrolled (in millions)	Benefit Payments (Part A-Hospital) (in millions)
1966	19.1	891
1970	20.5	5,124
1972	21.3	6,318
1974	24.2	9,099
1976	25.7	13,340

Source: Health Insurance Association of America, *Source Book of Health Insurance Data, 1984–1985,* p. 34.

Table 7-4. Number of Medicaid-Eligible Elderly, Relative to AFDC and Other Eligibles: 1975–1985

	1975		1980		1985	
Source	Number (thousands)	Dollars (millions)	Number (thousands)	Dollars (millions)	Number (thousands)	Dollars (millions)
65 and over	3,615	4,538	3,440	8,739	3,061	14,095
Blind	109	93	92	124	80	249
Disabled	2,355	3,052	2,819	7,497	2,936	3,210
AFDC	14,127	4,248	14,210	6,354	15,270	9,169
Other	1,800	492	1,499	596	1,214	799

Source: *Florida Statistical Abstract, 1989.* 23rd ed. Bureau of Economic and Business Research. Gainesville, FL: University Presses of Florida, 1989, p. 359.

As massive amounts of federal and state monies were infused into the health care system, the demand for new services increased among beneficiaries. The health care system expanded to accommodate the demand; it also began to transform itself to take full advantage of the reimbursement provisions of Medicare and Medicaid.

Medicare reimbursement under Part A favored inpatient services. It was not until the mid-1980s that Medicare, by way of reimbursement criteria, began to encourage ambulatory and outpatient care as both a cost-effective and setting-appropriate alternative to hospitalization.[20]

During the late 1960s and throughout the 1970s, the SNF industry began to grow along with hospital services, due in large part to Medicaid reimbursement for SNF care. Whereas Medicare reimbursement was limited for posthospital, SNF care, Medicaid payment for this service was subject principally to the economic qualifications of individual beneficiaries. Those elderly requiring longer-term skilled nursing care—for example, who did not have health conditions requiring further hospitalization but were disabled and could not be cared for at home—might become Medicaid eligible. The growth in Medicaid served as an important basis for the rapid evolution and financial successes of corporations such as Beverly, ARA, and Manor Care (a Maryland-based chain of nursing homes) during the 1970s.[21] By 1990, 67 percent of total Beverly corporate revenues were from government medical assistance programs.[22]

Once Medicare was implemented in 1966, hospitals found that it offered an attractive and fairly reliable source of payment for a rapidly expanding service base. Capital and educational pass-throughs and relatively generous *cost-based* (loosely interpreted, "charge-based") reimbursements under Part A helped to create the remarkable capital-intensive growth in all sectors of the health care industry through the end of the 1970s.

Under the provisions of Medicare Part A, hospitals were allowed to recover costs associated with capital improvement, acquisition of technology, and medical education. This recovery took place through the reimbursement process, whereby Medicare allowed hospitals to factor capital improvement and educational expenses into their operational costs. This created a virtual pass-through of capital costs from Medicare to the hospitals and reduced the hospitals' financial burden for growth—as well as the risks associated with financing this growth for banks and investors.

The legal basis for the reimbursement of hospitals for the "reasonable costs . . . of capital, primarily depreciation and interest expenses" was initially a virtual dollar-for-dollar pass-through.[23] The specific amount of capital cost pass-through, however, was subject to apportionment based on the percentage of Medicare patients using the facility.[24] In recent years, following TEFRA, the amount of capital costs passed through by way of reimbursement under Medicare has been less than the full costs. The Health Care Financing Administration (HCFA) currently is working to develop more appropriate mechanisms for incorporating capital costs into the prospective payment system.

Direct medical education costs also have been passed through by way of reimbursement—again apportioned relative to the percentage of Medicare patient volume.[25] In recent years HCFA has recognized that some teaching hospitals serve a "disproportionate share" of low-income patients and, as a consequence, HCFA has been less severe in its reduction of medical education–related pass-throughs to these facilities.[26]

The combination of Medicare and Medicaid reimbursement helped create a substantial revenue base for hospitals and established the foundation for the full emergence of the U.S. health care industry. Furthermore, as the federal and state programs grew, private employer–based health benefits also became more popular, and considerable growth occurred in the private health insurance industry.

Medicare Changes in the 1980s

By the 1980s many hospitals had become increasingly dependent on Medicare as a revenue source. Medicare patients represented, on average, about 40 percent of hospital inpatients.[27]

Prospective payment altered the reimbursement picture by literally changing the rules for hospital payment under Medicare. Prior to the introduction of prospective payment, hospitals were paid the entire cost of care (plus a portion of capital and educational expenses, as noted previously). Under prospective payment, Medicare created 468 distinct diagnosis-related groups (DRGs), and each DRG had a preset amount of reimbursement. As one observer noted: "Hospitals that could provide care within the price limit could pocket the savings. Those that could not had to absorb the losses. The payment change represented a significant environmental change for the industry."[28]

After the introduction of prospective payment in 1984, many hospitals experienced solid increases in their operating margins.[29] Prospective payment sets payment rates for a specific time period, regardless of costs. However, since 1986 hospital operating margins in general have declined, and by 1988 operating margins associated with Medicare revenues alone had plummeted. Data for Florida, a high-Medicare-user state, highlight these trends, showing that the Medicare operating margins after expenses for hospitals in Florida was 1.5 percent in 1989.[30]

The hospital industry's reaction to prospective payment was evident in several ways; for example, productivity improvements (increased efficiency) occurred almost immediately, resulting from a combination of staffing changes and a shift of care to outpatient departments.[31] Hours per discharge, hours per service unit, and service units per discharge all underwent sudden changes.[32] (See figure 7-2.) Thus hospitals tried to become more cost-efficient by reducing staffing, evaluating time spent caring for each patient (service unit), which led to a precipitous drop.

The declining operating margins from all payer sources—and from Medicare in particular—indicated that many hospitals must control costs and seek more patients with various payer sources.

Private insurers feared that prospective payment would encourage hospitals to "cost shift" losses or charge them more for losses sustained both in the provision of care to unprofitable or less-profitable categories of Medicare patients and to other, unfunded patients.[33] In this context *cost shifting* refers to attempts by hospitals to recover lower or lost profits by increasing their regular charges to private-pay patients and those covered by commercial insurance. Such increases in charges would have no effect under Medicare, but other third-party payers might pick up the tab. However, efforts to contain costs were implemented throughout the health care industry by third-party payers. The combined effects of prospective payment in Medicare and more aggressive cost-containment strategies among other insurers had their effects. Declining operating margins following the introduction of prospective payment are evident from most studies.[34] However, these trends should be considered within the broader context of other changes occurring throughout

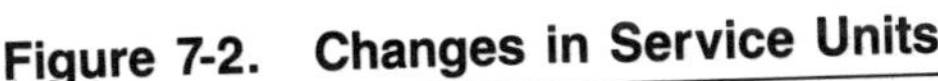

Figure 7-2. Changes in Service Units

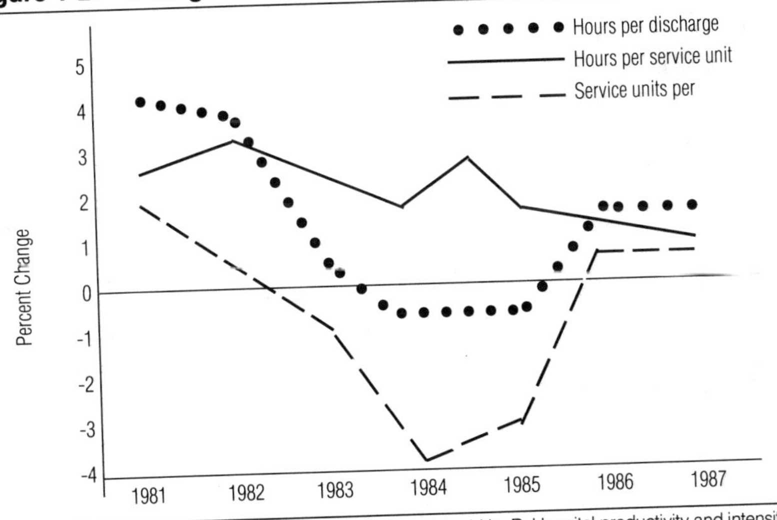

Source: Reprinted, with permission, from Cromwell, J., and Pushkin, D. Hospital productivity and intensity trends 1980–1987. *Inquiry* 26:373, Fall 1989.

Note: *Service units* refer to specific elements of care involved in patient services. They reflect diagnostic, medical, or surgical services, such as discrete categories of ancillary procedure per discharge. Reductions in these measures generally indicate productivity gains, since this would reflect fewer hours and resources consumed in the "production" of a discharge. Conversely, increases in these measures generally reflect declines.

the health care industry such as increased competition that were also contributing to reduced profitability.[35]

Both Medicare and other payers have made it increasingly difficult to successfully collect a higher amount in order to compensate for contractual allowance, bad debts, and charity care. Until recently it was possible to cost shift some losses to various payers, including Medicare; however, managed care and the use of DRGs have reduced this option.

Medicare reimbursement policies also have shifted more toward increased use of outpatient services. At the same time, in recent years a growing proportion of high-volume, good-profit inpatient services—such as cataract removal/lens implantation and a wide range of orthopedic and diagnostic services—have left the hospital, to be performed in freestanding ambulatory care centers. These services often compete quite successfully with hospitals for certain outpatient Medicare business.

These forces, combined with changing disease patterns among the elderly, challenge hospital administrators to stay current on Medicare policy and to consider additional services or programs that provide a continuum of care and can be developed using both inpatient and outpatient settings (as discussed in chapter 5). Planners will have to consider expanding their service base to the elderly along the continuum of care rather than concentrating on acute-care services.

Medicare Today

Many elderly have become increasingly concerned about the extent of their Medicare coverage. In early 1990, Medicare still had annual and lifetime limits on inpatient stays; a 100-day limit on skilled nursing care and a requirement that SNF services follow an episode of inpatient hospitalization; limitations on home care and hospice care; very limited prescription drug coverage; and no catastrophic component.

In 1988, Congress passed legislation intended to overhaul Medicare substantially and to create a catastrophic health insurance program. The changes were to have gone into effect in 1990, but they were repealed toward the end of 1989. Powerful national lobbying by interest groups representing the generally more affluent elderly rallied forces successfully to force Congress to repeal the entire package of proposed changes. The repeal signaled, among other possibilities, increasing bad debts and charity care write-offs for hospitals resulting from catastrophic-type situations beyond the scope of Medicare coverage.

Surprisingly, as third-party wizard Sam Kaplan has noted, business organizations were conspicuously absent during the death of the catastrophic bill.[36] Many business leaders simply did not think catastrophic care issues would affect them. However, they will because their financial burdens for retired employees under the Consolidated Omnibus Reconciliation Act of 1985 (COBRA) will increase, as will the costs of uncompensated catastrophic services in their communities. Among other requirements, COBRA expanded the commitment of employers to finance employee health benefits, including postretirement health benefits. Much of the catastrophic care issue relates to the long-term and skilled care needs of Medicare beneficiaries.

It is important to note that private, supplemental "Medigap" insurance protects many older Medicare beneficiaries, about 72–74 percent of whom purchase this coverage.[37]

The challenge posed by Medicare for hospital administrators is to stay current on the case/patient mix, DRG rates, and the behaviors of admitting physicians and other hospitals. Another challenge is to effectively manage the care provided to Medicare beneficiaries. More than anything else, this means having a management information, analysis, and reporting capability that effectively links clinical and financial information for internal use and analysis. However, it is also important to work with physicians to ensure that their practices and referral patterns are consistent with Medicare policies and to control Medicare admissions from other providers.

Medicare and Relationships with Physicians

Prospective payment has affected the relationships between physicians and administrators. Prior to prospective payment, many referring physicians who had patients with long lengths of stay and who required heavy use of ancillary services generally were viewed as the "good guys," especially relative to Medicare. But prospective payment and DRGs placed fairly well-defined reimbursement limits on diagnostic groups. Resource management became much more important. Longer lengths of stay and overuse of ancillary services became a financial detriment to the institution. Studies indicate there is considerable variation in physician practice patterns regarding those issues, even within very limited geographic areas.[38] This has been linked to physician training, habits, personal preferences, and other factors. Good communication between administrators and physicians coupled with clear hospital policies on these issues can be effective.

Under prospective payment and DRGs, hospitals must work with physicians and in some cases with local peer review organizations (PROs) to identify unusual and unexplainable variations in admitting and prescription behavior among physicians. Not only has this become a financial necessity, it could also have liability implications. For example, under the 1989 Medicare quality assurance guidelines, a third party can deny claim payment in its entirety if it is judged, upon peer review, that the services performed were not medically necessary. Consider the implications of this for a physician or a hospital denied payment for "unnecessary" or "inappropriate" service. Aside from the provider suffering potential loss of income from the denied claim, a far more pressing issue must be addressed. In each case of a denied claim, the beneficiary receives the standard explanation of Medicare benefits (EOMB), on which the Medicare third party notifies the beneficiary that the services were deemed unnecessary. On reading this many patients would be confused and angered, some to the point of seeking legal redress. How would the hospital protect itself from adverse reaction in a lawsuit against the physician? What would be the public relations and quality-of-care implications if such incidents were to occur frequently? Probably more than most hospitals could afford.

Medicare Admissions from Other Providers

A facility must keep careful watch over transfer policies of other nearby hospitals to prevent (when possible) the dumping of high-risk, high-cost Medicare patients into its care. Most well-managed facilities have mastered Medicare's product line management and selective marketing and admitting practices. Once it is determined which products are profitable and which are not, referral patterns are set, high-profit "products" targeted, and others discouraged (or skimmed) or even sent elsewhere—that is, dumped. Skimming and dumping have been discussed extensively in the professional literature.[39]

Institutions on the receiving end of dumping must strive to maintain close control over admissions, especially those that have already been admitted to another facility or stabilized in another facility's emergency room. Well-developed and tightly managed transfer policies, contractual relationships regarding stabilizing and returning patients to the original institution (especially patients on respirator care and transfers from local skilled nursing facilities) have become vital ingredients in the control of admissions and their costs.

Skilled nursing facilities often are unable or unwilling to care for residents experiencing an acute health care problem, and it is not uncommon for SNFs to send such residents to local hospitals for acute inpatient care. Hospitals acting as the receiving facility for such SNF patients should make certain that their transfer and care will be paid for by Medicare or Medicaid. Of greater importance, however, will be cautious treatment of the patient who is either on a respirator or may require respirator care during transport or once at the hospital.

Useful adjuncts to patient transport are *transfer centers.* These are formal units within hospitals whose responsibility is to manage (by establishing specific criteria and approving them) all in-transfers to the hospital. Among the characteristics of transfer centers are formal contractual transfer agreements, requirements for physician approval of transfers, and, where appropriate, conditions for return of the patient to the initiating hospital (for example, poststabilization).

Clearly articulated, contractual transfer and stabilization agreements must be in place between a hospital and any referring facility, whether it is another hospital in the area, a SNF, or an adult congregate living facility (ACLF). Without these agreements a hospital can become a repository of dumped patients who may become ineligible for Medicare, Medicaid, or other coverage. The results can be financially disastrous while at the same time raising central issues of ethics about patient care. The key is to establish and maintain well-defined relationships with physicians and to network with providers in the service area. In addition, institutions providing certain specialty services, such as heart transplantation and other open-heart procedures, should seek affiliations and referral arrangements with individual physicians, managed care and third-party organizations, and other hospitals in regions beyond their own service areas.

Medicaid

Many Medicare beneficiaries may find that a catastrophic, or extended long-term care, episode results in virtual impoverishment. This is especially true for those without Medigap coverage. Medicare's limited long-term care coverage and the relatively high costs of this care have caused many people to seek assistance from state Medicaid and public assistance programs.

Each state has different income and assets guidelines for Medicaid eligibility, and many elderly persons must virtually "spend down" their assets (excluding their homes and certain other property) in some states, to become eligible for Medicaid. Hospital admitting offices should maintain updated versions of state eligibility guidelines, along with specific county or city provisions for additional indigent care support. In many states, the county or the city may become the payer of near–last resort if Medicaid eligibility is not established. (Of course, in cases of wholly uncompensated care, the payer of last resort is the provider.)

Medicaid was enacted in 1965 and went into operation in 1966 as a joint federal and state program. Whereas states generally are required to accept the primary administrative responsibility, the degree of federal financial contribution will vary by state, depending on the percentage of people in that state who fall below federally defined poverty limits, or who are otherwise eligible for Medicaid services. Although the federal government establishes basic services a state must provide in order to be eligible to receive federal Medicaid monies, "States have wide discretion in the income levels used for eligibility determination; in the specific groups covered; in the amount, duration, and scope of services; and in reimbursement approaches."[40]

The Medicaid program was designed to assist families with dependent children (AFDC), as well as the elderly, blind and disabled.

However, the distribution of Medicaid resources is somewhat lopsided. More than 40 percent of Medicaid money provides care to the elderly population, which comprises less than 20 percent of all Medicaid recipients;[41] much of this pays for long-term skilled nursing care.[42] In 1986, more than 36 percent of all Medicaid monies paid for nursing home care.[43]

In general, because Medicaid is a *cost-based* form of reimbursement—that is, negotiated each year with the state Medicaid program—in some instances "cost-plus" factors must be built into the reimbursement. In areas of the country that have excess bed capacity, this means that Medicaid patients could provide sufficient cash flow to cover operating costs. This would be the case in areas where the census is low or where there is room for additional patients to fill vacant beds. As is the case in Medicare, "Even if these hospitals appear to 'lose money' . . . , these patients may provide a needed contribution to overhead costs—without which hospitals would be under even greater financial pressure."[44] By filling a bed with a Medicaid patient or by providing Medicaid-reimbursed outpatient services, some hospitals can help to offset their working capital problems, or at least provide a source of operating revenue that will help them meet fixed costs. Of course this will depend on the nature of the reimbursement contract with the state Medicaid program, the patient case mix, excess bed capacity in the area, and accuracy of cost data used to negotiate Medicaid rates.

Two issues regarding Medicaid must be addressed: patient eligibility and speed of payment.

Patient Eligibility

To receive Medicaid money for services provided, patients must be deemed eligible by their state Medicaid program. A substantial proportion of patients never attain Medicaid eligibility, often due to insufficient or inadequate documentation. Some hospitals now are implementing well-designed Medicaid eligibility protocols in the emergency room and for the regular admitting process. Patients sometimes require assistance from a case worker or volunteer to prepare materials for submission to the state's Medicaid program or the county's welfare program.

At larger urban hospitals that have a substantial number of Medicaid patients, investing in such protocols can be well worth the cost. At the Tampa General Hospital, a 1,000-bed tertiary care facility, the Medicaid program has offices and case workers adjacent to the hospital's outpatient area. In addition, the hospital employs case workers to drive to the homes of patients and their families to obtain necessary Medicaid eligibility data, such as rent and utility receipts, or to obtain other documents needed to process an application. These case workers are now equipped with mobile telephones and fax machines to expedite the process.

Speed of Payment

Some states (such as Massachusetts in 1989) essentially stopped paying Medicaid bills because no money was left. Others, however, have become notoriously slow in processing claims and appeals.

In a growing number of instances Medicaid has formulated HMO and PPO networks. The HMOs use modified forms of capitation, making utilization management essential.

Any facility going into the Medicaid business should establish a good working relationship with the Medicaid program office and with local welfare program staff to minimize payer–provider friction and help speed payment times. It is also important to make the most efficient use of reimbursable resources under Medicaid. As will be discussed later, alternative care settings, such as skilled care or home care, should be evaluated for Medicaid patients, so that economic exposure is minimized and reimbursement is maximized.

Private, Supplemental Insurance

As already noted, about 72 to 74 percent of Medicare beneficiaries purchase supplemental Medigap insurance, designed to help cover some of the costs not paid for by Medicare. The range and costs of these policies, which are advertised extensively, vary substantially.

Medigaps generally offer beneficiaries a range of coverage options, from basic assistance in meeting a percentage of Medicare unpaid expenses (a portion of deductibles and coinsurance), to additional coverage for pharmaceuticals, private duty nursing services, extended coverage for skilled nursing care, additional hospital care, and other features.

It is incumbent upon hospitals to determine the level and scope of private, supplemental Medigap coverage held by patients, for both inpatient and outpatient services. When possible, hospitals should arrange to receive assigned benefits, while at the same time keeping a close tab on the *net due from the patient* after all policies have paid their appropriate portions.

Some patients will have broad-based, supplemental coverage that includes additional days of skilled care, private duty nursing service, and so forth. Hospitals with affiliated services or swing bed–type arrangements will want to manage these cases carefully to ensure maximum reimbursement, minimum costs, and the best level and setting of care for patients. This will require management to conduct optimization analyses, product line cost and profit analyses, and to be able to determine the most appropriate type of care needed by each patient and juggle resources successfully to achieve this end. Again, ongoing communication with physicians is central to the success of these efforts.

Financing Alternatives for Eldercare Services

In the years ahead, a new and expansive range of supplemental, private insurance products might be available to assist elderly consumers accomplish two goals: protection against excess financial risk; and attainment of benefit levels beyond those offered in Medicare and other supplemental plans.

In addition to insurance plans, many older adults will have access to special annuity proceeds and, possibly, health individual retirement accounts (IRAs). *Health IRAs* could be created by Congress to allow people to place *tax-exempt* (pretax) portions of their earnings into separate, interest-earning accounts. If withdrawn for reasons other than a catastrophic health episode before participants reach a certain age, such deposits might be subject both to taxation and a "penalty" for early withdrawal. The idea would be that these accounts would be added to each year and mature over time to create a "health nest egg" to help pay for health care–related expenses later in life. Monies not expended might be rolled over to a spouse or a child for the same purpose—a "health bequest" in the form of a catastrophic insurance fund. More likely, the unspent assets might revert to the estate and become taxable as any other form of marketable security subject to inheritance.

Throughout the late 1980s there was serious discussion in Congress and in the health care industry about "universal" health insurance coverage for all persons in the United States. Canadian, various European, and even Japanese models have been examined and touted as including desirable features that currently are lacking in U.S. health care. These features include a basic level of guaranteed benefits available to all persons, regardless of ability to pay.

If the federal government finds an economic and politically viable vehicle by which it can successfully deploy a universal, national health care system—one that would include full coverage for long-term care—then fundamental questions about financing these services will become moot. At this writing, no sources of revenue have been identified to finance such a scheme, and the prospect of new taxes to finance one remains remote.

In the meantime, both the need for an expanded array of long-term health care services and marketplace opportunities to provide them face the nation's hospitals. How can these services be financed? No single financing alternative is likely to respond to all populations and service needs. For this reason, it is important to consider a variety of incremental programs and options designed to close the gap for both the elderly and providers of care.

Insurance and other programs may reimburse providers for a range of health care services delivered to older persons, but insurance does not cover certain costs (for example, catastrophic episodes and the myriad services associated with long-term care).

In addition to long-term care insurance, other financing options available now or on the horizon include annuities, employment-linked long-term care insurance, Medicare HMOs and PPOs, life care or assisted living arrangements, home equity conversions and reverse mortgages, and others.

Long-Term Care Insurance

Long-term care insurance, though available, is quite expensive and generally is purchased only by the more affluent elderly. Many insurers have been hesitant to develop and market long-term care insurance because of the problems of combined adverse selection of policy purchasers (that is, those with the greatest need, requiring the most costly care, might be most inclined to buy); and essentially undefined limits on liability (once people start using these insurance products, how long will they live, and what kinds of health care resources will they consume?).[45] The actuarial concerns here are not inconsequential.

Many long-term care policies require aggressive case-management programs by providers to ensure that the long-term care needs of elderly beneficiaries are most effectively and efficiently met in a combination of home and institutional settings, using a range of qualified health care practitioners in the care process.

Insurance products that will cover long-term health care needs of older adults are likely to become increasingly popular. Studies indicate that the private insurance marketplace will find the growing number of relatively healthy older persons to be an attractive market and a reasonable insurance risk pool.[46] But at present, the broad-based financial viability of long-term care insurance has not been demonstrated for the entire population.

It is important to distinguish traditional health insurance–type policies from the idea of long-term care insurance–type policies, a distinction that lies in the nature of the *event(s)* against which one seeks protection. Traditional health insurance is designed at best to assist in shielding specific population groups from untoward financial risks associated with the possible occurrence of acute-care problems generally requiring a combination of physician and hospital care. But traditional insurance and insurance systems generally are not designed or equipped to address the central element of long-term care, which is disability management.

Much of the long-term care needs of the aging, chronically ill involve the effective and careful *management of disabilities*—not the provision of unnecessary and costly acute-care services.

The present health care system, and the insurance vehicles (both public and private) that drive it, do not have the capability or the inclination to devote considerable resources to disability management. This will change, especially as hospital decision makers, policy makers, and insurers recognize the financial advantages of providing options for more independent elderly patients and managing disabilities rather than just attempting to cure conditions.

The growth and diversity of care settings outside the hospital and nursing home—specifically, home-based services, various community-based programs (day care, and so forth), and adult congregate living facilities (ACLF and other intermediate care environments)—will transform the present definition of long-term care insurance. As this occurs, managers will find it increasingly more sensible, profitable, and practical to learn how to manage disabling conditions most effectively to maximize independence. This may include greater use among the elderly of rehabilitation centers for outpatient and inpatient needs, already successful profit centers for many hospitals.

In lieu of expanded national health insurance coverage for long-term care, private products may become popular among those who can afford to pay the premiums. Even if the federal government were to expand the provisions of either Medicare or Medicaid to cover long-term care needs, private products will likely still be developed to fill gaps and to offer coverage for more expensive facilities for those wishing to pay the price. However, in these cases people might be more inclined to purchase various forms of annuities, or IRA-type products at an earlier age, in addition to basic insurance coverage.

Annuities

Annuities currently are used by many to defer tax liabilities and to produce a source of future income (generally for pension purposes or children's education). Most annuities are merely investment or insurance vehicles (with low-risk, guaranteed minimum rates of return, often backed by treasury bills or other government securities). These allow lump-sum or smaller deposits (depending on the product) into interest-earning accounts, wherein the interest earned is tax free. As with IRAs, the intent is that the funds will remain untouched until some future period (ostensibly for retirement), at which time annuity payments, like pension payments, would commence, and the income to the individual generally would be treated as ordinary income and may be used in a discretionary manner. In some cases, depending on the nature of the annuity product, the annuity may be borrowed against before the maturity date.

Employment-Linked Long-Term Care Insurance

Employment-linked long-term care insurance has the advantage of offering employees a low- or no-cost (if the employer pays) benefit. But the policy is generally available by way of employment, in addition to basic benefits, and employees may need to work a certain number of years to qualify. For many employee groups, the purchase of explicit long-term care insurance might involve a rider to an existing policy or the purchase of a supplemental freestanding insurance product. It would be useful for some hospitals to find out whether large employers in their service areas offer such coverage.

Some firms have begun to offer long-term care insurance for employee's *parents*. This innovative benefit recognizes the value of protecting the employee's family and of sheltering the employee from the time and expense burdens of caring for a chronically ill parent.

Although annuities, health IRAs, and long-term care insurance are attractive financing vehicles, they will likely appeal to the middle and upper middle class, leaving a substantial portion of the population without access to these "self-funded" methods of protection.

Medicare HMOs and PPOs

Medicare and Medicaid have each experimented extensively with versions of managed and prepaid health care. Medicare managed care programs, which differ little from other managed care products, appear in two forms: HMOs and PPOs.

Medicare HMOs involve explicit contractual relationships with formal health maintenance organizations, wherein annual capitated fees are paid to the HMO for each Medicare beneficiary enrolled. The HMO gets the advantage of a fixed, per-capita premium and then becomes responsible (generally with the back-up assistance of stop-loss insurance coverage) for effectively managing the health care needs of its Medicare enrollees. The HMO will use staff physicians and/or panels of physicians to provide care. As with other HMO arrangements, the specific reimbursement arrangements for physician and hospital care are subject to negotiated provisions between the HMO and these providers.

Medicare PPOs work the same as other PPOs, in that third parties contract with Medicare to provide services at prenegotiated and ostensibly discounted rates.

With Medicare HMOs and PPOs the principles of utilization management, emphasis on primary care, use of outpatient services, and incentives to keep patients out of costly inpatient and institutional care are the predicates to financial success. Except in cases of emergency or trauma, beneficiaries must use designated providers and generally should be required to seek care through a "gatekeeping" primary care physician who is responsible for managing and directing care according to protocols and guidelines of the HMO or PPO.

The problem with prepaid eldercare health services is that providers are at some financial risk, and in the case of long-term care there remain uncertainties about lengths of stay, scope of services to be used, and the adequacies of funding. These aside, the combination of Medicare and Medicaid HMO/PPO programs, and the social HMO (SHMO) does offer promise.

Many hospitals currently contract with Medicare HMOs, arrangements beset by at least the same challenge as any HMO contractual arrangement. Careful, clinically driven utilization management criteria must be in place within the hospital to ensure that unnecessary resources are not deployed during care.

The Health Care Financing Administration initiated demonstration projects for Medicare PPOs in the late 1980s. These projects, similar to other PPO efforts, seek to establish networks of "approved, preferred" providers to which beneficiaries are directed. The advantages in this can be patient volume and cash flow, but the basis for the PPO rate of reimbursement, which will be some rearrangement of DRGs, must be negotiated carefully (to the extent this is possible) to ensure affordability of care given the rate of reimbursement.

Life Care or Assisted Living Arrangements

In addition to HMO and PPOs, a variety of life care or assisted living arrangements offer a broad scope of "tiered" health and life care services to persons who can afford to buy in. These often involve a combination of housing and health care services and generally require the purchase of a real estate product, plus monthly maintenance fees.

A general principle of life care operation is the combination of financing and delivery of housing and long-term care services. Products may provide mixtures of insurance (or annuity) offerings for long-term care, residential services (apartments or houses), with ranges of social and health support services (recreational programs, physical therapy, levels of home assistance—especially for recuperation from inpatient acute care). These are paid for through a combination of Medicare reimbursement (where applicable) and private insurancelike products or annuities that pay for these services. Out-of-pocket costs are also common. In many life care arrangements, meals and other basic assisted living services also are available on an individual basis (personal care or assistance with medications), or in congregate settings (meals, recreation, physical therapy, and so forth).

These arrangements tend to be operated through the auspices of various not-for-profit corporations and may be affiliated with religious organizations.[47] Services are generally financed by an "entry fee," ranging from $45,000 (in Indiana) to $128,000 (in Massachusetts).[48] Depending on the nature of the contract, fees may be refunded to spouse or estate upon beneficiary's death or paid out as an insurance settlement to a named beneficiary. In addition, monthly fees (combinations of condominium-type maintenance fees and other assessments) cover housing, nursing, and social services;[49] these fees can average $1,327 for a couple.[50,51]

Some insurance company/long-term care company joint ventures for life care have worked out quite successfully. Many developers have gone into the senior housing business offering a whole array of personal care and support services, but not necessarily a life care contract. These have been found to be successful in many instances as well. The keys to success have been good case management and well-developed financial controls. There have been many failed plans that ostensibly left a number of elderly persons without coverage or assets. For this reason, state insurance commissioners have become increasingly involved in regulating these products.

However, a natural market exists for hospitals to develop a wide range of assisted living arrangements or ACLFs that are oriented toward intermediate care. They include support-type services designed to provide assistance in activities for daily living.[52]

Hospitals might own, manage, or joint venture life care arrangements. The captive market would be in the form of revenues gleaned from services provided to residents in the ACLF and also from inpatient and outpatient care provided by the hospital to these residents.

In 1988, St. Joseph's Hospital in Tampa, Florida, purchased a 1,500-bed, private, not-for-profit ACLF, which is adjacent to *another* community hospital about 10 miles from St. Joseph's campus. Each day, St. Joseph's buses transport ACLF patients past the neighboring hospital across town to St. Joseph's for inpatient and outpatient care. The investment has been successful thus far.

Home Equity Conversions and Reverse Mortgages

Home equity conversions and reverse mortgages have received increased attention in recent years as vehicles for financing long-term care. Each involves arrangements with banks and mortgage companies or other financial entities to use existing home equity to pay for health care services. Hospitals might link up directly with banks, mortgage bankers and brokers, or taxation/estate planning attorneys to develop these arrangements, which preferably should be made prior to the need for care. Hospitals might encourage their older consumers (and their families) to consider such forward thinking.

Both vehicles impose some limitations, principally relating to the value of homes held by elderly persons. Whereas some equity holdings may amount to hundreds of thousands of dollars—amounts that could sustain long-term care needs for several years—most homes in fact average much less in value and would afford only limited coverage of long-term care needs.

Many older adults own their homes, with little or no outstanding mortgages. An *equity conversion* involves the sale of the home to a third-party investor, with stipulations that allow the person to remain in the home for some set number of years into the future, or until death. Funds from the sale of the house are used to pay for a scope of long-term care needs, yet the terms for the sale of the house allow the person to remain in their home for as long as he or she is able.

Reverse mortgages involve the sale of a portion of the equity value of the home to a third party—or perhaps even the hospital or skilled care facility. The cash from the sale of these equity shares is used to pay for care. The loan might be repaid by heirs or through the decedent's estate.

Other Financing Options

Hospitals should become familiar with the various options available to finance long-term health care needs of the elderly. Every effort should be made to determine, either in advance or at the time of service, the scope of coverage held by each patient as well as the options that might be employed to finance care that lies beyond the scope of existing insurance provisions.

As part of this forward thinking about the financing of eldercare services, hospitals might consider cosigning loans for patients who have identifiable assets as collateral. These assets might include marketable securities, boats, or vacation homes, among other viable collateral. This at least would provide cash flow for services provided and, to the extent feasible, persons with liquid holdings may indeed pay all or part of the note, thereby reducing the probability of default to the hospital. But even a delayed default on a loan would provide the hospital with some cash and would forestall a bad debt.

Hospitals may want to work with family members to secure long-term care loans through local provider cooperation. A particularly innovative approach would involve a group of local hospitals forming a captive financing company designed to provide low-interest, secured loans to patients and/or their families. These aggressive financing ideas, however, would place hospitals firmly in the business of financial services and could also create perceived conflicts of interest and ill will regarding bad debts.

Another innovative financing method involves the use of existing life insurance policies. Older adults who have life insurance policies in force may "sell" these policies to a second or third party for cash, for example at 70 percent or 80 percent of the face value of the policy; proceeds would pay for long-term care. The policy is "sold" in the sense that the new beneficiary would be the party purchasing the policy (similar somewhat to a reverse mortgage). These policies will become increasingly popular.

In addition to long-term insurance, annuities, and other such products, "community investment" models have been proposed for health services, to include long-term care.[53] In one of these models, care financing is achieved through a combination of bond proceeds, dedicated Medicaid and local tax dollars, tax-deductible contributions from relatives and others, and premium contributions scaled to means.

For example, tax-exempt bonds would be issued locally and sold to a variety of corporate and individual investors. Existing Medicaid and local tax dollars used to support long-term care in the community would be diverted to a fund into which a portion of the bond proceeds would also be placed. Local health care providers requiring capital to develop or support long-term and chronic health care services for the elderly would compete for low-interest loans from a portion of the bond sales. These same providers would be eligible to receive market-rate payments for well-managed, long-term care and disability management services provided to community residents who lack the means or insurance to cover such care. Residents could buy in to the risk pool, financing the care at premium levels scaled to their assets and income. Relatives and others could contribute set amounts to the program and be eligible for a tax deduction. The Medicaid, local, and county funds would be guaranteed and would serve as part of the revenue stream against which the bonds would be issued. Interest revenues generated from loan repayments by providers, and funds from bond proceeds that have been invested and even arbitrated, also would serve as a revenue stream.

In this model, long-term and other eldercare becomes a community asset, and investors are given financial incentives to support this essential infrastructure item. Corporate and individual investors would be encouraged to purchase these bonds for the same reasons they choose to purchase municipal and industrial development bonds.

Evaluation of Eldercare Products

For each DRG or other category of illness, the specific range of care options (product lines) offered by the institution should be considered with respect to the average percent operating margin generated from *that* service and the dollar profit generated from an average case in that setting. This becomes very important when considering the merits of transferring a patient in need of less than acute care to a less-intensive, less-costly—but possibly more profitable—care setting. Increased profitability may result from optimizing available resources. *Opportunity costs*—the costs of selecting a decision that is *less than* the best economic alternative—must be calculated in each case. Therefore in all cases of decision analysis, managers should state the best possible *economic* alternative, along with other options, and specify in dollar terms the cost of not having selected the best financial decision.

Of course, the best financial decision may not be the best clinical decision or even relate to the purpose of a health care organization. The reason for conducting this kind of analysis is to establish a purely economic benchmark against which decisions can be compared. For example, assume that limited expendable resources are available for a capital/program decision and that there are four options for spending the money. Assume as well that each option carries with it projected revenues and benefits, as shown in table 7-5. In this example project A would break even; project B would result in a net loss of $20; project C would cause a net gain of $20; and project D would gain a net of $5. Recognizing that the best *financial decision* is not always the operative decision of choice for the hospital (relative to its strategic plan, environment, and patient mix), assume that project D is selected by management, yielding a net gain of $5. The opportunity cost in this example would represent the *difference* between the *best* identifiable *financial* option and the option selected. In our example the *best* financial option would yield a net of $20 whereas management's (or the board's) decision would yield only $5. Therefore the opportunity cost (financial benefit foregone from not having selected the best financial option) would be: $20 – $5 or $15.

If the best identifiable financial decision had been selected (project C) the opportunity cost would have been zero.

To conduct this kind of analysis most appropriately, substantial information must be obtained about the nature and scope of projects, services, and programs. For example, make the following determinations by major category of care or patient:

- What kind of care does the patient need, and what setting options are available to satisfy this need?
- What is the maximum, necessary, and reimbursable scope of services and procedures needed to provide to this patient (for example, ancillaries)?
- How much additional revenue might be generated if a patient is transferred to another revenue-generating setting and the acute-care bed filled with a new patient?

Table 7-5. Opportunity Costs by Option Analysis

	Project A	Project B	Project C	Project D
Revenue	$100	$ 80	$120	$105
Cost	100	100	100	100
Net	$ 0	$–20	$ 20	$ 5

By asking these questions managers address the opportunity cost issue of trade-offs between types of care. The goal is to maximize revenue from existing resources (beds, services, staff) while at the same time ensuring that patients receive the most appropriate level of care. Therefore, if a postsurgical or posttreatment inpatient can be treated successfully in a less-restrictive setting—even if that setting may not generate revenue for the hospital (for example, an outside SNF or home care service)—the hospital may benefit from freeing up the bed for a new patient who will be generating significantly more revenue from services received.

This type of resource optimization requires good case management and discharge planning at the time of admission and carefully developed networks of linked services, either within the structure of the hospital (owned or managed) or with neighboring providers of these services. When patients are placed in the most appropriate settings and their care is most effectively managed, the result in most cases should be a combination of cost savings (for the institution and for the payers) and revenue enhancement.

Table 7-6 shows an analysis of the profits associated with three product lines: inpatient care, skilled nursing, and home care. In this example home care seems to afford the lowest profit margin of the product lines. Home care would be less profitable than, for example, inpatient care and may seem to warrant less emphasis by the hospital. But in the context of high hospital occupancy, demand for beds, and the importance of "most appropriate" care, the hospital might select the home care product on a case-by-case basis. When this is done the inpatient bed is made available for more intense, revenue-producing services, and the discharged patient produces $850 per case in a more appropriate care setting. The result is enhanced revenue and better care. Similarly, because in this scenario the SNF product provides the best profit margin, it might be more profitable to turn some inpatient beds into skilled nursing beds, which generate a better profit margin per case than inpatient beds.

The idea is to maximize available resources and minimize the use of higher-cost services when patients can continue to receive an appropriate level of care in another setting.

Hospitals must be in a position to determine which of the health care products, services, or facilities they might want to purchase, develop,

Table 7-6. Profit Margin and Average Charge per Case by DRG or Other Category of Illness

Product Line	Inpatient care	Skilled Nursing	Home Care
Profit margin percent	3	8	2
Average dollars per case	1,000	3,000	850

lease, or manage for the provision of care along the continuum of elder-care. To do this, it is essential to incorporate at least two key financial management techniques in the decision process: product line analysis and present value/opportunity analysis.

Product Line Analysis

Product lines in health care can be defined as services (specific or grouped procedures or current procedural terminology–CPTs) or as diagnostic groups (major diagnostic categories or diagnosis-related groups–MDCs or DRGs). Managers must have the ability to determine the actual costs of each health care product and establish parameters for these costs (on a per-unit, aggregate, and per-department basis) based on ranges of projected volume. Managers can use product line analysis information to perform more effective strategic financial analyses of profitable and unprofitable services and products, and to conduct meaningful financial evaluations of existing and proposed services and products.

For example, personnel costs, supply costs, overhead, and other costs, direct and indirect, associated with the provision of a multiple coronary bypass admission should be obtained. Cost accounting and cost finding methods can be employed to determine the *fixed* and *variable* portions of these costs. Management should be prepared to generate these data for major product lines that contribute substantially to the operation of a hospital.

A *contribution margin* for each of these procedures or product lines is then calculated as total revenue from a specific product, minus the calculated variable cost per unit of service for that product:

Contribution margin = Total revenue from product – Variable cost per unit

Contribution margins are the difference between revenues from the sale of a product and the variable expenses attributable to that product. The costs associated with any health care product are assumed to be a combination of fixed costs (those remaining unchanged relative to volume) and variable costs (those fluctuating with volume, either directly or inversely). Some costs are essentially fixed, meaning they remain the same regardless of volume or use. Examples are annual insurance expenses; preset leasing costs for space, equipment, or furniture; and, in many cases, substantial portions of administrative and staff salaries (to the extent they are not affected by overtime or productivity bonuses).

Variable costs will fluctuate with volume. Dietary department expenses, lab supplies, maintenance costs, and linen and laundry are examples. Variable costs behave differently for specific expense items and are measured in terms of total variable costs for a service or product (in dollars and percent) and in terms of variable costs *per unit of service.*

Generally speaking, variable and fixed costs are analyzed within "relevant ranges" of activity. This means that costs must be studied to determine when and how they react to changes in volume or demand or to changes in the mix of services or products. For example, nurse staffing costs in an outpatient eldercare center may be related to patient volume in the following, hypothetical way. (The example is represented in figure 7-3.)

> Assume that 3 RNs and 5 LPNs are able to provide outpatient clinical services for a *maximum* of 50 patients each day. Assume further that the "relevant range" of volume is 0–50 patients per day, assuming that the base staffing patterns for the facility consists of 5 RNs and 5 LPNs.
>
> If RN salaries and benefits total \$60,000 per employee, and LPN salaries and benefits total \$35,000 per employee (exclusive of overtime), then the nursing costs for the unit, given 0–50 patients per day, would be:
>
> | | | |
> |---|---|---|
> | \$60,000 × 3 (RNs) | = | \$180,000 |
> | \$35,000 × 5 (LPNs) | = | \$175,000 |
> | Total nursing salary and benefit costs for 0–50 patients | | \$355,000 |

What happens, however, if volume *exceeds* 50 patients per day—if it leaps to 70 patients per day?

> Assume that the *incremental* nurse staffing needs are 1 RN and 1.5 LPNs for each increment of 25 patients beyond 50. Therefore, to meet the new demand effectively, add 1 RN at a total incremental cost of \$60,000 and 1.5 LPNs at a total incremental cost of \$52,000—a total additional volume-related cost of \$122,500. The "relevant range" of activity (volume capacity relative to nurse staffing alone) has now risen to 75 patients per day (giving a margin of 5 additional patients before having to revisit staffing numbers).

This example shows that even some fixed costs can be subject to the effects of volume, within measurable and defined ranges of activity. This behavior is generally called *step-variable,* or *semi-fixed* costs. Unless variable and fixed costs within relevant ranges of activity are known, profitability or loss associated with specific products and services (as indicated in part by the contribution margin) will not be known.

In health care, as in other ventures, the contribution margin is the amount from each unit sale that goes toward meeting fixed costs. Once

Figure 7-3. Example of Step-Variable Staffing

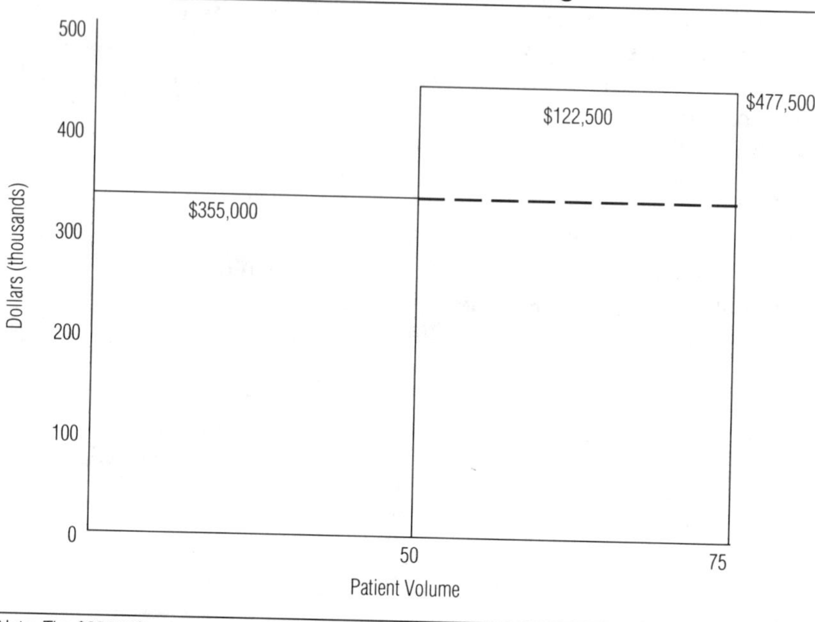

Note: The $355,000 represents total nursing salary and benefit costs for 0–50 patients. For each increment of 25 patients beyond 50, it would cost $122,500 to provide nursing staff to handle the additional patient volume.

fixed costs have been met, the contribution margin essentially represents incremental net income—the first step toward profitability.

The contribution margin is becoming increasingly important for health services administrators as they seek to determine how best to survive the vicissitudes of a volatile health care marketplace. The importance of contribution margins lies in the fact that different health care products contribute in very different ways to the financial well-being of a health care organization. Some products are very profitable, though their volume is relatively low, whereas others have low margins of profit and depend on high volumes to produce desirable financial results. The product line analysis approach has gained considerable currency in health care management. Surprisingly, few organizations have successfully developed their financial information systems to produce accurate analyses of product lines.

Specific health care products can be analyzed to reveal their fixed/variable cost components and, subsequently, their relative contributions to profitability within relevant ranges of activity. For almost any health care provider, from small practitioner settings through complex managed care–related systems, this information is essential to sound strategic planning, fiscal analyses, and the evaluation of program performance. If contribution margin analysis is conducted for each product line, it becomes clear that each behaves and contributes to the hospital's financial welfare in a different way. Some products may contribute directly, whereas others may "feed" patients into different lucrative product lines, though contributing little in direct dollars. Relative contribution margin data provide managers with information about the profitability of *each* product, as well as information about the percentage of profit (or loss) that each product contributes to the bottom line.

This kind of product line analysis provides baseline data for managers to identify the relationship of each product line to the production of bottom-line profits. At the same time it provides an important framework for examining possible changes in service mix that might come about due to reimbursement system changes, retirement of a referring physician, or some other factor. The relative contribution of each product line must be carefully considered when making product decisions.

Table 7-7 shows a simple contribution margin analysis across three product lines. For each product line, data are presented, obtained through careful cost finding and cost behavior analyses, displaying charge per service; total revenue for the period (monthly, quarterly, or annually) for each product; variable cost in dollars per service, and percent and total variable cost per product; the contribution margin, reflecting the difference between per service and total revenues, and per service and total variable costs, respectively; the fixed costs; and the resulting contribution margin percentage for each product line and for the total scope of products offered. Should changes occur in the proportion of one or more product lines (in terms of volume), the total contribution margin may be affected.

For example, as shown in table 7-7, a change in the proportion or number of knee replacements provided relative to herniorrhaphies could have significant effects on the bottom line. Each knee replacement in

Table 7-7. Contribution Margin Analysis by Product Line

	Bypass		Herniorrhaphy		Knee Replacement		Total of All Three Services
	per Service	Total	per Service	Total	per Service	Total	
Revenue	$10,000	$500,000	$2,000	$100,000	$5,000	$150,000	$750,000
Variable cost	20% 2,000	100,000	25% 500	25,000	30% 1,500	45,000	170,000
Contribution margin	8,000	400,000	1,500	75,000	4,500	105,000	630,000
Fixed cost		350,000		70,000		100,000	450,000
Total contribution margin		80%		75%		90%	84%

this example contributes 90 percent of its revenue toward meeting fixed costs, *after which* 90 percent of knee replacement charges go directly to the bottom line. The remaining 10 percent will continue to pay variable costs; this is a very profitable situation. Herniorrhaphies, on the other hand, contribute only 75 percent of each revenue dollar toward meeting fixed costs, and *thereafter* only 75 percent of revenues to the bottom line. Again, the remaining 25 percent pays for variable costs. Were knee replacements to decline substantially relative to herniorrhaphies and bypass procedures—even if the total revenue were to remain the same—the result would be considerable, because profitability would be much harder to achieve.

This kind of comparative product analysis can help managers appreciate the relative contribution made by each product line to the total profitability of either a cost center or an entire institution.

However, this form of analysis can be misleading unless it takes into consideration the relationships that often exist between and among product lines in the production of revenues. To examine this, we advocate the use of "linked" product line studies, which can be especially important in eldercare services (see figure 7-4).

A specific example of such a linked contributor to other hospital services would be especially well-managed aeromedical transport services. The transport service (air-taxi service), when viewed separately, is a clear loser in that it does not contribute directly to the bottom line and may not even pay entirely for its own costs. It cannot win, unless it depends considerably on private pay, fee-for-service, actual-cost, transport fees. But if the transport service is responsible for bringing in patients who have insurance and who represent a profitable product line for the hospital, then the service has contributed substantially to the success of those product lines. Extensive well-developed and cultivated referral networks between a hospital and local as well as other providers (both institutions and individual physicians) would be key to a successful aeromedical transport service; and elderly patients would be central benefactors in such arrangements. Hospitals in other nearby areas that do not possess

Figure 7-4. Product Lines and Linked Contribution Margins

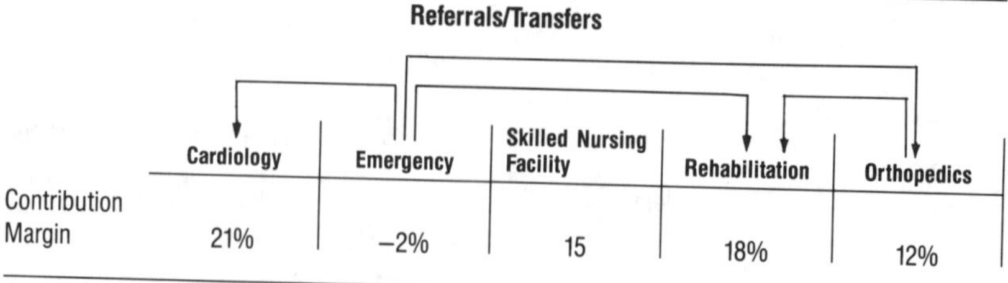

Referrals/Transfers

	Cardiology	Emergency	Skilled Nursing Facility	Rehabilitation	Orthopedics
Contribution Margin	21%	−2%	15	18%	12%

Note: Orthopedics can link to rehabilitation; emergency can link to cardiology or orthopedics to improve the contribution margin.

the level of medical services capable of supporting full cardiovascular services should be prime targets for collaborative agreements. Similarly, physicians in nearby as well as distant areas, especially primary care practitioners, should be the targets of aggressive negotiation and contracting.

Linked product line analysis also should help to determine the relationships that do or could exist between various services such as the emergency room and orthopedics; or between swing beds or freestanding SNF and rehabilitation services. More interesting would be the linkages between other seemingly unrelated services that exist within the continuum. The contribution of many services generally is not recognized, because they are not analyzed as feeders into more profitable services. Linked product line analysis, or at least understanding of such linkages, allows managers to view the continuum of care as a set of manageable, interrelated revenue producers.

Present Value/Opportunity Analysis

The second technique used to assess new or expanded products is basic present value/opportunity analysis, whereby hospitals must examine the costs and benefits that might accrue as a consequence of developing a new or expanded product for the elderly. This requires the same kind of cost and financial data produced in product line studies, but it may often be based on prospective data rather than an actual or historical data.

To accomplish this prospective product line analysis, detailed information must be obtained about all prospective costs, revenues, and projected savings associated with each project, product, or program. The purpose of this analysis is to generate empirical information about the financial performance of existing or proposed relative products.

Detailed analyses of costs, presumed benefits, resources needed, capital as well as working capital issues, and specific, expected measures of success must be articulated in advance. In addition, the sources of funding for each such project—"Who will pay?"—must be identified though the potential contribution of a "loss leader" to the bottom line should not be forgotten.

In addition to carefully estimating and analyzing costs and benefits, managers should be encouraged to consider variations of each idea. Given resource limitations, what other uses of existing resources could be considered that would yield equal or better financial results? Once options have been reviewed, cash inflow and outflow associated with each project should be analyzed for an extended period of time, usually for the "life" of the major capital assets involved in the project.

All prospective setup costs, repair and maintenance costs, cost savings, and other cash flow-related factors should be subjected to a basic present value analysis. The net present value of each option provides objective, purely financial information about its long-term contribution and its permutations to the financial success of the institution. The following are factors in the present value analysis model:

- Initial project and project component costs
- Life of proposed project or asset
- Year(s) of cash flow associated with aspects of project
- Actual annual cash flow (inflow and outflow)
- Salvage value of proposed project and those to be replaced
- Rate of return to serve as present value analysis base

This model is played out in the following case example of Northside Community Hospital:

> One of Northside's departments proposed to purchase a piece of lab equipment that will cost $494,100. After five years, the equipment will have no salvage value. During its five years of expected productive life, it will reduce labor costs by $180,000 each year. Northside's investment policy has been that it will generally require a 20 percent return on projects. Should the new piece of equipment be purchased?
>
> The first step in calculating the present value of the decision is to identify each category of cash inflow and cash outflow that would be associated with the project. In this example, assume that only one of each occurs: a cash inflow or annual cost savings of $180,000 each year for labor cost reductions (savings are considered cash inflows in present value analysis); and a cash outflow of $494,100, which will occur at the time of purchase.
>
> To determine whether the proposed project meets Northside's investment criteria, measure the present value of the *stream* of cash inflows and outflows for the period of the project (five years):

Initial cost	$494,100
Life of project	5 years
Annual cost savings	$180,000
Salvage value	$0
Desired rate of return	20%

These data can be inserted into the format displayed in table 7-8.

To conduct the analysis consult present value tables, available in most accounting and finance textbooks. These tables represent calculations of the *current* value of a dollar that is received at some *future* point in time, given a stated rate of return. Two tables are used traditionally, one for single-event cash flows (such as single payments or cash receipts expected at some future date) and the other for multiple cash flow events associated with annuities. Both tables are used to analyze cash inflows

Table 7-8. Present Value Analysis for Purchasing Laboratory Equipment, Northside Community Hospital

	Year(s) of Cash Flow	Annual Cash Flow	20% Factor	Present Value of Cash Flow
Annual savings	1–5	$180,000	2.991	538,400
Initial investment now		(494,100)	1.000	(494,100)
Net present value				443,000

and outflows associated with most complex projects. The *factor,* the multiplier against cash flows, based on an analysis of the institution's general investment policies or the return on the institution's current financial portfolio. In lieu of this, current market rates for stable investments (such as treasury bills or CDs) could be used. These rates serve as the basis against which the proposed project and its estimated cash inflows and outflows are measured. Anything less than the optimum level of return would be an opportunity cost. Anything beyond this level would be desirable in terms of the proposed project's ability to compete favorably with other alternatives.

In any present value analysis, a net present value of zero would indicate that the proposed project meets the investment criteria exactly, a positive net present value would suggest that the project exceeds the investment criteria; and a negative number would indicate that the project performs at a level below that prescribed in the investment criteria. As the table in the example indicates, the investment would probably be a good one.

The example shown here is expandable to complex, multiple-facet projects and to comparisons across proposed projects. Critical to the effectiveness of such analyses are valid cost data and valid information about true contribution margins, including "linked" contribution margins.

Hospitals and Their Communities

A final issue relating to the financing of health services for the elderly is that of the hospital's role vis à vis the community. Hospitals are, and must remain, providers of care to and for their communities. Aspects of this mission may have become displaced during the 1970s and 1980s, as hospitals reacted to changes in the financing and reimbursement rules, to new technologies, and to perceived marketplace opportunities. As we approach the 21st century, hospitals should recognize that they must forge strong relationships with others in their communities—of consumers and payers—to bridge gaps and to create new awareness about the importance of hospitals to the health and welfare of people.

This mission is especially important in the care and financing of health services to older adults. As society ages and the needs of patients and care givers alike increase, hospitals have a special opportunity to position themselves as a central resource for care and services, not only to the ill but to the healthy elderly.

It is incumbent upon hospitals to find innovative and progressive ways to survive and thrive in the health care marketplace of the future—a marketplace that will be profoundly affected by the needs of a rapidly growing aging population. Toward this end, hospitals will want to determine which services they can/must provide or manage, and with which they should affiliate.

Currently there are several vital missing links in the health care system that stand in the way of developing and delivering high-quality and profitable health care services to the elderly. Among the most pressing of these is the lack of a reliable, well-trained, well-paid work force to care for the many noncritical care needs of older adults. Turnover in SNFs is very high, and many health care institutions have great difficulty recruiting and training less skilled support staff so critical to the management of aging patients.[54]

Another problem hospitals have to face is that the educational programs currently in place in most U.S. communities do not cultivate career interests in caring for the elderly. High schools, vocational schools, and junior colleges could develop training programs that are linked directly to the providers of long-term related eldercare services, and they could encourage the acquisition of basic skills and knowledge that would lead to a qualified work force. States with the highest proportions of elderly persons (such as Florida, Arizona, and California) will need to develop more active plans within their educational systems to fill this rapidly growing marketplace gap.

Innovative educational programs could certify people in basic areas of patient care and support in long-term care, individuals who might then have access to higher-level educational and training programs that are designed to enhance their skills by way of modular learning programs. Completion of each module would lead to some advanced certification, which would be recognized and valued by the health care industry. By piecing together a number of modules, these health care workers might earn special certifications, such as LPN status or associate of arts degrees. The use of computerized self-instructional learning programs, intensive seminars, and other innovative teaching methods could be employed in these efforts. But providers as well as communities must be committed to creating such a work force, one that is central to the successful future of extensive long-term care arrangements.

Future Directions in Eldercare

The health care system of the future will contain more explicit classes of service and care. Regardless of the direction taken by the federal government to create some form of "universal" health benefit, three facts must be faced. First, the United States cannot and will not pay for "gold-plated" comprehensive services to all people by way of publicly financed and managed health benefits program. Care protocols, forms of rationing, and other tough choices will be made by public and private sector payers—if not by some hospitals (especially publics and not-for-profits) shouldering high uncompensated care loads.

Second, a sizable proportion of health services for the elderly will consist of disability management and rehabilitation programs. Among other things, disability management recognizes the important difference between efforts to cure and services that promote care and ensure independence. Disability management coupled with utilization management will drive a substantial portion of the future market in eldercare health services.

Third, the aging population comprises a sizable and growing number of upper-middle-class people, many of whom will choose not to partake of generic, prepackaged, limited health insurance benefits. Instead this population will demand and find a range of services that may not be paid for by insurance and that offer them both freedom of choice and virtually "customized" products and services—for which they generally will be prepared to pay. Others will purchase private, supplemental insurance and insurancelike products (for example, annuities) that will afford them greater latitude in provider selection, product scope, and amenities of comfort and special services. Congress may also reverse itself on tax-exempt IRAs, allowing "categorical" health IRAs, to stimulate savings and to provide a buffer against future government costs.

There will, however, be a vast population divided into holders of basic benefits—perhaps privately enhanced—and those less fortunate who will rely exclusively on prevailing social welfare income and services. Older adults will constitute a sizable proportion of this financially limited group.

Short of a virtual social reordering and enforced redistribution of wealth and power, expect more disparities in health care needs in the future and more demand for expensive, "boutique," and other products by a well-heeled, aging population that grew up in the 1950s, 1960s, and 1970s—not in the Depression era.

Services to the disabled, sick, and dying elderly will continue to demand hospital attention. The healthy elderly, however, are potential customers.

Summary

The basic reimbursement funding programs for eldercare services are Medicare, Medicaid, and private supplemental insurance or "Medigap" policies. For each, hospitals must carefully manage resources and match care, whenever possible, to reimbursement policies. Other financing alternatives include long-term care insurance, Medicare HMOs and PPOs, life care or assisted living arrangements, and home equity conversions and reverse mortgages.

It is important to maximize resources and, hence, reimbursement by determining operating margins. Health care products and services for the elderly can be evaluated using product line analysis and present value/opportunity analysis. Finally, hospitals must consider their role with regard to the communities which they serve and work.

References

1. Zuckerman, S., Feder, J., and Hadley, J. Hospital responses to Medicare's Prospective Payment System. *Bulletin of the Academy of Medicine* 64(1):52–62, 1988.
2. Guterman, S., and others. The first 3 years of Medicare prospective payment: an overview. *Health Care Financing Review* 9(3):67–76, 1988.
3. Thompson, J. D. DRG prepayment: its purpose and performance. *Bulletin of the New York Academy of Medicine* 64(1):28–51, 1988.
4. Hadley, J., Zuckerman, S., and Feder, J. Profits and fiscal pressure in the prospective payment system: their impacts on hospitals. *Inquiry* 26:354–65, Fall 1989.
5. Aiken, L. H., and Flynt-Mullinix, L. The nurse shortage, myth or reality. *New England Journal of Medicine* 317(10):641–45, 1987.
6. Roberts, M., Minnick, A., Ginsberg, E., and Curran, C. What to do about the nursing shortage. *Hospital Topics* 67(4):8–20, 1989.
7. Serow, W. J., and others. Beyond shortage: nursing personnel in Florida. *Florida Health Care Cost Containment Board,* Feb. 1990.
8. Rogers, B., Sweeting, S., and Davis, B. Employment and salary characteristics of nurse practitioners. *Nurse Practitioners* 14(9):56–63, 1989.
9. Starr, P. *The Social Transformation of American Medicine.* Lexington, KY: Basic Books, 1982.
10. Shain, M., and Roemer, M. I. Hospital costs related to the supply of beds. *Modern Hospital* 92(6):73, 1959.
11. Guterman and others, pp. 52–62 and pp. 67–76.
12. Shortell, S. M., Morrison, E. M., and Friedman, B. *Strategic Choices for American Hospitals.* San Francisco: Jossey-Bass, 1990, p. 4.
13. Shortell, and others, p. 4; Wolfson, J., and Levin, P. J. *Managing Employee Health Benefits.* Homewood, IL: Dow Jones-Irwin, 1985.
14. Wolfson and Levin; Hadley, and others, pp. 354–65; Guterman and others; and Frech, H. E., and Ginsburg, P. B. Competition among health insurers,

revisited. In: W. Greenberg, editor. *Competition in the Health Care Sector: Ten Years Later.* Durham, NC: Duke University Press, 1988, pp. 57-79.

15. Koff, T. H. *New Approaches to Health Care for an Aging Population: Developing a Continuum of Chronic Care Services.* San Francisco: Jossey-Bass, 1988, p. 118.
16. Health Insurance Association of America. *Source Book of Health Insurance Data, 1984*–1985. HIAA: 1986, p. 34.
17. HIAA, pp. 34, 39.
18. HIAA, pp. 4, 34.
19. HIAA, p. 34.
20. Hadley and others, pp. 354–65; Guterman and others.
21. *Value Line,* Nov. 10, 1989, p. 1280.
22. *Value Line,* p. 1280.
23. 42 CFR, 412.113 (a)(1), 413.130.
24. 42 CFR, 413.50.
25. 42 CFR, 412.113(6), 413.85.
26. U.S. Department of Health and Human Services. *Prospective Payment Assessment Commission Report and Recommendations to the Secretary.* Washington, DC: HHS, Mar. 1, 1990, p. 71.
27. Shortell and others, pp. 4–5.
28. Shortell and others, pp. 4–5.
29. Hadley and others, pp. 334, 362.
30. Florida Hospital Association. *Florida Hospitals 1989* FHA, 1989.
31. Cromwell, J., and Pushkin, D. Hospital productivity and intensity trends: 1980–87. *Inquiry* 26:366–80, Fall 1989.
32. Cromwell and Pushkin, p. 373.
33. Shortell and others, p. 6.
34. The Hospital Research and Educational Trust of the AHA. *Economic Trends,* reproduced in: *Health Care Management Review,* Summer 1989, p. 50; Hadley and others, pp. 354–65.
35. Zuckerman and others, pp. 52–62.
36. Kaplan, S. Trends in health cost management. Seminar sponsored by the Gulf-Coast Health Care Coalition and the University of South Florida College of Public Health, Tampa, Feb. 1990.
37. Health Insurance Association of America, *Sourcebook on Health Insurance Data,* 1989.
38. Wennberg, J., and Gittelsohn, A. Small area variations in health care delivery. *Science* 182(117):1102–8, Dec. 14, 1973.
39. Friedman, E. Problems plaguing public hospitals: uninsured patient transfers, tight funds, mismanagement, and misperception. *Journal of the American Medical Association* 257(14):1850–57, Apr. 1987.

40. Howell, E. M., Baugh, D. K., and Pine, P. C. Patterns in Medicaid utilization and expenditures in selected states: 1980–1984. *Health Care Financing Review* 10(2):1, 1988.

41. HIAA, p. 33; Howell and others, pp. 1–15.

42. Employee Benefits Research Institute. *Facing the Costs of Long-Term Care.* EBRI, 1990, p. 27.

43. EBRI, p. 27.

44. Hadley and others, p. 362.

45. Ginsburg, J., Eisenberg, J. M., and others. Financing long-term care. *Annals of Internal Medicine* 108(2):279–88, 1988.

46. Meiners, M. R. The case for long-term care insurance. *Health Affairs* 2(2):55–79, Summer 1983.

47. EBRI, p. 92.

48. EBRI, pp. 92, 93.

49. EBRI, p. 92.

50. EBRI, p. 93.

51. Raper, A. T., and Kalicki, A. C., editors. *National Continuing Care Directory: Retirement Communities with Nursing Care.* 2nd ed. American Association of Homes for the Aged, 1988.

52. Skinner, J., Levin, P. J., Wolfson, J. *Financial Viability of Adult Congregate Living Facilities in Florida.* Florida Department of Health and Rehabilitative Services, Sept. 1989.

53. Wolfson, J., and Levin, P. Linking health care for the poor to health care for profit. *Health Affairs* 6(1):129–35, Spring 1987; and Brown, J. B. *Health Capital Financing.* Ann Arbor, MI: Health Administration Press, 1988.

54. Serow, W. J., Cowart, M. E., Chen, Y. *Results of Nursing Home Shortage Study: Hospitals, Nursing Homes, Home Health Agencies, and Hospices.* State of Florida, Feb. 1990.

Chapter 8

Hospitals, Corporations, and Eldercare

Nancy Alfred Persily and Sonya R. Albury

Recent demographic trends have generated a diverse team of players who are becoming involved in eldercare activities and initiatives. Health maintenance organizations, long-term care providers, and even nonhealth-related industries are taking on roles in the healthcare arena that traditionally were held by hospitals. Because of this, hospitals may be missing out on opportunities to develop new markets and linkages with corporations and others.

Rather than feeling threatened by the influx of corporate players into the health care field, hospitals must recognize that industry represents many market opportunities for providing services for the elderly, as well as a large potential patient population comprised of employees and their families. Corporations are attempting to respond to their employees' health care needs through a variety of initiatives.

Corporate interest in eldercare is the result of two major trends in the United States. These trends, which will be discussed in this chapter, are among care givers and government initiatives. Hospitals can provide leadership in making these efforts successful while also identifying potential partners in health care delivery and gaining access to new patient markets by developing links within health systems and with corporations, insurers, and HMOs. These links can help hospitals improve the continuum of care and maintain a competitive position. Hospitals can help ensure the availability of needed services, and they have the expertise to design high-quality care programs that foster continuity of care at all levels across the health care continuum for corporate employees and their families.

Forces Driving Corporate Interest in Eldercare

Corporate interest in eldercare is mainly a result of trends among care givers, specifically employees who must care for older relatives, and trends in government initiatives in eldercare.

Corporate Response to Trends among Care Givers

This book has gone into great detail describing the graying of America and the swelling ranks of older adults in the health care marketplace. Another major demographic shift within the industry is represented by the ballooning number of care givers as baby boomers reach middle age. Many middle-age workers have elderly parents who become unable to care for themselves, a fact that has helped interest U.S. corporate decision makers in eldercare services and care-giver needs. The baby-boom generation comprises a large share of the work force. The first boomers turned 40 in 1986, and an additional 4 million will cross that threshold every year through 2004.[1] By the year 2000, nearly 35 million people over age 65 will live in the United States; almost half of these will be over age 75.[2] Much of the care-giving responsibilities for this elderly population will fall on middle-age workers.

A 1988 study of care givers who provide assistance to their elderly relatives found that:

- 64 percent are women
- 57 percent are primary care givers
- 34 percent have lost time from work or have come in late as a result of care-giver duties
- 33 percent are unable to take vacations
- 22 percent provide 21 or more hours of care each week
- 14 percent of part-time workers gave up full-time work
- 12 percent have had to quit their jobs
- 9 percent have taken a leave of absence[3]

Compounding the impact of this trend is the mobility of the U.S. population. Although some workers reside in the same area as their elderly parents and provide assistance directly, others live in different locations, necessitating long-distance care arrangements. Regardless of geographic location, both types of arrangements can be taxing on family life.

Because working care givers may be less productive and under more stress than their non–care-giving peers, corporations are beginning to realize that tremendous amounts of time and money are lost as employees are forced to use company time to arrange for the care of their elderly relatives. In a study of its employees by the Travelers Corporation, 28 percent said they spent an average of 10.2 hours a week caring for elderly relatives or friends, and that 60 percent of employee care givers suffer from increased stress, which interferes with their social and emotional needs. General Telephone of California estimated that the cost of days lost from work for care givers in 1988 was at least $2 million a year.[4]

Care-giving duties also can limit career ambitions by reducing the ability of workers who relocate to seek better jobs or accept promotions.

This could affect many care givers who work in managerial positions, an issue attracting attention from concerned corporate executives who themselves have frail elderly relatives.

The impact of these care demands has been particularly acute for women. Whereas availability of child care has helped increase the number of women in the work force, the demands of eldercare threaten to take them out again. The major problem is that these women are already serving a dual role as career person/mother. Increasingly, many are becoming part of the "sandwich generation," those who provide care for their children *and* aging relatives. The average woman can expect to spend as many years caring for a dependent parent (or spouse) as she does in caring for a dependent child.

Care giving, however, is more an economic issue than a women's issue. The family or informal support system provides more than 80 percent of the health care to the elderly disabled.[5] Family members are the primary providers of thousands of dollars worth of health care services each year, and the emotional stress to these families is immeasurable. In addition, it is very difficult to locate qualified help even for publicly financed home health. Often, the wages are too low to attract trained personnel, and service dollars are limited, which results in lengthy waiting lists for care. Families frequently must provide most—if not all—the care required. Given the rise in two-income families, the impact on business is sure to mount.

Corporate Response to Trends in Government Initiatives

Another factor attracting corporate interest in eldercare issues is government's efforts to shift primary health benefits away from Medicare and other government programs toward corporate health care programs. Employers today provide health insurance coverage for more than 80 percent of the nonelderly population, representing 160 million Americans.[6] Those over 65 and retirees still rely heavily on Medicare as their primary health care benefit source.

Retirees often are covered by "Medigap" insurance provided by their former employers. However, those over 65 who are currently employed on a full- or part-time basis must receive the same insurance package offered to those under age 65.[7] These new federal efforts, coupled with the repeal of the Medicare Catastrophic Coverage Act (1989), have intense consequences for the corporate bottom line. More corporations are renegotiating their benefit care packages, seeking alternative methods of health care delivery and financing.

The Consolidated Budget Reconciliation Act of 1985 (COBRA) is another recent effort to regulate benefits through the use of legislation that will continue to affect employers' costs for years to come. Under COBRA, unemployed people may now continue insurance coverage through their former employer's health plans. Even though former employees pay for coverage they may end up being heavy users of benefits. Their utilization patterns will continue to impact the experience rating imposed by insurance companies on their former employers. Faced with soaring costs and the threat of mandatory employer-sponsored health care, employers are being forced to include additional cost-containment strategies in their plans.

Some employers now believe the key is healthier employees. They have come to understand that healthier employees function better and use the health care system less, resulting in lower costs. Investments in wellness will be offset by reductions in health care costs, absenteeism, and tardiness, followed by increased productivity.

Corporate Initiatives in Eldercare

For years retail and other business interests have viewed the elderly as a viable market for services and products. Extensive market research routinely conducted by large corporations has shown what much of the country is only now learning—that older consumers account for one-half of the country's discretionary income. Coupled with this finding is the observation that the 55 and over age group is expected to increase 41 percent by the year 2010, compared with 13 percent for the total population.[8] These demographic and economic trends point to a strong older consumer market that is expected to gain even greater strength in the years to come.

Sears Roebuck and Company, for instance, is tapping the elderly market through an unusual cooperative effort with a group of Chicago developers who build retirement communities. Sears offers residents of Active Life retirement communities a one-stop package of financial services, real estate advice, travel packages and an array of products designed for these communities. The company's merchandising arm is even involved in decorating some of the project's apartments.

The Hartford Insurance Group is identifying itself with elderly concerns with its Hartford House, a model home that exhibits home modifications that could keep the elderly living in their homes longer. The model, to be demonstrated at home shows, includes more than 100 design modifications such as extra lighting for decreased visual perception, contrasting colors for difficulty in distinguishing colors, translucent shades and matte finishes to reduce glare, carpeting and fabric treatments to reduce echo, smoke detectors, electric appliances to avoid unnoticed gas leaks, lower water temperatures, and other safety features.

Other corporations, however, are seeking more than a high profile within the older adult market. Faced with the prospects of economic pressures due to eldercare issues, many corporations have initiated efforts to curb absenteeism and improve worker productivity among those caring for aging relatives and friends. Morgan Guaranty Trust Co., American Express, and Phillip Morris Companies, Inc. have given nearly $250,000 to New York City's Department for the Aging to develop and run a pilot program that will operate a special telephone number for corporate employees to call with questions about the needs of their elderly relatives. In another instance, IBM has contracted with a private agency to set up an information and referral service to help their employees select eldercare services. The program was established under a contract with 175 community agencies located in areas served by IBM. Aetna Life and Casualty has developed a similar program that provides information on nursing homes, other housing arrangements, medical services, in-home services, community programs, and transportation. Remington has set aside $10,000 in matching funds to help employees pay for home nursing services.[9]

The Travelers Corporation, which may have been the first major employer to examine the issue of adult care through a wide-ranging survey, provides seminar series, support groups, a library, and a Caregivers Fair for its employees. The Travelers also initiated the Older Americans Program, which funded a $1 million grant to found the Travelers Center on Aging at the University of Connecticut Health Center and established a retiree job bank through which retirees are hired for part-time and temporary work.

Many companies are setting up dependent care allowance plans whereby employees can set aside pretax dollars for dependent care. These plans take advantage of a federal law that allows employees to direct up to $5,000 of their salaries, tax free, toward the care of a dependent. The law requires that the care giver provide at least 50 percent of the older adult's support and that the older adult spend at least eight hours a day in the care giver's home.[10]

Links between Hospitals and Others in Health Care

In order to expand their market base and develop a continuum of care for the elderly, hospitals should develop links with others in their service area. These links can form the basis for referrals and networking relationships and provide hospitals with critical ties to other organizations that affect health care in the community. Service opportunities between hospitals and corporations in eldercare, as well as links with insurers, create opportunities to improve services to the elderly. Links with HMOs can help maintain markets, and links within a health system can strengthen resources for hospitals with this relationship.

Links between Hospitals and Corporations

With increased competition, changes in financing, and pressure from employers, hospitals are learning to streamline their operations, many times drawing on corporate experience. Hospitals and corporations have recognized that they can learn from each other. Both groups, for example, have joined health care coalitions, using increasing health care costs as a rallying point.

In the past (and to some extent today) hospitals and corporations mainly have ignored each other, and some have even been adversaries. The corporate sector has long held the perception that hospitals did not fall under the same financial scrutiny that most industries do and therefore did not consider them as having to operate as "real businesses."

In previous years hospitals tended to be insular, focusing on acute care without a strong marketing approach. They rarely worked with corporations in establishing new health care programs or managing patient care outcomes but rather communicated through third-party administrators or insurers.

Direct relationships between hospitals and corporations have been primarily for the provision of specific services: executive fitness programs, wellness programs, or substance abuse counseling. Most of the services that hospitals provided to corporations focused primarily on health needs of employees. Few looked at eldercare issues, such as the stress associated with care-giving demands, or targeted subgroups such as the families of corporate employees. Given the numbers noted earlier in this chapter on the impact of care giving on the workplace, there would seem to be service opportunities hospital administrators need to consider. There are many services that hospitals can provide to corporations and their employees and many ways that hospitals can develop relationships with corporations.

The hospital setting can serve as the central access point for an entire network of care to serve the corporate market, with a full range of services including those for the elderly and their care givers. The hospital has the expertise and resources to address needs from the top of the corporate ladder to the lower echelons. A full spectrum of care can be developed ranging from executive health screening to long-term care insurance for older persons. In this arrangement the hospital would become the preferred provider for health and social services. A centralized access system would provide integrated services that are coordinated with health insurers as well as community-based service organizations. Through an information and referral program and a comprehensive case-management system, service arrangements can be facilitated readily, whether it be for a work-hardening program for employees or adult day care for employees' elderly relatives.

By utilizing eldercare as a foundation for developing a strong corporate interface, the hospital will be positioned to establish a variety of opportunities and activities, thereby bonding the entire corporate community to the hospital and its network of care. For example, hospital-based adult day care can provide a place for elderly parents, older spouses, siblings, or significant others to be cared for during the day while the employee is at work. Adult day care services can contribute to easing of stress experienced by the care giver, as well as a reduction in lost time and productivity at the workplace. Such programs can also ensure a bonding between family and hospital; for, as mentioned before, a hospital that provides high-quality services to an elderly parent will likely be perceived as a good hospital for the entire family.

Through its volunteer department, a hospital can offer a telephone reassurance program for employees who have elderly relatives staying at home alone. Such a program could be jointly sponsored by the employer and the hospital. A telephone reassurance program relieves the care giver from being preoccupied during the workday and needing to make frequent telephone calls. Similarly, information and referral programs can reduce the time needed by care givers to evaluate and make service arrangements.

Case-management programs go one step further and translate into "one-stop shopping" where one call puts the care giver in touch with a case manager who contracts with the family to assume responsibility for all service arrangements. The case manager monitors the care provided to ensure that all services are delivered appropriately based on the changing needs of the individual client. Through a centralized case-management system, family care givers are relieved of making care arrangements for elderly relatives while on the job, thus alleviating some of the stress that prevents them from performing effectively at the workplace. This program can be jointly funded by the employer and the employee. Consultation by the case manager can be provided before and after work hours and during lunchtimes, if necessary. Additionally, programs can be available to company retirees and their spouses who are in need of this type of assistance.

Senior membership programs can be marketed to care givers and employees in the "senior" age group. They can provide financial/insurance counseling, express admitting and discharge, transportation services, or a personal customer service representative who can run interference on bureaucratic problems. Senior membership programs are discussed in chapter 4.

Not all services offered to employers need to be newly developed programs. Hospitals already offer a host of educational programs that easily can be taken to the work site. These might include classes on safety, stress, nutrition, cardiopulmonary resuscitation, or care giving.

In addition, a hospital generally has access to a wide range of health and support services information that could be retrieved by a variety of methods: computer, a telephone/audio cassette program, newsletters, and so on. Ryder System provides its employees with a computerized system by which the employee can choose a physician or hospital based on location, specialty, certification, fees, and a number of other criteria. A hospital could provide that type of information directly to corporations over the telephone or through on-line computer systems.

Links with Insurers

Insurers need case-management and assessment services to keep costs down, and they are increasingly contracting with private companies to provide those services. Hospitals have many advantages over other companies in providing case-management programs. They are the place where large numbers of elderly go for health care and where the necessary elements of staff and information are available in one place. Hospitals also have existing networking and referral relationships with nursing homes, legal services, home health agencies, and other groups that are essential parts of the case-management system and service network.

Long-term care insurance can be marketed to groups such as retiree associations, unions, senior membership programs, and retirement facilities as part of a membership package. In addition, long-term care insurance can be jointly marketed to corporations and their preretirees by a hospital and an insurance company, in an arrangement wherein the hospital becomes the preferred provider and the coordinator for assessment and case management. Other services can be included in such a program, including retirement housing, skilled nursing home care, home health and support services, adult day care, and health education, among many others. Developing groups large enough for preadmission assessments and case management keeps costs down for insurance companies and links hospitals with members for acute care and other services.

Links with Health Maintenance Organizations

Health maintenance organizations are another possibility for linkage and need not always be viewed as more competition. Health maintenance organizations in an area may need appropriate and cost-effective skilled nursing facilities (SNFs). Hospital facilities that offer short-term rehabilitative and convalescent care are particularly attractive. Hospital-based SNFs are convenient and often offer a higher level of care than other nursing homes. Linking up with HMOs can provide opportunities for offering all sorts of short-term inpatient and ambulatory rehabilitation services to HMO clients.

Links within Health Systems

Health systems present a myriad of opportunities for the development of joint initiatives between corporations and hospitals. These opportunities lie in the large network of facilities owned by these health care organizations. Affiliated hospitals located in various communities throughout the United States can serve as the hub for eldercare services, ranging from preventive educational programs to long-term care.

Health care systems could offer eldercare information and referral services and much more to the major businesses located in the communities they serve.

Religious-affiliated hospital systems, for-profit chains, teaching hospitals, and nonprofit/voluntary hospital systems and alliances would be prime candidates for this type of eldercare network. They may have a variety of acute and long-term care providers strategically located throughout the United States. These providers could develop a continuum of eldercare programs to be marketed directly to employers and their employees. The system would realize economies of scale by sharing program development and management resources across multiple sites. Replication could be achieved easily from one location to the next.

Hospital/health systems could go well beyond the information and referral level. Many have both hospitals and long-term care facilities along with other support services within a single community. Designated hospitals could serve as the fulcrum of eldercare services around which other services could revolve. A centralized case-management system would serve to coordinate a full range of care including information and referral, home health, acute care, and long-term care services. By building on the network concept, the system can enhance its visibility and influence the delivery of care within each of its service areas. The program can also lead to increased patient referrals and added revenues for the hospital system.

Hospital systems can offer services directly to corporations and their employees or develop joint venture arrangements with other providers. The provision of long-term care services can be delivered in coordination with a community-based agency. The hospital can offer a diverse spectrum of geriatric programs including day care for the frail elderly, an Alzheimer's Respite Care Program including day care and inpatient care, and specialized geropsychiatric and rehabilitative programs. In addition, the hospital can provide private case-management and home health services. By forming links with other providers such as nursing homes and senior centers, as well as offering services directly, the hospital is able to expand its referral base, extend its market penetration, and become the focal point for eldercare-related activities in the community.

An added spin-off for hospitals would be increased utilization by non–care-giving employees who seek care at the hospital because of its heightened visibility. Through these initiatives, the hospital will establish a strong presence as a caring institution for the entire family's medical needs. The attraction for corporations will be a coordinated system of care for their care-giving employees and their families, resulting in greater productivity and cost savings.

Summary

A variety of innovative cooperative relationships are possible between hospitals and corporations. As the demands mount for employee care givers, corporations will become increasingly sensitized to the need for specialized programs that address the stresses experienced by their employees. Hospitals and other health care systems should have a major role in this process by ensuring continuity of care by linking with corporations to meet health care needs of employers and elderly relations. By becoming the centralized coordinating entity for a wide spectrum of eldercare initiatives, the hospital can foster various spin-offs from such programming.

Major benefits to the hospital are bonding the corporations and families with the health care organization, increased market share, and increased private pay sources. Businesses can project curbed absenteeism, reduced stress, and higher staff retention, all of which translate into increased worker productivity and cost savings with higher profits for the corporation.

A combination of hospital initiatives to corporations, care givers, the elderly themselves, and the community will ensure that hospitals are prepared for the changes that the growth of the elderly population will bring.

References

1. Wessel, D. One sure fact: baby boomers are aging. *Wall Street Journal,* Jan. 3, 1989.
2. Special Committee on Aging. *Aging America: Trends and Projections.* Washington, DC: U.S. Government Printing Office, 1989, p. 4.
3. *National Survey of Caregivers Final Report.* Opinion Research Corporation for the American Association of Retired Persons and the Travelers Foundation, Nov. 1988, pp. 11–14, 43–51.
4. Persily, N. A. Opinion. *Florida Medical Business,* Jan. 31, 1989.
5. Brody, S. J. Geriatrics and rehabilitation: common ground and conflicts. Presented at the conference on *Rehabilitation and Geriatric Education: Perspectives and Potential,* Arlington, VA, Dec. 4–7, 1988.
6. Bubb, H. G. Startling resurgence in costs require new national policy. *Financier* 12(12), Dec. 1988, p. 29.
7. Meier, E. The future of early and late retirement. *Business and Health* 4(8):18, June 1987.
8. Special Committee on Aging, p. 4.
9. Lund, D. S. Caregiving plans seen as boon to worker productivity. *Health-Week* 2:12, Feb. 1, 1988.
10. Lee, E. D. Firms begin support for workers who look after elderly relatives. *Wall Street Journal,* July 6, 1987.

Part Two

Innovative Programs in Eldercare

Chapter 9

Geriatric Program Development at a Community Hospital

Robert R. Fanning, Jr., Linda J. Cragin, and Paul J. Lanzikos

Introduction

The North Shore region of Massachusetts, the primary service area for Beverly Hospital in Beverly, Massachusetts, is composed of 16 cities and towns, with about 250,000 residents. The 1980 census reported that 14 percent of these residents were over age 65. This compares to a state average of 13 percent and a national average of 11 percent. During 1990, the older adult population on the North Shore is expected to rise to 17 percent.

The North Shore, like the rest of the state, has a variety of services for the elderly, but there remain many significant gaps. The North Shore area is faced with a severe nursing home bed shortage. On any given day at Beverly Hospital, approximately 10 percent of the beds are occupied by patients waiting for placement in a nursing home, with projections that during the early 1990s this number will increase to 12.5 percent. This shortage has a significant effect on the hospital's lengths of stay for elderly patients. Similarly, appropriate housing for the elderly is also in short supply. Many elderly are forced to leave the area when they can no longer care for their often large, multifloor, single-family homes. Home support services in the area are also very fragmented by the numerous agencies that provide the services and are restricted by the type of funding received. Home care corporations, funded by the state through the Executive Office of Elder Affairs, provide home support services such as Meals on Wheels, homemakers, and help with chores, but are limited by client income eligibility rules and by a defined geographic service area. Not-for-profit visiting nurse associations and for-profit home health agencies receive Medicare and Medicaid reimbursement or private payment for those elderly who meet specific acuity levels and service requirements. Local boards of health and councils on aging also provide services but are limited to their township or city limits and provide services only to those over 60. This fragmentation makes access to service by the elderly and their families frustrating and confusing.

In FY 1986 approximately one-quarter of Beverly Hospital's admissions (26 percent) were paid for by Medicare, accounting for almost one-half of all patient days (45 percent). Medicare accounts for 46 percent of the hospital's inpatient revenues. Thus the population of Medicare recipients is a significant factor in the hospital's planning and program development.

The Planning Process

In May 1982, the hospital held a planning retreat for its senior management, board of trustees, and medical staff. The focus of the retreat was to outline steps the hospital would need to take to survive in the 1980s and 1990s. Several major directions and opportunities were identified. The first was the need for corporate restructuring and flexibility to diversify into other areas of the health care continuum. This diversification, both horizontal and vertical, would become increasingly important with the changes in reimbursement and other factors in the external environment. In Beverly's case horizontal integration was the further development, expansion, or acquisition of programs and services that were similar to those already offered by the acute-care community hospital. The corporate restructuring was organized under a parent holding company, Northeast Health Systems, Inc. Examples of horizontal integration included Beverly Hospital's affiliation with the Center for Addictive Behaviors, a company providing inpatient and outpatient treatment of substance abuse; or the joint venture with four other area institutions to develop a freestanding magnetic resonance imaging center. Vertical integration included further development, expansion, or acquisition of programs and services that varied in their acuity and which, particularly in reference to the elderly, allowed for the more complete management of care in a variety of settings, from the acute-care hospital to home services.

The other major outcome of the planning retreat was board and medical staff support for a new senior management position—the director of geriatrics and long-term care programs—with responsibility for developing programs for the elderly. This position was the first of its kind in any hospital in the state.

During the summer of 1982, the hospital conducted a geriatric services survey of the needs and perceptions of service availability of the elderly on the North Shore. Survey results, compared to actual service availability, clearly identified a major need for information, referral, and outreach services. Many existing information/referral programs were community programs and were town or city specific; providers often did not know about resources that were available and accessible in neighboring communities or from other agencies. This fragmentation also was felt by hospital staff in attempts to seek information or to refer patients.

Meanwhile the North Shore, with little prior HMO involvement, became an attractive and fertile area for both staff and physician independent practice models and, within 18 months in the early 1980s, six HMOs extended their service area and targeted the North Shore market. Since then more HMO and preferred provider organizations (PPOs) have moved to the area. Beverly Hospital became the exclusive or semiexclusive hospital for four of the HMOs, participates in a contractual relationship for some services with four more HMOs, and participates with eight PPOs. Currently, more than 32 percent of the hospital's admissions are from HMO and PPO sources.

Combining the HMO growth and their increasing enrollment of Medicare-eligible participants with the concurrent changes in overall Medicare reimbursement strategies, the hospital began to identify the areas of diversification that would become important for clinical and financial reasons. It also helped respond to the needs identified in the geriatric services survey.

Among the issues identified were a shortage of area nursing home beds, duplication and fragmentation within home care services, and a complete lack of affordable and appropriately designed housing for middle- and upper-income elderly. Areas spotlighted for diversification included nursing home development, home care services, and housing.

Goals

Following the internal and external assessment of the environment and trends, a board-level committee was formed to direct the hospital in its program development efforts. The Health Care Services for the Elderly Committee included members from the Beverly Hospital Planning Committee, medical staff, senior management, and directors of community elderly service providers. This committee was charged with continuing to assess the environment and to make recommendations to the Planning Committee regarding opportunities for program development.

Several goals were identified as desirable and necessary. The first and most important was to collaborate and support other agencies currently providing services to the elderly, without appearing as a competitive threat. It was very quickly understood that these agencies provided many high-quality services efficiently and effectively, yielded a great deal of influence within the community, and provided direction to the elderly seeking assistance and services.

Related to this first goal—but also an important second goal—was the expansion of the hospital's market share, both in market penetration and in geographic expansion. Goal attainment would rely on strong relationships and support/referrals from community agencies, as well as programs designed to reach and serve the elderly directly. Vertical diversification was most appropriate when considering service development for the over-65 population. Care from hospital to nursing home to home health care, with ongoing social, support, and outreach programs, would meet several goals and needs simultaneously. The HMO movement and other reimbursement changes made it important to have a system of care approach that would allow care to be provided in the most efficient, economical, and appropriate setting. The hospital also had the opportunity and resources to develop programs that reached across city and town lines, providing a networking opportunity from community to community.

Development Process

In the development of geriatric services at Beverly Hospital, the decision was made not to centralize the development and management of each service within one department but, wherever possible, to have departments within the hospital or the separate corporations assume the responsibility. The director of geriatrics and long-term care programs is responsible for coordination of all of the services.

The decision to decentralize geriatric programs operationally for development and management has resulted in a great deal of enthusiasm and creative effort throughout the hospital. Instead of a few select people being responsible, everyone throughout the hospital is encouraged to consider the needs of the elderly and how best to respond to those needs. This philosophy has resulted in the development of new programs by those most skilled to do so. An example is the Sunday Brunch Program, suggested by the manager of the hospital's food service department. Once a month, 30 to 40 older adults attend a brunch in the hospital cafeteria, listen to a lecture on a medical/health care topic, then go shopping at a local mall. This program, including the reservations, lecture, and transportation, is organized by the Beverly Council on Aging. The food service staff prepare breakfast and the $1.25 charge covers the cost of the meal.

Another example is the Liberty Stroll, a three-quarter-mile walk mapped out in a local shopping mall. The program, enthusiastically supported by the shopping center, was developed by the manager of the bioenergetics department, who has a very strong interest in fitness and the elderly. The program was developed concurrently with a psychiatry department–sponsored support group for adults with aging parents. Also at the same time, the respiratory department was assisting with the expansion of Harbor Home Care, the hospital's home health agency. If all these efforts had to be centralized and were the responsibility only of a geriatrics department, time constraints and other priorities would interfere and most of the programs would never get under way.

As a result of this hospitalwide effort, the geriatric services at Beverly Hospital do not have the negative image often found in other institutions. For example, the hospital's physical therapy staff, who provide contracted services to Ledgewood Nursing Care Center (the Beverly-owned nursing home), find the time spent providing care in that facility to be a rewarding change of pace.

Although Beverly Hospital is committed to serving the elderly population and is gaining community recognition in this area, services to other age groups also are vital, and new programs are always under exploration. Recently, the maternity service expanded its number of beds and the birth center, staffed by nurse-midwives, is one of two freestanding centers in the state. The hospital sponsors an occupational health program, a sports medicine clinic, a women's health service, and a dialysis program, and it runs a children's day care center on the hospital campus.

Innovative Services

When seeking information, obtaining services, and obtaining coordinated ongoing care, family members or the elderly themselves can experience frustration and confusion when they discuss their needs with providers. Beverly Hospital has several programs in place to address this confusion at these three stages.

Seeking Information

To simplify the search for information, several programs have been implemented. Often the hospital is the place where a family member goes to obtain information, especially if he or she does not live in the community and is not familiar with other local services. However, depending on the questions and their interpretation by the telephone operators, the family member may be referred to any of many departments. This was the case at Beverly Hospital: if a physician was needed, the call was connected to the medical staff secretary; if the name of a nursing home was requested, the call went to Social Services/Continuing Care; if the issue was Medicare coverage, the business office became involved. This was frustrating for staff, who were interrupted constantly, and for the family members, who were getting incomplete answers.

The development of Timely Information on Programs and Services for Seniors–TIPS®–was in response to this need. Staffed by trained older adult volunteers, TIPS offers several programs. The TIPS Line is a telephone information and referral service that directly addresses a scenario like the one depicted above. Telephone volunteers have a resource file that provides information not only about the hospital's services but also the myriad of services available in the community. Periodically this information is summarized and written on the TIPS Sheets according to topic and is then mailed out following an incoming request on the TIPS Line or in conjunction with *Living Right Along (LRA®)*, a newsletter that is distributed to over 25,000 area elderly each month. Each issue of *LRA* contains two articles dealing with concerns of older adults and a question and answer section that prints a frequent request from the TIPS Line. The editor of *LRA*, an older adult volunteer, requests articles from the hospital staff, medical staff, or professionals in the community, and each article is then reviewed by the hospital's medical education director. Every other month *LRA*, with a TIPS Sheet attached, is distributed by the local councils on aging; is available in physicians' offices, banks, libraries, churches, and pharmacies; and is directly mailed to many homes. A recent addition to the TIPS service line is a Medicare/Insurance Counseling Group. This program, also staffed by trained older adult volunteers, is available in the hospital lobby to anyone with questions about Medicare coverage, a bill, or HMO services. During its first four months the program successfully handled over 100 inquiries, was instrumental in recovering refunds totaling almost $2,000 from Medicare, straightened out questions about bills from other hospitals in the area, and provided guidance on supplemental insurance policies or HMO benefits. In 1990 the 1000th elder was served, and the service is now offered in two other locations, a physician office building and an elderly housing complex.

Obtaining Services

Obtaining services and, more important, obtaining the most appropriate service are other steps fraught with confusion and frustration. Often a family member has determined that nursing home placement is the only alternative for a loved one.

The Stay at Home Program, offered by Bay Area Visiting Nurse Association ([Bay Area VNA] a corporate affiliate of Beverly Hospital), offers an 11-step assessment of an older adult's capacity to live independently. Assessment categories include the following:

- Evaluations of physical and emotional health
- Ability to function in the home (with suggestions for modifications in the home to facilitate independence and improve safety)

- A financial/insurance review
- A resource evaluation that includes available assistance from family and other providers

A plan is developed that is discussed with the elderly client and family and referred to the client's physician for approval and implementation.

The Stay at Home Program works in conjunction with the hospital's department of Social Service and Continuing Care (SS/CC). This department, staffed by nurses and social workers, assists with nursing home placement, including establishing levels of care, and has access to all community services, including home health care, home care, Meals on Wheels, respite, Lifeline (a personal emergency response system), transportation, and many other support programs. The staff develop a plan of care to coordinate all the necessary services. Then this plan is discussed with the patient and family and approved by the patient's physician. Once the required paperwork is accomplished, the referral is made. The SS/CC staff expend a great deal of effort to make the most appropriate placement or referral, matching client needs and financial resources with available community services. The discharge planning process has become increasingly difficult as hospital lengths of stay decrease, benefits and coverage restrictions increase, and the labor pool diminishes for semiskilled/paraprofessional services. The SS/CC staff participate in many community activities, provide several ongoing support groups, and offer community educational sessions to inform themselves of needs within the community as well as inform the community of the services they provide.

Obtaining Coordinated Ongoing Care

Once service needs are identified and services provided and coordinated to ensure maximum benefit, the elderly and their families must be assured of obtaining coordinated ongoing care. The development and continued strengthening of a vertically integrated health care system at Beverly will address this need.

Corporately related to Beverly Hospital and constructed on its campus is the Ledgewood Nursing Care Center, a 122-bed skilled nursing facility that opened in December 1985. The administrator at Ledgewood reports to the director of geriatrics. The Bay Area Visiting Nurse Association is an 85-year-old certified home health agency that joined the corporate structure of Northeast Health Systems, Inc., in November 1985. The executive director of Bay Area VNA also reports to the director of geriatrics. A year later, in December 1986, Harbor Home Care Supply Company was formed. This durable medical equipment (DME) company is a partnership between Northeast Health Systems (representing Beverly Hospital and Bay Area VNA), two other North Shore VNAs, another local hospital, and a local DME provider that serves as the operating partners.

In 1989, the Hospice of the North Shore Collaborative, Inc., was developed to provide Medicare-certified hospice services to terminally ill patients on the North Shore. This venture, like Harbor Home Care Supply Company, was the joint effort of several health care providers in the area. Such joint efforts provide programs such as a hospice or a DME provider with the expertise to develop a high-quality program, as well as a significant, immediate market.

The latest enterprise, The Spectrum Center, is an adult day care program managed by Bay Area VNA and offered on the site of an elderly congregate housing program, Cable Gardens. The Spectrum Center works collaboratively with the Garden Preschool, a day care program for toddlers and preschoolers run by Beverly Hospital. This is the first intergenerational day care program on the North Shore.

The corporations, although legally and financially separate, have a close working relationship with Beverly Hospital and with each other. The home health agency employs a liaison nurse who works in SS/CC and fully participates in the development of care plans; the home health agency and hospice also share staff and provide coordination from acute care to terminal care. Meetings are held monthly with key staff from each corporation to discuss operational issues and how to improve the coordination and linkage between separate services. These meetings focus on administrative concerns—reimbursement and joint recruitment and training for staff, for example—but also on particular patient concerns. Ongoing planning to ensure a smooth discharge from one setting to another, to maximize insurance benefits, and to reduce patient and family anxiety is each staff person's objective.

Beverly Hospital patients are also cared for by many community agencies, and it has become increasingly important for hospital staff to know these agencies and the issues they are grappling with. Similarly, it is important for the staff of the community agencies to understand the issues facing the hospital. Senior Network (SEN-NET) evolved to address this concern. Every other month, representatives from over 60 community agencies serving the elderly of the North Shore meet at the hospital for brunch to hear a lecture on a timely topic, announce their new programs, raise their concerns, and discuss areas of cooperation. This program provides an ongoing forum for staff to keep current on the many issues within the eldercare network in housing, health and medical care, social programs, insurance, and so on, and also to ask how referred patients are progressing or find out whether a program has the capacity for a new referral.

It is at this point of coordinating services that the TIPS program again becomes involved. A TIPS team member sends a postcard to former patients inviting them to call the TIPS Line if they have any questions.

The TIPS volunteers also make reassurance calls to each elderly person who has been discharged with a care plan set up through SS/CC. The purpose of the call is to determine whether services have been received as ordered in a timely manner and if the patient is pleased. Any problems are referred back to SS/CC. A unique aspect of these reassurance calls are the calls made to family members of an elderly person placed in a nursing home. The family is asked about various aspects of the relative's placement: comfort, atmosphere, quality of care, food service. This feedback from families has helped to ensure smooth transitions to the most appropriate facility.

Financing

Financing is an important consideration in the development of any new service. Beverly's geriatric program development efforts have approached this issue in several ways.

The TIPS program is a low-cost, high-return program. By using the resources and skills of older adult volunteers, components of the TIPS services have developed at little expense. The TIPS team occupies an office equipped with basics and receives administrative support from the hospital. An office has provided the TIPS team with an identity and a sense of permanency.

An example of TIPS's cost efficiency is the budget for *LRA®*. The only expenses incurred by the newsletter are the printing costs; the authors, the editor, and the advisory board are volunteers. Distribution is accomplished through hospital staff on their way home or by volunteers to the sites in each local community where *LRA®* is available. In almost every North Shore community, the council on aging staples it to their monthly newsletter. This ensures that *LRA®* is mailed to the home of every person over the age of 60, at no additional cost to the council, and at no cost to the hospital.

The few expenses that are incurred by the TIPS program are funded by revenues from the Lifeline Program, a personal emergency response system. The program employs a part-time coordinator and uses 10 older adult volunteers for office work and installation of the Lifeline equipment. The program, which initially received contributions from the hospital's women's auxiliary and local companies and churches to buy the hardware, now bills the users, Medicaid, and other insurers monthly. Program revenues cover the salary expenses of the TIPS and Lifeline coordinators and office expenses and completely fund the purchase of new Lifeline equipment.

The Lifeline response center is located in a freestanding emergency center operated by the hospital. The Beverly Hospital Lifeline program is a national demonstration site for the use of an IBM computer system to improve the response time and compile data. The program currently has over 350 active participants and is one of the largest in New England.

Ledgewood Nursing Care Center is a joint venture with the Hillhaven Corporation. Northeast Health Systems and Hillhaven contributed equally to the capitalization of the facility, located on hospital property and leased from the hospital by Ledgewood. This arrangement greatly reduced the land acquisition costs and also provided a revenue stream to the hospital for land that had been vacant. Ledgewood is licensed for both Medicare and Medicaid reimbursement, has several HMO contracts, and plans are under way for a 41-bed addition.

The Bay Area VNA provides yet another example of financing strategy. The Bay Area VNA is a United Way–funded agency and receives private, third-party, Medicare, and Medicaid reimbursement. It has sought and received grant support for some of its services. Changes in reimbursement have affected the cash flow within the agency, and the hospital has provided financial and managerial expertise and secured a line of credit to assist the agency through some difficult times.

Perhaps the most creative financing is the package used to develop Cable Gardens. In 1979, the Cable Hospital in nearby Ipswich, Massachusetts, closed, and the land and building were given to Beverly Hospital. In 1987, $2.24 million of federal housing development action grant funding was received by Beverly Hospital and its joint venture partner, Harbor Development Company, to renovate the facility into 70 units of elderly congregate housing. This funding was combined with a mortgage from Massachusetts Housing and Finance Agency, a rental subsidy from the Executive Office of Communities and Development, and historical preservation tax credits for the hospital (built in 1916) and tax credits for low-income housing. The result was an $8-million housing project that serves as a model for mixed-income rental housing, with a range of support service for the frail elderly. Included in the monthly rental fee is a monthly on-site wellness clinic. A service manager provides residents with assistance in obtaining services, a nurse is on call for residents, and a van provides local transportation. Additional services include a noontime meal, adult day care, and the full range of home support services through Bay Area VNA. Within three months of opening, 60 of the 70 units were rented.

This mixture of financing methods has allowed the hospital to develop new programs and services without draining reserves, totally relying on grant funding, or being restricted by reimbursement limitations. Program administrators have been as creative in developing the financial support needed for their programs as they have in developing the service.

Planned Services

The list of program development opportunities is endless. Major program development efforts for the future include the expansion and strengthening of all current programs. Ongoing evaluation efforts and measurement systems provide feedback and indicate new directions to explore. Additional appropriate housing for older adults is a significant need, and several plans are under way to fulfill it.

Laurel Ridge, a continuing care retirement community, currently is in the design stage. This 190-unit complex will be located on 40 acres of ocean-view property in Beverly, about four miles from the hospital. The property was previously owned by a college and is adjacent to its campus. The college is actively developing programs and services for future Laurel Ridge residents.

The complex will include one- and two-bedroom apartments and suites with one or two bathrooms, full kitchens, and living and dining rooms. In the core of the complex will be common spaces for meals, recreation, health services, mail, library, and other services.

Unlike many continuing care communities, Laurel Ridge will not have an on-site nursing home facility. Laurel Ridge will be a joint venture by Beverly Hospital and Hillhaven, and residents will have access to the beds operated by Hillhaven, including Ledgewood. Nursing services will be provided at Laurel Ridge by the Bay Area VNA, and several units will be in an assisted living area, where nursing assistance is available.

Residents will pay an up-front, reimbursable fee and a monthly fee related to the menu of services they choose. A long-term care insurance program, custom-designed for residents, will be offered to cover a full range of long-term care services.

The initial response to Laurel Ridge has been positive and has illustrated the great demand for housing on the North Shore. Another program under exploration is an assisted living facility to be located on the land adjacent to the hospital and nursing home. Although only in the early planning stages, the proposed facility already is being evaluated by staff from Beverly Hospital, Ledgewood Nursing Care Center, and Bay Area VNA. Currently under construction on land also within the hospital campus is the senior center for the Beverly Council on Aging. This center will provide the social and recreational programs needed to balance the range of health and medical services and to offer a complete continuum of on-campus services.

Conclusions

The approach to geriatric planning and program development at Beverly Hospital is predicated on the assumption that increasingly greater proportions of acute-care hospital resources will be necessary to meet the chronic medical needs of an ever-aging population. Increasing financial and societal incentives also will promote as much high-quality care as possible in the least restrictive and least costly setting. To meet these demands, the community hospital must expand its traditional outlook and mission. Beverly Hospital anticipates the formation of a managed, capitated health care system for large portions of the elderly population. With the development of a multicomponent geriatric service and a strong network of support from community agencies, Beverly Hospital is preparing for this future.

Chapter 10

Geriatric Program Planning at a Public Hospital

Kathleen J. Farkas and J. Dermot Frengley, M.D.

Introduction

How could a public teaching hospital respond to the health care needs of the elderly without adding staff or obtaining additional resources? Cleveland Metropolitan General/Highland View Hospital of the Cuyahoga County Hospital System faced that question in 1981 and developed a program to meet the medical and social needs of the frail elderly by reorganizing and refocusing the hospital system's resources.

The Cuyahoga County Hospital System, now known as the Metro Health Medical System, is a public hospital system that provides multiple levels of health care across Greater Cleveland. The system is centered on Cleveland Metropolitan General/Highland View Hospital (CMG/HVH), a modern combined facility with 550 acute hospital beds and 180 rehabilitation hospital beds, as well as comprehensive outpatient services. This combined hospital provides tertiary services as well as primary care. The primary care services are largely provided within the 98 outpatient clinics. Regional specialized services such as a trauma center, a burn unit, intensive rehabilitation, and a perinatal unit are part of this hospital's clinical services.

Cleveland Metropolitan General/Highland View Hospital is one of the two principal teaching hospitals of the Case Western Reserve University Schools of Medicine and Dentistry, also located in Cleveland. All of the hospital system's physicians are faculty members of Case Western's School of Medicine. Physician training at graduate and undergraduate levels is conducted largely by a full-time faculty of approximately 275 instructors. In addition, there are about 200 house staff in the hospital's residency and fellowship training programs. These programs encompass internal medicine and all its major subspecialties, including geriatric medicine; surgery and its subspecialties; obstetrics and gynecology; pediatrics; orthopedics; psychiatry; anesthesiology; family medicine; dentistry; dermatology; neurology; and physiatry.

Other institutions in the Cuyahoga County Hospital System include a 350-bed skilled nursing facility, a satellite comprehensive primary care clinic, and an in-home support service for the chronically ill. The system is county owned and operated. Ten appointed trustees govern the system through a mandate from the three elected county commissioners.

Cleveland Metropolitan General/Highland View Hospital is located three miles south of downtown Cleveland on the city's near west side. Traditionally, the near west side was the home of Eastern European families who had come to Cleveland to work in the steel and manufacturing industries. As the city grew and jobs moved to the suburbs, younger members of these families moved, the older people tended to stay, and other ethnic groups, such as blacks and Hispanics, moved in. The neighborhood, although now of mixed ethnic groups, has as the majority of its elderly population European descendents.

The 1988 planning figures for the four neighborhoods that surround the hospital (Clark/Fulton, Tremont, Old Brooklyn, and Archwood/Denison) showed 16 percent of their residents as age 65 or older. Seven and one-half percent of the population were older than age 74. Over half of these elderly residents (60 percent) were female and 7 percent lived alone. The area is economically poor, with 12 percent of elderly householders below the poverty level. The housing stock is largely of modest single or double frame houses, most two-storied and built 65–85 years ago.

The hospital is the largest single employer in the neighborhood and is seen by community residents as the major provider of health care and health-related services for all age groups.

Planning/Development Process

The first step in planning geriatric services was taken in 1980 when 10 rehabilitation beds were set aside as the beginning of the medical unit for the elderly. These 10 beds were reserved for exclusive use of patients age 70 and older. The idea was to group people by age to observe more readily the medical, nursing, and social problems associated with old age. The hospital administration appointed an existing full-time staff member as the director of geriatric medicine.

The medical unit for the elderly was supported by an interdisciplinary team made up of CMG/HVH employees who were interested in working with the elderly and in creating an innovative service. Over the next several years this unit expanded to incorporate an entire floor of 28 rehabilitation beds. Staffing on this floor did not change after it was converted to an all-elderly unit. As a consequence of developing the medical unit for the elderly within the rehabilitation area of the hospital, the unit became Medicare DRG-exempt but had to meet Medicare regulations for rehabilitation hospital beds.

The medical unit for the elderly provided a rehabilitation setting for geriatric services, but the acute-care floors of the hospital had few formal resources in geriatric services. In 1981, an acute-care consulting service was begun with the idea of offering physicians expert help with problems they experienced in caring for elderly patients. The service was expanded quickly to include consultation to nursing as well.

The emergence of the medical unit for the elderly and the acute-care consulting service further emphasized the hospital's recognition of the elderly as a growing target population and deserving of special services.

In 1981, the board of trustees appointed an interdisciplinary geriatric task force representing the hospital's professional staff. The group was charged with strategic planning for comprehensive long-term care services involving all the hospital system's components. The task force issued a report in February 1982 outlining three broad recommendations:

1. The development of a major geriatric center at CMG/HVH for service, education, and research
2. An in-depth study of program capabilities of the system's skilled nursing facility
3. The development of a curriculum in geriatric nursing at the system's Diploma School of Nursing

It was a serendipitous event that in 1982 the Robert Wood Johnson Foundation (RWJF) should issue a request for application for the *Hospital Initiatives in Long-Term Care* program. The hospital system was already moving toward a coordinated model of care for frail elderly people and found that the RWJF guidelines were consistent with the system's current ideas and innovations in geriatric services. The system's proposal to the RWJF initiative was facilitated by the blueprint developed by the geriatric task force.

Through the geriatric task force report and the designation of geriatric medicine as a center of excellence, the Cuyahoga County Hospital System had set the field of geriatrics as a priority, at least conceptually. The actual programmatic effort, however, was initially not given additional funds to add staff, to secure resources, or to expand services. The foundation grant allowed the system to accelerate its plans and also to gain some recognition for the work already in progress.

The geriatric program's outpatient and community thrust that followed was designed to maximize the health and social service resources to area residents. The target population initially selected were people age 70 years and older who lived within a two-mile area of the hospital and who had no regular source of medical care. By selecting this group, program adherents hoped to serve local elderly who had chronic health problems and were in need of comprehensive primary care services.

The system already offered many specialty clinics and a large general medical clinic. However, only an older adult adept at navigating a complex bureaucracy could fare well in arranging multiple clinic appointments. There was no one place that afforded all the necessary services for a *comprehensive* primary eldercare package. Consequently, the geriatric ambulatory clinic was begun late in 1983. Similar to the inpatient unit, clinic team members were recruited from existing staff interested in eldercare. Thus an outpatient assessment clinic began to evolve without the addition of new staff.

By the time the RWJF grant was awarded in 1984, the hospital system had three distinct services for the elderly:

1. A medical rehabilitation unit
2. An acute-care consulting team
3. A fledgling outpatient primary care clinic

However, the problem was that there was no clear way for elderly people to gain access to these services or for various staff members to interrelate for coordinating care.

Goals

With the help of the RWJF *Hospital Initiatives in Long-Term Care* program (RWJF Initiatives Program), the hospital began the Geriatric Program. Using three organizing principles, staff devised a network of five interlocking interdisciplinary teams to improve and expand services to the elderly. The three organizing principles were:

1. Any new effort should begin with a review of existing services, resources, and current service users.
2. Reorganization of existing resources should result in less fragmented and more efficient services.
3. Each new service component should be securely established prior to development of the next one.

During the initial year of participation in the RWJF Initiatives Program, the hospital system set forth five principal objectives, drawn from the task force's recommendation for development of service, education, and research programs for eldercare.

1. To develop, refine, and integrate geriatric services into the hospital system's acute care and rehabilitation hospital

2. To provide within the hospital system a replicable model of coordinated, multilevel long-term care services that are responsive to the elderly's medical and social needs
3. To extend the hospital system's medical and social resources for the elderly into the local community
4. To educate medical, nursing, social work, and other health professionals to provide high-quality medical and social services to the elderly
5. To study the impact of the program on the health and well-being of community elderly and on the administrative staff and financial structure of the hospital

The CMG/HVH Geriatric Program, designed to meet these goals through the five-team network and the central coordination office, provided a focal point for systemwide service and teaching efforts in geriatrics.

The Geriatric Program at CMG/HVH

The four components of the Geriatric Program at CMG/HVH are interlocking interdisciplinary teams, a central coordination office, outpatient services, and inpatient services.

Interlocking Interdisciplinary Teams

Five teams of various combinations of physicians, nurses, social workers, rehabilitation therapists, and nutritionists made up the nucleus of the Geriatric Program. The teams are "interlocked" in that members belong to several teams. Continuity among teams has been furthered through the efforts of the intake process, which also has a coordinating function for referrals and planning.

Each level of care component has been envisaged as a model program for teaching as well as for services. Each program team has participated in residency training for physicians and, as practical, for students in nursing, social work, rehabilitation therapy, nutrition, and pharmacy.

Each team is specially tailored for the level of care in which it operates and provides direct patient care. The teams are intentionally interdisciplinary and focus on the needs of the patient with the intent of bringing resources to the patient in order to meet needs. For example, the core team for the outpatient clinic consists of physicians, nurses, and social workers. However, the team also includes a nutritionist, a pharmacist, a podiatrist, a dermatologist, a dentist, and a physical therapist who are on call during clinic hours. If an elderly person in the clinic needs the services of one of these professionals and pages the provider, the service provider responds to the page and comes to the clinic–this in lieu of having the patient schedule an additional appointment in another part of the hospital.

Collectively the team members contribute the skills and knowledge of their respective disciplines in order to better define the needs of the patients and marshal the resources needed both within the hospital and in the community.

Central Coordination Office

The central coordination office is staffed by the program's administrative coordinator, the intake social worker, and a secretary. The community outreach team is also located in the central office. The functions of the central coordination office are to provide a continuing link between and among teams, to complete intake procedures, to assign patients to the community team, and to schedule clinic appointments. The research and evaluation tasks of the program have remained in the purview of the director of geriatric medicine and the administrative coordinator. Figure 10-1 shows how the central coordination office links patients within the Geriatric Program.

Admission to the Geriatric Program can originate at any of the levels of care. Generally people from the community are referred to the program's outpatient clinic or to the community outreach team. Admissions to the Geriatric Program can also originate when someone is admitted to the medical unit for the elderly. All admissions to the program are completed through the central coordination office staff.

Once accepted into the Geriatric Program, a person is sent a welcoming letter and a service information card, which explains the type of service to be expected. Service packages are tailored to the needs of the individual. Typically, program clients receive primary care in the geriatric outpatient clinic and a home assessment and/or monitoring visit(s) from the community outreach team.

Service management has been a team process performed by people involved with the client. The community team, for example, meets to share their assessment perceptions and write a service plan. The intake social worker sees that plans are up to date, carefully constructed, and clinically sound. Because the intake social worker has sat on both the community and clinic teams, the position has become a conduit for the information and service links between these two services.

When a person is admitted to the hospital, service management shifts to the appropriate team in the hospital. For example, for acute-care admissions, the acute-care physician, nurse, and social worker become directly responsible for care and service planning. The Geriatric Program's acute-care consulting services provide assistance in medical management and nursing of older people. The community team comes

Figure 10.1 Geriatric Program: Cleveland Metropolitan General/ Highland View Hospital

CENTRAL
COORDINATION
OFFICE
COMMUNITY
OUTREACH
OUTPATIENT
ASSESSMENT
CLINIC
CONSULTING
SERVICE
INPATIENT
ASSESSMENT
UNIT
LONG-TERM
SKILLED NURSING

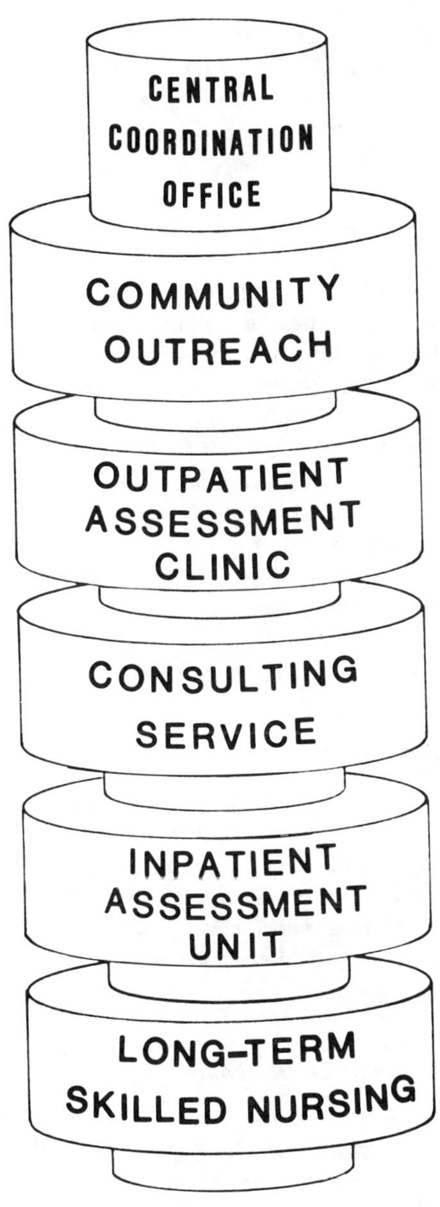

into play as the discharge plans are started, because these team members have information about the person's family, home environment, and community resources.

The program has employed low technology to help speed the flow of information among teams. One low-tech method used involves stamping each patient's chart with the program office extension so that if someone is admitted or is seen in the emergency room, the program office is called. Another method is to have the secretary review the daily admission sheets to double-check whether any clients were admitted overnight.

Outpatient Services

Outpatient services—the community outreach team and the outpatient assessment clinic team—have been structured as tightly articulated services designed to provide coordinated primary care and social services to a specific target group of elderly. The staff and resources were limited, so logically the target population also had to be limited. Geographic location and age were the criteria used to define the population. Frail people age 70 and older who lived relatively close to CMG/HVH were accepted for outpatient care.

The program's outpatient services not only reached out to the community but also developed a supportive relationship with other ambulatory units. These services have taken on the care of frail elderly patients of other clinics if they were considered to benefit from the program, either at a consultation level or a primary care level.

Community Outreach Team

The community outreach team provides in-home nursing assessment and psychosocial assessment as well as ongoing monitoring and counseling for program clients. The team, made up of a master's-level social worker, a registered nurse, and a specially trained geriatric outreach worker, refers clients to the geriatric clinic. Team members meet daily with the intake social worker to develop plans and monitor progress. Over 250 patients and their families have received services from the team.

Outpatient Assessment Clinic Team

The outpatient assessment clinic or, as it sometimes has been called, the geriatric ambulatory clinic, provides both primary medical care and a consultation and referral service. The core clinic team is composed of five geriatricians, a social worker, a nutritionist, a registered nurse, a pharmacist, and a psychiatrist. These team members meet weekly after each clinic session. The intake social worker has been active in the clinic as part of the clinic team. Other specialists who have provided services or conducted subclinics have been a podiatrist, an audiologist, a neurologist, and a urologist. By September 1989, 850 patients had received outpatient services.

Inpatient Services

The geriatric inpatient services that have been developed within the hospital system have a countywide referral base. Therefore these units have served mainly elderly patients who have not been clients of the outpatient and outreach components of the program. These inpatient services have made up the three more-restrictive levels of the program's vertical components and extend the continuum of care to focus on the needs of the elderly. Three inpatient services form part of the geriatric program—a consulting service, an inpatient assessment team, and a long-term skilled nursing team. These services have been available, when appropriate, for the community-supported clients who require more intensive management. In this way, the intrahospital divisions have been able to provide specialized medical and social services for the program's community levels. These intrahospital components have been guided by the same geriatricians as those working in and guiding the outpatient and outreach activities. Moreover, other members of the interdisciplinary teams also have crossed these levels of care, adding more cohesiveness to the program.

Consulting Service

The consulting service provides a tie between the geriatric program and the hospital's acute medical sections. The consulting team makes weekly rounds and sees all program patients hospitalized for acute medical problems; it accepts referrals from other physicians caring for elderly people. The consulting team refers patients to the outpatient clinic and to the community team. Residents and other staff physicians have participated in consulting rounds, which have been viewed as important for the teaching of geriatric medicine. The consulting team has included physicians and a clinical specialist in gerontological nursing with backup support from a senior social worker.

Inpatient Assessment Team

The inpatient assessment team, composed of health service professionals caring for elderly rehabilitation patients on the medical unit for the elderly, has been responsible for the development and implementation of detailed rehabilitation and discharge plans. Formal interdisciplinary team rounds have been held weekly and have included geriatricians, social workers, nurses, occupational therapists, physical therapists, and speech therapists. This team has also referred patients to the outpatient clinic and to the community outreach team. The intake social worker has participated in the formal interdisciplinary team meetings when appropriate. As of October 1989, the medical unit for the elderly had served close to 1,600 patients. An evaluation of the unit's efficacy showed that patients were discharged at a higher level of independence than case-matched controls.[1]

Long-Term Skilled Nursing Team

The Geriatric Program and the hospital system's long-term skilled nursing facility, Sunny Acres, have collaborated in establishing a geriatric unit to provide long-term skilled nursing care and related social services. This unit has included physicians, nurses, social workers, and rehabilitation specialists and accepted referrals from the other program teams.

Professional/Clinical Staff Responses to the Geriatric Program

The geriatric program has been well received by the physicians of the hospital who for some time had felt that improvements could be made in the care of the frail elderly. The program has not been seen as being competitive for patients but as an additional resource for the care of the frail elderly; therefore, it has been actively supported by the chairman of the department of medicine. Evidence from this comes from the subspecialists of the hospital who have referred a small number of elderly patients for more global assessments and evaluations. More important, the departments of medicine, psychiatry, and family medicine have included mandatory rotations in the geriatric program for all their residents. This is a notable endorsement of the program by the hospital's physicians.

The department of nursing has found the program valuable and actively supported it by adding clinical nurse specialists in gerontological nursing. All the students of the hospital's School of Nursing have had their clinical practice with the program's inpatient and outpatient services as well as with the community outreach team.

The social work department has actively supported the program, for the department has a long history of strong advocacy for the frail elderly. Students of social work from Case Western's Mandel School of Applied Social Services gained clinical experiences across the continuum of the program.

Others interested in the care of the elderly, especially those professionals involved in rehabilitation therapies and pharmacy, have joined the program for their own enrichment. The program has in turn encouraged younger professionals to attend appropriate continuing medical education courses in which the needs of the elderly are addressed.

Financial Impact

The precise financial impact on the hospital is unclear. Because only two new staff positions were added (a secretary and a nurse) and no new facilities built for the program, it can be assumed that the effect of reorganizing services to focus on the frail elderly has been positive in terms of hospital revenues. A conservative accounting shows that 233 patients have been referred to the hospital because of the Geriatric Program. In 1988, the program generated $5,630,000 in patient charges for all of the services received at the hospital.

On the other hand, the costs of providing these services is unknown. The fact that the medical unit for the elderly lies outside the Medicare diagnosis-related groups (DRGs) and within the rehabilitation beds has allowed the hospital to provide cost-reimbursed restoration of independence for frail elderly patients. Both patients and the hospital clearly benefit. The patients benefit from the enriched levels of acute and rehabilitation services and by avoiding being discharged "sicker and quicker." The hospital benefits through reimbursement for appropriate care within the acute and rehabilitation beds.

Conclusions

The care of the frail elderly provided by the Geriatric Program appears to have enhanced the image of the hospital. Younger family members of clients in the program have chosen to come to the hospital for their care. The program can continuously assess the changing needs of frail elderly persons and has extensive resources to meet those needs. Although it is possible that individual components of the geriatric program may not "make money"–for example, the community outreach team–the program does well for the hospital through effective management of patients across a long-term care continuum.

This model hospital-based geriatric program used the extensive resources of a major public hospital system to form a coordinated service program via five different interlocking programs. The program was designed to capture the existing strengths of the institution as well as to develop new services needed by elderly people. This organizational repackaging of clinical services has used existing staff more efficiently and improved the hospital's ability to care for more frail elderly people.

The principle of reorganizing existing fragmented services to provide a coordinated clinical service for the frail elderly patient may well be applicable to all hospitals that care for older adult patients. To do so does not necessarily entail the addition of significant numbers of new staff or the creation of new buildings. It does require an understanding of how the needs of the frail elderly can be appropriately met by the existing resources of the hospital. Furthermore, it requires support from the highest level of administration and governance of the hospital. Inevitably the repackaging must cross established authority lines of various hospital departments. Equally important is a group of clinicians who are willing, eager, and competent to care for frail elderly patients. Without such a group, no amount of planning will lead to a successful program.

The Geriatric Program has become deeply embedded in the hospital by being modeled on other subspecialty services. Therefore it has become a hospital service that has provided care for a specific group of patients who needed the services provided by the program; that is, the frail elderly. It differs from the other subspecialty programs by having already addressed the continuum of care and by having provided care through interdisciplinary teams.

Reference

1. Lefton, E. L., Bonstelle, B., and Frengley, J. D. Success with an inpatient geriatric unit: a controlled study of outcome and follow-up. *Journal of the American Geriatrics Society* 31(3):149–55, 1983.

Chapter 11

A Patient and Family Services Department in a County Hospital

Anne H. Williams

Introduction

Craven Regional Medical Center (CRMC) is a 301-bed, not-for-profit, county-owned hospital located in New Bern, North Carolina. Craven Regional Medical Center serves 91,145 residents in Craven, Jones, and Pamilco counties. The residents of this rural (primarily agrarian) area are poor, with 31.5 percent having a 1980 income of less than $7,000; minorities comprise 30.6 percent of the population. Figures also show a rise in the percentage of older adults, with 8.8 percent of the population over 65 years of age in 1980. Utilization at CRMC by Medicare beneficiaries age 65 years and older has decreased from 40 percent in 1982 to 34 percent in 1989, with a decrease in total patient days from 84,000 to 82,299 annually.

The Patient and Family Services Department (PFS) at CRMC, which provides services to the elderly, serves two target populations. The first is the Medicaid-eligible population, clients who either must be elderly or disabled (minimum age 18 years) and meet the requirements for a skilled nursing facility (SNF) or intermediate care facility (ICF). The second population is clients who are 65 years of age or older, have at least two chronic illnesses, and are not otherwise eligible for Medicaid.

Goals

Craven Regional Medical Center is committed to the development of a community-coordinated, hospital-based case-management program of care for the elderly. The goals of the institution are twofold:

1. To develop a comprehensive hospital-based health care program for the elderly that will deter unnecessary institutionalization or hospitalization and improve the quality of life for elderly persons
2. To provide ongoing training and experience to improve the capabilities of those involved with elderly persons during hospitalization and community placement

These goals are being achieved by:

- The development of linkages with existing physicians, agencies, and services in order to establish a countywide system of coordinated, community-based, long-term care following the case-management model
- The establishment of a Medicaid waivered project at CRMC for disabled adults and elderly at risk of institutionalization
- The development of a fee-for-service case-management system for the non–Medicaid elderly
- The development and implementation of educational projects on aging, the elderly, and long-term care issues for the medical and hospital staff as well as the community
- The development and implementation of a community outreach, a wellness project for the rural areas of Craven County
- The development of hospital-based services for the elderly

Figure 11-1 lists the hospital goals at the time of program initiation. Each goal has been met, with the exception of number 17, which will be reviewed in 1991.

The goals in long-term care for CRMC and PFS have been maintained constantly. The Patient and Family Service Department gained acceptance in the community as a provider of eldercare services, and PFS staff were committed to specific goals. Through this commitment, to date the principal accomplishments of the project have been achieved. New ideas and new objectives are now on the horizon, such as contracting to perform initial assessment on all home health clients and providing the client with the case management team approach of a registered nurse and a social worker. Needs for the home health staff or possible further case-management involvement will be identified.

Planning/Development Process

A growing need and demand for geriatric and long-term care services was identified during the development of the 1982 hospital strategic long-range plan. Because this need centered on community and in-home services for the aging population, the hospital's administration believed it

Figure 11-1. Craven County Hospital Corporation's Long-Term Care Proposal for the Robert Wood Johnson Foundation

Goals

1. To develop a system for a continuum of coordinated care for elderly patients, which will include preventive, diagnostic, therapeutic, medical, rehabilitative, supportive, and maintenance service addressing health, social, and personal care needs. These services will be provided in the least-restrictive environment possible, selected by the patient.
2. To develop a CRMC Corporation Long-Term Care network, which will be based on a local, state, and private partnership for the planning, delivery, and evaluation of long-term care services.
3. To provide a hospital-based, long-term care program accessible to all persons in need of care across the county, regardless of ability to pay.
4. To develop a model project at CRMC Corporation, which demonstrates the rule, "Hospitals can provide comprehensive programs to better meet the health care needs of the elderly."
5. To help elderly persons obtain maximum independence of functional ability and avoid unnecessary use of hospital and nursing home services.
6. To assist physicians and hospital administration in the education of all personnel relative to geriatric needs, thereby improving total geriatric patient care.
7. To develop appropriate alternatives of care for the elderly to avoid institutionalization, achieve independence, and retain the comfortable standard of living of their choice.
8. To provide coordination of the array of long-term care services available in the tri-county area for elderly individuals.
9. To provide comprehensive medical and social services for the elderly through continuity of care beyond the hospital's walls by coordination of community services.
10. To marshal and direct long-term care resources in this community to contain overall costs.
11. To increase access to a wider range of services currently available.
12. To stimulate the development of needed in-home and community services, which do not now exist or are in short supply.
13. To promote efficiency and optimum quality in community long-term care delivery systems.
14. To promote a reasonable division of labor between informal support systems (including families, neighbors, and friends), privately financed services, and publicly financed care.
15. To develop a community-based wellness program for adults in the area, aimed at enhancing the later years.
16. To develop case-management data systems, including monitoring and evaluation, for the care of elderly patients and for patient plans.
17. To lower the cost of Medicaid and Medicare services for Craven County. A review of Medicare and Medicaid cost will be done in 1991.
18. To develop and manage a volunteer system of telephone reassurance through the Patient and Family Services Department or an efficient community agency (auxiliary persons).
19. To develop management and transportation systems that will relieve case managers of this time-consuming activity.
20. To develop alliances with community organizations—for example religious community services and so forth—through communication and explanation of long-term care activities.

was important to enter the long-term care and aging services market. Several factors influenced the decision to diversify into these fields:

- Numerous older adults who moved into the retirement communities in the area had moved away from a family support system or primary care givers who would have been available to assist with providing home care.
- Few organizations in the region had the resources to meet the emerging need for community long-term care services. Although the services available were excellent, a coordinated continuum of services was not in place, and there were many gaps in the existing service system.
- A severe nursing home bed shortage contributed to longer hospital stays, especially for Medicaid patients. State policies regulating nursing home construction made it difficult to alleviate this situation.

These factors made it apparent to the hospital administration that greater private investment in the development of community long-term care services was needed.

One of the first steps CRMC took was to hire an employee with a doctorate in gerontology. The duties of the new director of geriatric services included developing a department of geriatrics, directing PFS, further examining the needs in the long-term care area, and developing resources to meet these needs.

Goals and objectives were established. Next, CRMC conducted a door-to-door countywide needs assessment statistical survey of older adults, using over 250 volunteers who were trained by the PFS staff. Volunteers familiar with the area for which they were responsible were recruited, training classes were conducted by precinct, and a questionnaire was developed (figure 11-2). The county was divided into sections, each having a chairperson who was responsible for the volunteers and for completion of the survey. The resultant information was compiled and service gaps were noted.

The survey, which was shared with each area agency, revealed the following areas of need among the elderly: Lifeline, transportation, respite care, and telephone reassurance.

Instead of pointing a finger at different agencies for not providing these services, PFS formed an elderly action committee, which consisted of at least one member from each agency that provided services in the community. The purpose of the committee was to review the services available and to find out how PFS could complement services already in place. The committee determined service gaps, working as a unit to meet these gaps instead of having one agency identify needs and try to point out deficiencies throughout the county. This may appear to have been an easy task, but agency "turfism" was a great dividing element. Some of these agencies had not met together in years, and there was fear that PFS would take over some of the community agencies' functions.

Figure 11-2. Geriatric Services Survey of All Persons over Age 60 in Craven County

RESOURCES AND NEEDS

Area: ____________________ Date of survey: ____________________
Name: ____________________ Age: ________ Date of birth: ____________
Address: ____________________ Telephone number: ____________________
____
Physician: ____________________ Telephone number: ____________________
Nearest relative: ____________________ Telephone number: ____________________
Address: ____________________

1. *How do you spend your day?*
   A. In bed ☐
   B. Up in a chair part of the day ☐
   C. Up in a chair all day ☐
   D. In home, passive activity ☐
   E. Active exercise ☐
   F. Watching TV ☐
   G. I'm just bored ☐
   H. Unknown ☐
   I. Other ☐
   Explain: ____________________
2. *Are you feeling well, or is there something you need to make you feel better?*
   A. I feel fine. ☐
   B. I need transportation to do any type of errand. ☐
   C. I need transportation to the doctor's office. ☐
   D. I need daily telephone contact. ☐
   E. I need daily visits. ☐
   F. I need home-delivered meals. ☐
   G. I need someone to cook for me. ☐
   H. I need help with shopping. ☐
   I. I need help with housekeeping. ☐
   J. I need speech therapy. ☐
   K. I need adult day care. ☐
   L. I need legal services. ☐
   M. I need Lifeline. ☐
   N. I need financial (or other) counseling. ☐
   O. Other: ____________________
   ____
3. *Are you living alone or with family or friends?*
   A. Alone ☐
   B. With a friend ☐
   C. With family ☐
   D. With one child for a time and then with another child ☐
   E. Pay someone to stay with me ☐
   F. Other: ____________________
4. *Do you have any housing needs?*
   A. Repair ☐
   Explain: ____________________
   ____
   B. Heating ☐
   C. Cooling ☐
   Other: ☐
   Explain: ____________________
   ____
   D. Do you have any problem getting around? ☐
   Problems with stairs? ☐
   Small bathroom? ☐
   Safety problems? ☐
   Getting to the telephone? ☐
   Getting to the shower or tub? ☐
   Getting to the toilet? ☐
   Other: ____________________
5. *Do you like to cook?*
   A. No, I can't. ☐
   B. Yes, I do. ☐
   C. I eat out. ☐
   D. I get Meals on Wheels. ☐
   E. My family cooks for me. ☐
   F. I have a chore worker. ☐
   G. I eat with a group. ☐
   How do you manage on weekends?
   Explain: ____________________
   ____

Continued on next page

Figure 11-2. (Continued)

6. *Would you enjoy going to a senior center to be with others and to take part in different activities?*

   A. Yes ☐ B. No ☐

   What activities are you interested in?

   A. Sewing ☐
   B. Crafts ☐
   C. Stamp collecting ☐
   D. Cooking ☐
   E. Cards ☐
   F. Bible study ☐
   G. Educational classes ☐
   H. Exercise classes ☐
   I. Nutrition classes ☐
   J. Other ☐
   Explain: ______________________
   ____

7. *Would you like to participate in volunteer activities in the community?*

   A. Yes ☐ B. No ☐

   If "yes," what would you like to do?
   1. ______________________
   2. ______________________
   3. ______________________

8. *Do you feel that we need a "life care" type of community housing in this area?*

   ("Life care" would provide housing options for older adults. The choice in housing would range from the single, independent resident to the more protected, dependent group housing, that is, with planned activities, meals, security, and so forth.)

   A. Yes ☐ B. No ☐

Name of Interviewer: ______________________
Telephone number: ______________________

After many meetings, PFS was able to reassure the different community agencies that the purpose of the newly formed hospital department was to coordinate the services of the different agencies. The staff of PFS, by being honest and sincere, have gained the trust and respect of the county agencies. The committee now meets quarterly to discuss problems, and it works as a unit to provide the best possible community in-home care.

Many achievements were gained by Craven County residents through the joint efforts of this elderly action committee. Patient and Family Services, working with the local chapter of the American Red Cross, obtained a grant in 1984 from the Public Welfare Foundation for transportation services for the elderly. The Craven County Council on Aging and PFS developed a telephone reassurance service in Craven County. The Craven Regional Medical Center auxiliary, in a combined effort with PFS, set up a growing Lifeline system or telephone alert system in two counties. Respite care is provided by the Council on Aging through the adult day care and senior companion program. The centerpiece of the CRMC program is the case management and assessment system, which includes case management, education programs, and a wellness program. The providers and their various responsibilities include the following:

- Craven Regional Medical Center auxiliary provides clients with the telephone Lifeline units (Lifeline is staffed by volunteers).
- Craven County Council on Aging builds patient ramps and steps and provides Meals on Wheels, transportation, and adult day care. It also has the telephone Lifeline units and a senior companion program, which provides respite for care givers free of charge. The Council on Aging is funded by various organizations, which include the ACTION group and the United Way, and by federal, state, and county sources; private contributions; fundraisers; and foundation contributions.
- Craven Regional Medical Center Patient and Family Services Department provides clients with telephone reassurance services. Volunteers make "friendly calls" to the sick and shut-ins.

Case Management and Assessment

Craven Regional Medical Center has two long-term care programs based on type of funding; the Medicaid Waiver Program, funded by Medicaid, and the Community Care Program, funded by the Robert Wood Johnson Foundation and by private pay and other insurance reimbursements. Although CRMC has two programs, case management is the same. The system used for case management is referred to as *phases.*

First Phase of Case Management: The Plan of Care

The first phase of case management includes the following:

- *Referrals.* Referrals are obtained in two different ways: (1) Adults who qualify for ICF or SNF levels of care and are Medicaid-eligible recipients able to purchase services privately, or have other insurance that reimburses for in-home care; and (2) those referred by physicians, nurses, discharge planners, family members, community agencies, and prospective clients.
- *Comprehensive screening/evaluation.* This includes a home visit conducted by the case-management team, composed of a social worker and a nurse, to determine each client's medical, functional, psychosocial, financial, and environmental status.
- *Development of a plan of care.* This is completed by the case-management team in consultation with the physicians and community agencies to determine whether in-home care would enable the client to be maintained in the home or community safely.

- *Implementation of the plan of care.* With the client, his or her family, and the physician's approval, the care plan will be implemented by various formal and informal support services within the community.
- *Monitoring the plan of care.* The plan of care will be monitored, coordinated, and reevaluated by the case manager as the client's needs and adjustments indicate.

Second Phase of Case Management: Geriatric Education

An integral part of case management is to develop educational programs for physicians, nurses, hospital staff, community agencies, and family members who provide care for an elderly or disabled adult. In-services to the medical staff, nurses, and community are performed on a regular basis. These in-services inform those in attendance of community services and how case management can coordinate the services with different needs of the elderly.

Third Phase of Case Management: Health Promotion

The third and final component of case management is a community-based wellness and health promotion program aimed at long-term health care planning and fitness. A monthly meeting is held that stresses health topics related to older adults. Fitness programs are offered by the CRMC cardiac rehabilitation program to those interested.

The Role of the Case Manager

The case manager becomes a statistician who completes monthly analyses to track the client's progress or declining condition. The case manager tracks hospital admissions and discharges, DRG-assigned hospital stays, emergency room visits, ambulatory care visits, and nursing home admissions, as well as the number of professional home visits and paraprofessional health visits. Utilizing this method, case managers can determine the effectiveness of care to the client.

Case management is an ongoing learning experience. One need being met is for the elderly to organize their finances to pay their bills. All case managers are now bonded so they can assist clients in writing checks. Attempting to work up a budget for a client is difficult when that client receives only $336 per month, for example, in Social Security benefits. Case managers also act as patient advocates, performing a continuous comprehensive evaluation of health status and sometimes fighting to keep a late-stage AIDS client from being evicted from an apartment complex. The case manager learns to wear many hats and to improvise care when the client's home environment is below standards.

Case management can be frustrating but, generally speaking, the most rewarding work a professional can experience. Cooperation and communication with the various formal and informal supports and services in the community are the keys to success for case management.

Innovative Services

At the beginning of CRMC's program of case management, nursing services and aide care were provided only by the existing County Home Health Department. However, after recognizing the need to service a larger area, the hospital's administration pursued a certificate of need for a hospital home health agency—for which licensure was received in November 1985. As of this writing the referrals have tripled the anticipated growth pattern; the County Home Health Department also has grown. In 1986, PFS applied for a grant to the Duke Endowment through the Kate B. Reynolds Care Trust and received $60,000 as startup funds for the hospital home health agency. The two exceptionally good home health agencies now in existence in Craven County provide patients with a choice.

Transportation in this rural area has always been a problem, although some agencies provide transportation on a limited basis. If a client lived 15 miles outside the city limits, a trip to the physician's office was difficult to manage. This problem was resolved when PFS obtained a grant to provide transportation for elderly adults for shopping and physician office visits.

Bereavement counseling for hospital home health patients is being provided by PFS social workers. Social assessments are also being contracted through PFS to the Hospital Home Health Program.

A two-county Lifeline unit program has been established by the hospital auxiliary and the Council on Aging. Approximately 60 percent of all case-managed clients have Lifeline units in their homes. A Lifeline unit, placed in a client's home, has a direct line to the emergency department at CRMC and is connected to the client's telephone. A distressed client only has to push the button on a bracelet or necklace he or she wears; this signals the Lifeline unit itself. Once the emergency department responds to the signal, help is on the way. This unit helps to ensure client safety while in the home. The program is staffed by auxiliary volunteers at CRMC.

Community support groups, although a challenge to initiate, have been developed for Alzheimer's disease, stroke, and care givers. Patient and Family Services works with the County Health Department and the arthritis support group, sponsored by the health department. Each of these groups meets monthly during the day. The education coordinator has a caseload of 28 to 30 clients, works with all support groups, and handles education emphasis. Participants are contacted on a regular basis regarding newly developed programs each month.

Gold Care, a program initiated solely by CRMC for older adults, currently has in excess of 700 members. Monthly meetings stress various topics of interest to older adults, from health to gardening and travel to living wills. Gold Care has helped to promote health and overall well-being among the elderly.

Craven Regional Medical Center implemented a personal care program effective in 1987. Personal care provides care for those still living at home who are unable to provide their own care. Personal care aides assist patients with light housekeeping, laundry, meal preparation, as well as any personal care needs the patients may have. The program has its own monitoring system in that a registered nurse makes a home visit to each client every 60 days to see that the personal care aide is performing his or her duties. A contract is signed between the supervisor, the aide, and the patient stating what services the aide is to render. Personal care is also offered to the private pay sector at the same rate that the state reimburses for this service through the North Carolina Division of Medical Assistance.

Support for Elderly Services

Competition for services was nonexistent at the beginning of the CRMC case-management system; however, PFS welcomes competition, and each agency provides its own service. Now CRMC has two home health agencies, several medical equipment stores, and two personal care programs. Craven Regional Medical Center Corporation has established a home health department. The case manager has been able to broker home health services at a better price, to the advantage of both private-pay clients and the state program, because it saves Medicaid monies. Competition also exists between area medical supply companies, thereby reducing the cost to clients served by PFS. Because PFS personnel probably have not had time to determine whether competition is friend or foe, the case manager must monitor closely to ensure that clients do not suffer because of possible inadequate services attributable to lower prices.

Support from administration and physicians has been excellent. Patient and Family Services operates fairly independently—a morale booster for the staff. Confidence in CRMC administration and physicians also is evident in the community, resulting in better working relations with other community agencies.

Physician participation for the CRMC case-management program has been overwhelmingly good, although encouraging physicians to utilize a new system had its problems. During the developmental process, questions arose as to who should refer. The decision was made to accept referrals from all physicians, the hospital, agencies, and the private community. Priority referrals, however, are from physicians and hospital clients. The rationale was to provide assistance quickly to the physician with a problem client and to provide the hospital with a process to follow the client back into the community with the assistance of a case manager.

Referrals from within the hospital were a problem at the beginning of the program. Referrals were to come through the discharge planning department to the intake worker in PFS. Although criteria were established for all referrals, some appropriate referrals were falling through the gaps. The hospital administration was approached with the problem, and the discharge planning department was placed under the PFS director, a decision that has proved effective. The discharge planners are now part of the case-management program, working with the short-term acute needs of all patients. If a patient has long-term care needs—for example, for nursing services, performing chores, telephone reassurance, or aide services—the patient (with physician approval) is referred to a case manager.

Physicians' offices were visited and advised of the programs available. Materials were distributed to each physician's office. Physicians serve on advisory committees and constantly consulted for their ideas about the program. Physicians have been the key factor in any measure of success attained by these programs.

Financing

Craven Regional Medical Center Corporation was fortunate in receiving grants from public and private sources to provide additional resources for program development. The hospital's program has two major components: a state-supported Medicaid Waivered Program and the Hospital Initiatives in Long-Term Care Program, part of a national demonstration (model) program that includes private and insurance reimbursement. The Medicaid Waivered Program receives monies from the state for assessments and case management. The community care program has developed a sliding-fee scale for private-pay clients. The Medicaid Waivered Program has received $25,000 for three years in succession to pay the social worker's salary. The four-year RWJF grant pays the salaries of other employees—the program director, two registered nurses, one social worker, the educational coordinator, and an administrative assistant.

At present, a personal care program initiated by the division of medical assistance of Medicaid is being implemented. This program functions under the Hospital Home Health Program and PFS and will give PFS better control of patient care. Ninety-five percent of program funding is under the division of medical assistance (Medicaid), and 5 percent matching county funds comprise the remainder. The social worker and registered nurse team from PFS have assumed the responsibility of completing the initial comprehensive assessments for the newly organized Hospital Home Health Agency. This comprehensive assessment by a social worker and registered nurse team—unique for home health programs—has provided a more comprehensive assessment for each client and identified needs of clients, while simultaneously serving as another referral source for private-pay, case-management services and medical social worker assessments.

Data are stored regarding all clients who left the hospital early, with case-management system support, due to lack of ability to place the client in an ICF or an SNF. These data will serve to assure administration of the cost-containment aspects of case management.

Conclusions

Craven Regional Medical Center's excitement with the patient and family services department should be apparent, despite its ups and downs. One recommendation to other projects for the elderly would be to start small and grow strong.

With all the discussed services in place and the case-management system available for coordination of these service, CRMC has become a comprehensive health center providing and coordinating a range of services for the elderly.

The demand for long-term care services will grow as the number of older adults in the community increases. Craven Regional Medical Center is an example of a rural hospital that has taken the initiative to develop a long-range strategy recognizing the importance of focusing on services for older adults.

Chapter 12

The Continuum of Care for the Elderly Concept

Elaine M. Frank and Michael Gordon Sorohan

Introduction

The Greater Southeast Healthcare System is a comprehensive community-based health care network operating in southeast Washington, D.C., and southern Prince Georges County, Maryland. Despite the generally low socioeconomic status of its catchment area, Greater Southeast is committed to providing high-quality, innovative services to its community.

A primary focus at Greater Southeast is the development of a *continuum of care,* designed to address the changing needs of the area's elderly population. Activities are focused in the Center for the Aging, though geriatric programs and services operate throughout the system. Figure 12-1 depicts the range of gerontologically oriented programs in operation at Greater Southeast.

Goals

The continuum of care for the elderly at Greater Southeast has two goals. First, it seeks to improve the quality of care provided to older adults and eliminate existing gaps in available services. Area older adults are better served as Greater Southeast continues to increase case-management activities and eliminate the difficulties that usually accompany transfers among facilities or programs. The holistic approach to the needs of the elderly at Greater Southeast improves the continuity of care.

Second, the continuum of care provides a means for the Greater Southeast to improve the efficiency with which it operates by allowing maximum use of scarce resources. By coordinating services among the

Figure 12-1. The Continuum of Care at Greater Southeast

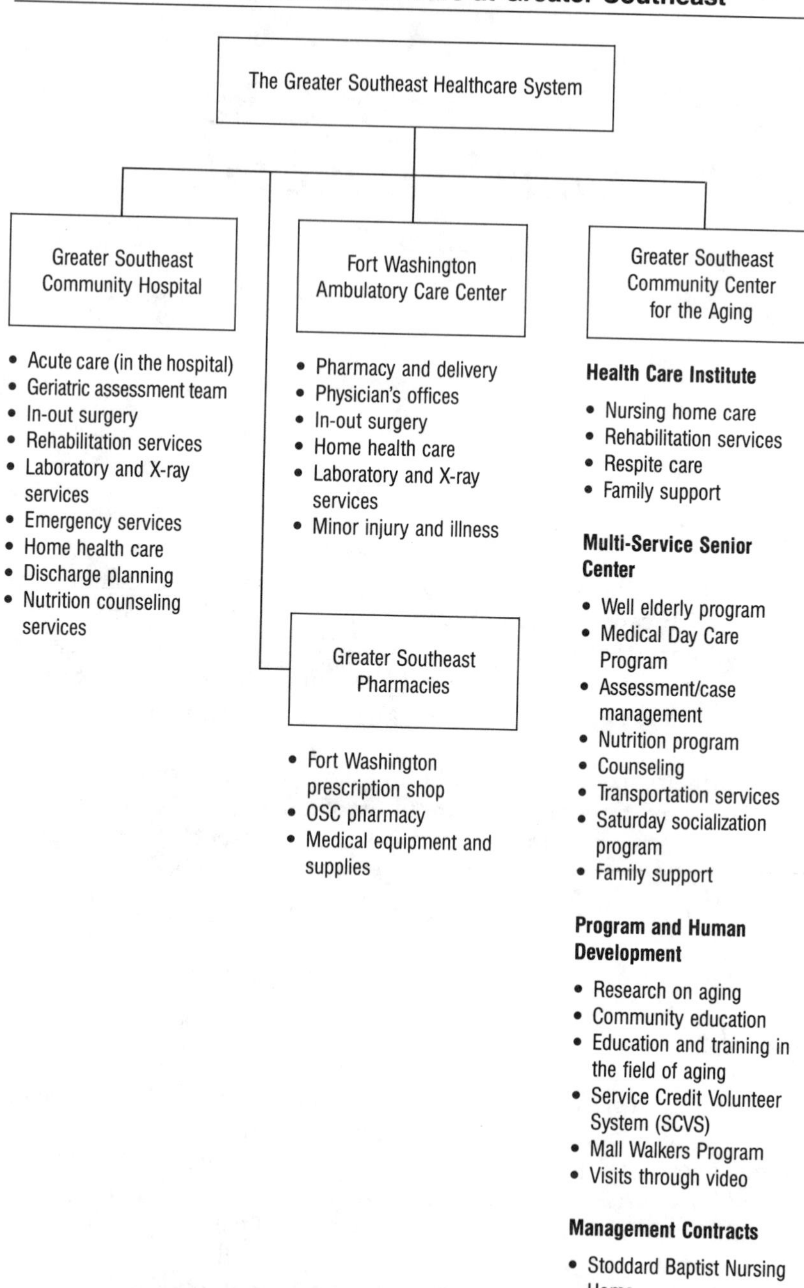

various levels of care and consolidating some administrative and management tasks, Greater Southeast's multifacility system gains economic and other advantages. Through this concept, Greater Southeast has made it possible to bring innovative health and related services to its community.

Internal/External Environment

The Greater Southeast Healthcare System is a private, not-for-profit organization, which owns and operates several facilities in southeast Washington, D.C., and suburban Prince Georges County, Maryland. The 450-bed Greater Southeast Community Hospital is the largest entity. The System also includes the Center for the Aging, the 33-bed Fort Washington Medical Center, several medical office buildings, two pharmacies, and an ambulatory care center. Financially each entity operates inter-independently, with a common budget process but independent management and operations.

The Center for the Aging, which focuses on the System's geriatric programs, was founded in 1978. It is the second-largest entity within the System. The Center for the Aging currently includes the 180-bed Health Care Institute, a skilled- and intermediate-care teaching nursing home; and the Multi-Service Senior Center, which provides area elderly persons with senior center activities, a medical day care program, a nutrition program, assessment/case-management services, transportation, a Saturday socialization program, and other counseling services. Also, Greater Southeast Consulting offers extensive hands-on experience in developing and operating long-term facilities and programs and senior day care programs. The Center for the Aging also manages the Stoddard Baptist Nursing Home and the Brentwood Adult Day Care Center.

The Center for the Aging's service area reflects many of the demographic changes that have shaped American society, particularly the growth in the number of elderly Americans in the past few years. The area's older population continues to grow—nearly 35,000 residents over age 65 live within a few miles of the Center. Seventy-five percent of these residents are members of minority groups, and a significant proportion are considered low income. The result is a poor payer mix. For example, more than 96 percent of the Health Care Institute's revenues come from Medicaid, creating a dependence on public funding, with few private-pay patients to supplement.

Planning/Development Process

The System began to broaden its services from a freestanding community hospital to a multifacility system in the mid-1970s. The expansion was in response to the unmet service needs of the community and recognition of service gaps that existed in the District of Columbia and Prince Georges County. The continuum of care concept evolved in an effort to fill those gaps. The Health Care Institute opened at a time when a significant shortage of nursing home beds existed. The Multi-Service Senior Center's day care program was the first of its kind in the city.

Since the Center's development, other facilities have been established, and the resulting competition has strengthened the effort toward development of a systems approach to geriatrics. Despite the competition and increasing reimbursement pressures, some of the needs of the area's elderly population remain unmet. For example, inadequate medical transportation still exists between health care facilities even with the Greater Southeast System. To move a resident of the Health Care Institute at 1380 Southern Avenue, S.E., to Greater Southeast Community Hospital at 1310 Southern Avenue, S.E. (a mere 100 yards), an ambulance must be dispatched, because neither facility has a vehicle that will meet the stringent requirements for medical transportation. The trip costs $120.

Continued service gaps have encouraged development and use of innovations that can meet the community's needs. The Center for the Aging and the System have moved toward a system of vertical integration (continuum of care), wherein a person's comprehensive health care needs can be met within the Greater Southeast Healthcare System. An elderly patient at Greater Southeast Community Hospital may be treated for urgent or acute care and later transferred (if need be) to the Health Care Institute for nursing home care. In the alternative, the patient may be rehabilitated through the programs offered by the Multi-Service Senior Center, the Hospital's Home Care Service, or a combination of programs and facilities.

The continuum of care serves both patients and providers. By simplifying interfacility transfers and reducing the replication of efforts commonly associated with these, the quality of care and the efficiency of the entire system will improve.

The continuum of care concept at Greater Southeast is an ongoing developmental process based on meeting the community's changing needs while *maintaining* the System's viability. For example, the Multi-Service Senior Center's day care program emerged from several community needs. Today's working society, with more women in the work force and more multiple-income households, makes it increasingly difficult for families to care for the daily needs of their elderly relatives. Yet many people are uncomfortable with placing a family member in a nursing home.

The day care program has dealt with these community concerns and in turn has demonstrated advantages for the overall system. Day care is a cost-efficient program that has given the Center for the Aging an advantage under the prospective payment system (PPS) by its ability to discharge patients who otherwise would use long-term beds. The day care program reinvolves its participants in community activities. The program also allows the "formal" system (the Center's personnel and services) to work more closely with the "informal" system (the patient's family and friends).

A variety of internal and external barriers can prevent the System from running optimally. The financial autonomy of each entity within the Greater Southeast Healthcare System leads to problems involving cooperation, logistics, and structure. Interfacility/program cooperation can be difficult; getting a committee to meet or to develop a systemwide form can take months. Some internal barriers are physical; for example, the problem of moving a patient from the Health Care Institute to the hospital. Many barriers are a matter of logistics, resulting from differences in policies and orientation. For example, no common admissions or discharge forms exist between the hospital and the Center for the Aging. A resident of the Health Care Institute who needs acute care has to complete discharge papers there, as well as complete admission forms at Greater Southeast Community Hospital. Improvements have been made in this area, though a systemwide admissions form has yet to be developed. Other logistical problems remain.

External barriers, which are more difficult for the System to control or change, have proven even more troublesome. Medicaid's confusing eligibility guidelines is one such example; Medicaid allows for a person to receive full-time nursing home care, but the same person might not be financially eligible to receive home care benefits. A related problem is Medicaid's institutional bias of reimbursement. For instance, Medicaid might agree to pay an institution $300 per day for an elderly person's hospital care but will not pay $40 per day for that same person to live at home and have someone come in to perform light housekeeping—despite the obvious savings to Greater Southeast or to Medicaid and the improved functioning of the individual.

Such barriers have encouraged varying expectations within the Greater Southeast Healthcare System. Some programs, such as the Health Care Institute's Respirator Unit, currently operate at a loss. This is acceptable, however, as long as the combined activities translate into increased overall revenues for the System.

Case Management and Assessment

A key element in the development of an effective continuum of care is the existence of a coordinated case-management program operating throughout the System; at present, Greater Southeast has several such activities. In addition, efforts are underway to coordinate these various aspects more closely.

The Multi-Service Senior Center, through a contract with the District of Columbia Office on Aging, operates an *assessment/case-management program.* The program serves more than 100 older adults living in the community who, because of multiple health and other problems, are "at risk" of institutionalization. Once referred, the individual receives a comprehensive assessment, examining not only medical needs but also economic, social, psychological, and spiritual needs. Following an assessment, a trained social worker manages the client's case. The social worker ensures that needs are met as efficiently as possible, while encouraging the individual to maintain maximum independence. To be successful, program staff must use all available resources, formal and informal, and those within and outside the Greater Southeast System, to assist the older person to remain in the community.

Another important case-management component is *discharge planning,* which is carried out at both Greater Southeast Community Hospital and the Health Care Institute. Both facilities work toward maximizing use of resources as well as the individual's functional level. Staff at both facilities identify potential clients early in their stay, so that discharge planning efforts take place in a timely manner. The staff coordinates efforts through regular interfacility meetings.

These case-management steps attempt to give physicians and other health care professionals more involvement in the care of elderly patients. Although recognizing the importance of nursing management in the long-term care of older adults, there is increasing awareness of the value of a multidisciplinary approach to eldercare. By including the perspective and expertise of these professionals, nursing care quality can improve to the benefit of both patients and care givers.

Innovative Services

At present the System includes a variety of innovative programs that comprise its continuum of care for older community residents. Several additional services are in planning.

The Service Credit Volunteer System (SCVS), operated by the Center for the Aging, is sponsored by the Greater Southeast Management Company (a subsidiary of the System), the Meyer Foundation, and the Robert Wood Johnson Foundation (RWJF). Through SCVS, older adults (and handicapped people of any age), their relatives, and organizations concerned with the well-being of older adults earn service credits by performing a range of predetermined tasks for other program participants. These tasks are divided into four major categories—personal care, home management, cleaning and other environmental services, and transportation/escort. To qualify for the program, the services must increase an older adult's ability to remain in the community and at home. The earned credits may be used in the future to "purchase" services performed by persons who themselves are being "paid" with service credits. Thus service credits become a form of insurance against future needs. A literacy component has also been added, and tutors earn credits for teaching, while students provide transportation and other services in exchange.

In addition to the direct benefits accruing to the recipients of services, SCVS can also make significant contributions in maintaining the physical and psychological well-being of the providers. Further, it converts the elderly from being simply consumers of services to being both providers *and* consumers and assists in repudiating the image of older people as societal burdens.

Greater Southeast sees SCVS as an important innovation in filling the gaps throughout the system and in fostering volunteerism within the community. The Service Credit Volunteer System promises to be an exemplary model of how the private sector can cooperate with the government to revitalize the spirit of neighbors helping neighbors, the strength of our communities in the past.

The Center for the Aging's Medical Model Day Care Program, the first and only such program in the District of Columbia, has operated since 1981. The day care program is licensed by both the District of Columbia and Maryland Medicaid programs, and its services are reimbursable through both of these third-party systems. To be admitted to the program, an individual must qualify for intermediate-level nursing home care. Thus the program is geared toward the frail elderly population.

The day care component is an essential link in the continuum of care concept. It offers a full day of supervised activities as well as any necessary health monitoring and therapies. Thus an individual can participate during the day and return home in the evening. It allows participants to live with family members who have other daytime responsibilities or to live alone while receiving stimulation and needed nursing/medical care. The program provides an alternative for individuals who may need significant services on a daily basis but can avoid institutionalization through day care and other resources available to them.

The day care program is directed by a full-time, on-site registered nurse. The director provides hands-on nursing care and handles all administrative duties, including monitoring of clients, recruitment and screening of new participants, supervision of staff, and preparation of budgets.

This program is particularly innovative in one other respect. Unlike most such programs, Greater Southeast's operates at the same time and place as the Senior Center program, which is designed for the community's well elderly. This offers both populations an opportunity to interact and assist each other, which also broadens the resources available to each group.

From its inception the Health Care Institute (HCI, the extended-care facility) operated as a *teaching nursing home* through a grant from the

Robert Wood Johnson Foundation. Since completion of that project, HCI maintains affiliations with Georgetown University's Schools of Nursing and Dentistry and other educational institutions. The project concentrates on providing students with clinical experience, but has also influenced research and practice.

As a teaching nursing home, HCI and other components of the Greater Southeast System have served as the primary geriatric clinical site for students in both graduate and undergraduate nursing programs at Georgetown. Dentistry students have also used the facility for clinical experience, with emphasis on the elderly. By extension, and because of its experience, reputation, and philosophy, HCI and the Center for the Aging have provided students in many disciplines and at many levels with hands-on experience with the elderly throughout the continuum of care. Undergraduate and graduate students in social work, physical therapy, recreational therapy, health administration, and medical records from many different colleges and universities come here to learn. In addition, through affiliation with the local school district, licensed practical nurse and nursing assistant students have rotated through the Health Care Institute.

A Young Look at Aging is a unique program developed with a local high school as part of an elective course in aging. Through this program, high school students and Center participants interact at least once per month, at the nursing home, the senior center, or the high school. Through the exchange each group gains understanding of another generation. The students also are exposed to a variety of career options in the health and human services fields.

These programs are designed to teach geriatrics and to stimulate interest in the field among today's students. They also serve a valuable secondary purpose. The presence of students has encouraged staff to examine their own practices and the policies they follow and to keep staff current with advances in the field.

The affiliation with Georgetown University and the RWJF grant have also stimulated research at the Center for the Aging. To date, projects have included a study of falls among the elderly and how to minimize them; an examination of patient behaviors that are disruptive to both staff and residents; and an examination of the turnover among staff at the Center for the Aging.

Greater Southeast Community Hospital has developed a multidisciplinary Geriatric Assessment Team to improve the care provided to its older patients. The team consists of a physician, a nurse, a social worker, a dietitian, and a pharmacist, with other disciplines brought in as needed. All patients over age 65 are screened at the time of admission for signs of functional dependency. If necessary, they are referred to the team, where each member then carries out an independent patient assessment. Once these are completed, the team meets to agree on a single set of recommendations to improve the patient's overall care and prognosis.

Based on its effectiveness as demonstrated during a pilot research phase, the team has become an official hospital consultative service. Many patients appear to benefit from this multidisciplinary approach to their cases, particularly with regard to medications and nutritional issues. Team members, and by extension their colleagues, have indicated that they learn a great deal about the multiplicity of factors affecting their elderly patients. The Geriatric Assessment Team thus appears to have a two-pronged positive impact on the care provided to older patients.

The Greater Southeast Healthcare System has also begun to alter the traditional distinctions between acute care and long-term care. The first step has been to develop a *respirator care unit* in the Health Care Institute. Although the unit is still small, it is evident that with proper skilled nursing care, respirator patients can be maintained effectively in the nursing home at much lower cost than in the hospital. Therefore plans are under way to expand the unit.

The System has also developed significant housing opportunities for community residents, including the Robert L. Walker House, with 69 subsidized units for the elderly and handicapped. This offers another important element to the continuum of care.

Financing

Each subsidiary of the System operates as a separate financial entity. However, there is an integrated concern for achieving systemwide efficiencies and maximizing overall reimbursement. As a result, the System will subsidize programs that are not self-sustaining, provided they contribute in some demonstrable way to the overall positive flow of resources.

The respirator unit is one example of such subsidization. Another example involves the decision to continue the teaching nursing home program beyond the funding period provided by the RWJF. With the introduction of the prospective payment system, Greater Southeast Community Hospital, along with other hospitals, faces increased pressure to discharge its Medicare patients in a timely manner. Through its influence on the availability of nursing home beds, the level of nursing care provided to residents, and alternative placements, the Greater Southeast Healthcare System can mitigate the negative fiscal and quality-of-care impacts of PPS. Whereas continuing some aspects of the teaching nursing home program will result in some nonreimbursable expenses, the continued availability of high-quality, skilled nursing care required by discharged patients will be ensured.

Other programs financed by the Greater Southeast Management Company are designed to increase public awareness of services offered and to fill existing gaps. These include SCVS, the Neighborhood Blood Pressure Watch Program (which works with area churches and barber shops in increasing awareness of the dangers of hypertension), the Mall Walkers Program (an exercise program at a local shopping mall), and health fairs.

Under the current reimbursement system, expenditures of Medicaid funds at the Health Care Institute in any one year determine the reimbursement rate for the following year. The Center for the Aging has done marginally well under this system–*marginally* because of its commitment to the teaching nursing home program. The financially driven reimbursement system provides little if any incentive for such innovations. The Greater Southeast System, however, has made community development and high-quality health care part of its mission and sees the necessity of these non–revenue-producing programs.

Vertical integration is a means by which the Greater Southeast Healthcare System can help contain overall costs and avoid the negative effects of a DRG-based reimbursement system. By offering and controlling a complete range of services for the elderly community, the System can provide needed services at lower cost to reimbursement programs. Medicaid will save money if a person's health care needs can be met through one system. At present, the Greater Southeast Healthcare System can provide treatment to elderly patients at any level of acuity, from urgent care to long-term nursing home care to home-based care.

Conclusions

The continuum of care concept developed by the Greater Southeast Healthcare System has made great strides in addressing the continually changing needs of its service area population. The System has worked around restrictive Medicaid regulations to encourage innovation among its subsidiaries.

New programs such as the Service Credit Volunteer System and the Medical Model Day Care Program have filled critical service gaps in the community and allowed the subsidiaries within the System to further improve both the quality and continuity of care provided to area elderly residents.

Within this environment, Greater Southeast expects to continue taking steps toward providing a comprehensive range of services.

Chapter 13

Senior Care Program Development

David R. Cornell

Introduction

Montana Deaconess Hospital in Great Falls, Montana, was originated in 1897 by Reverend William Wesley Van Orsdel as an institution to care for the "sick and infirmed" residing in the Great Plains along the Missouri River in the territory called Montana. Since that time, Montana Deaconess has continuously upgraded and expanded its services to carry out its mission and has positioned itself as a diversified health services corporation that is financially strong, influential, and recognized as a leader in the delivery of health services in the northern Rocky Mountain region.

Internal/External Environment

Montana Deaconess Medical Center is a not-for-profit health care corporation that consists of a 288-bed acute-care general hospital, a 124-bed skilled nursing center that is physically attached to the main structure, a large home health agency, and a for-profit subsidiary that deals in home oxygen services and durable medical equipment sales. A freestanding outpatient surgical facility is attached to the main hospital structure by means of an underground tunnel, and an addition to the main complex houses a magnetic resonance imager. Montana Deaconess also operates a large and diverse clinical services division that provides contract services such as computerized electrocardiographic interpretation, computerized pulmonary function interpretation, electroencephalography, laboratory management, respiratory therapy management, and dietary management to over 60 hospitals in a seven-state surrounding area. Additionally, Montana Deaconess offers broad programs in health promotion through its Wel-Fit center and has utilized this mechanism as the initial step in forming preferred provider organizations with community businesses.

Great Falls has a metropolitan population of approximately 60,000, with the total population in Cascade County approximating 83,000. Nearly 7,500 individuals, or 14 percent of the population, are over age 65. Additionally, Medicare patients over age 65 account for 36 percent of Montana Deaconess' admissions and approximately 42 percent of its total patient days. Further review of the data indicates that approximately 27 percent of surgery is performed on Medicare patients over age 65, and that group provides Montana Deaconess with 36 percent of its total revenue.

Montana Deaconess recognized that the aging population represented a large market and has positioned itself to capture the majority of this market. As such, Montana Deaconess has seen its market share of elderly patients increase. This chapter details the steps taken that assured Montana Deaconess' leadership in the aging and long-term care service market in north/central Montana.

Planning/Development Process

Being the largest hospital in Great Falls, as well as in the state of Montana, and a major provider of health care services to the elderly, Montana Deaconess Medical Center was "targeted" in late 1984 by a small group of senior citizens to "lower the health care costs in Montana."

In the fall of 1984, Montana Deaconess was approached by the Montana Senior Citizens Association (MSCA), a small organization (representing less than 3 percent of the total older adult population in Great Falls), who demanded a discount program for their members based on a scale to be determined by them. Furthermore, they proposed the administration of the program would be handled solely by their organization. After the initial contact, Montana Deaconess learned that this organization had received a $40,000 grant from the Villers Foundation in Washington, D.C., and that they would use AFL-CIO tactics in their negotiations with Montana Deaconess. This was evidenced by their hiring of a professional organizer to manage the campaign.

Montana Deaconess administrators also learned that the hospital was singled out because it was the largest medical center in the state and because MSCA perceived a trend toward declining inpatient admissions as a sign of weakness for negotiation purposes. In reality, the organization's representatives did not fully understand the nature of the health care business in that the prospective payment system had altered physician practice patterns whereby fewer patient days were utilized, but an increase in outpatient business was also materializing.

Several meetings were held between hospital representatives (who included the chief executive officer, the senior vice-president of finance, the public relations director, and the administrator of the nursing home) and a team from MSCA. After a few meetings it became evident that MSCA was seeking more than lower health care costs for the elderly. The group wanted the program to increase their membership and political power base as a representative organization for senior citizens in Great Falls, Cascade County, and the state of Montana.

Because MSCA did not represent a majority of the older adult population in Great Falls and surrounding Cascade County, Montana Deaconess representatives met with several other senior citizen groups, including the Cascade County Council on Aging, the two local chapters of the American Association of Retired Persons (AARP), and the Retired Teachers Association to determine the health needs for the elderly that were not being met by the provider network.

During these discussions it became evident that four areas concerned older adults:

1. Payment of the Medicare deductible, which was a burden for those living on fixed incomes
2. Education on the Medicare program and the rights of beneficiaries
3. Health-screening programs that were expensive when performed at private physicians' offices or other clinics
4. Transportation to the hospital or to physicians' offices

It appeared that a number of the elderly were not gaining access to health care because of these barriers.

After gaining insights and information from various senior citizen groups, Montana Deaconess devised an alternative program to that proposed by MSCA.

Montana Deaconess formed its own ad hoc committee consisting of representatives of all the above-mentioned senior citizen groups in Great Falls. The ad hoc group was charged with creating a senior care program that would meet many of the unfulfilled needs of the elderly. Montana Deaconess also appointed a coordinator of the Senior Care Program, a nurse with specialized training in psychiatry and geriatrics and who was already on staff at Montana Deaconess Medical Center.

Because other providers in Great Falls had not demonstrated an interest in developing an all-inclusive eldercare program, Montana Deaconess Medical Center, through its ad hoc advisory committee, initiated its Senior Care Program in February 1985.

Two financial feasibility strategies were employed in the design of Montana Deaconess' Senior Care Program. The first centered on the breakdown of the income levels of senior citizens in Cascade County to arrive at a meaningful discounting strategy. The second strategy entailed determining the break-even analysis necessary to ascertain the required number of new patients that would allow the program to "pay for itself" or actually contribute incremental revenue and margin to the medical center.

First, planners determined the percentage of older adults residing in single-person households and those residing as couples. It was found that approximately 63 percent of the elderly in Great Falls and Cascade County were singles, and only 37 percent were couples. Then they broke these two groups down by level of income to arrive at a sliding-scale discount. The planners next took the historical Medicare deductible and coinsurance amounts and factored that total by the percentage discount to be applied to the various income levels to arrive at a potential total discount for the Senior Care Program. A measurement of the actual first-year cost of discounts proved that Montana Deaconess overestimated the amount of discount related to the 100 percent discount category and underestimated its amount of discounts required in the 50 to 100 percent categories. Planners were very accurate in their projection of discounts based on the 10 percent level. In general, they slightly overestimated the total discount commitment for the first year of the Senior Care Program.

The second financial analysis related to the number of new patients necessary to help the program break even and above which it would provide incremental revenue and incremental margin to the Medical Center. This was done simply by taking the average gross revenue per Medicare patient, subtracting the amount of contractual allowance (or the difference between the actual charge and the amount Medicare pays under the DRG system), and dividing that number into the proposed total discount for the program. This calculation demonstrated the need for approximately one new patient per week to make the program break even. During the first year of operation, Montana Deaconess averaged slightly more than one new patient per week and, therefore, has added incremental margin to its corporate operations.

Although Montana Deaconess had always served the needs of elderly patients, the advent of the Senior Care Program brought about a change in orientation of the goals of the corporation as well as a reorganization to meet those goals. It was necessary for Montana Deaconess to redevelop a portion of its strategic plan to deal specifically with the eldercare market. In the past Montana Deaconess had dealt with health care for the elderly in the same way as health care for anyone else, namely, by disease or by service, using this same strategy in marketing. With the understanding that new care systems for the aging population are present today and a distinct market exists to be tapped that will only grow in the future, Montana Deaconess changed its plan by reallocating and redeploying resources to capture that market.

Implementation

After the reorientation of the strategic plan and its goals related to the aging market, it was then necessary to effect an organizational change to carry out the plan. Montana Deaconess Medical Center named a coordinator of its Senior Care Program, a specially trained nurse in psychiatry and geriatric care. Finally, to complete the transportation portion of the plan, it was necessary for Montana Deaconess to act as dispatcher for the system. (This system includes Montana Deaconess' wholly owned wheelchair vans, as well as the local taxi company and the local transit authority.)

In carrying out its strategic plan, Montana Deaconess found few barriers to implementation. The Montana Senior Citizens Association initially could have become a barrier due to their antagonistic approach. However, through meetings with the major senior citizen groups, including MSCA, that potential was averted. Some concern was expressed over the cost of the program and whether the cost/benefit ratio would be exceeded. After careful financial analysis, it was proven that the program would pay for itself as well as add incremental revenue and margin with the addition of only one patient per day to the inpatient census.

Finally, as seen throughout the first year of operation of the program, although not a barrier to program implementation, some other Medicare beneficiaries do not participate in the program (for example, those on Medicare disability). However, the Medical Center has maintained that the program is for older adults and not just for Medicare-eligible recipients.

Innovative Services: The Senior Care Program

Montana Deaconess' Senior Care Program consists of the following five categories:

- *Discount scale.* The discount scale is applied to the amount of the bill that the patient must personally pay after Medicare and supplemental insurance payments have been applied. This usually results in a discount of the $592 inpatient Medicare deductible by a percentage factor based on level of income.
- *Senior Card.* The Senior Card ensures quick access to Medical Center services by cutting the time spent on paperwork.
- *Educational benefits.* The Medical Center provides *The Handy Guide to Medicare,* which explains Medicare coverage in simple terms for program participants. The Medical Center also holds educational sessions to help older adults deal with the myriad of insurance forms and the claims-filing process.

- *Clinical screening programs.* Montana Deaconess, through its Home Health Care Division, organizes and operates many clinical screening activities (for example, for blood pressure and diabetes) in the various senior citizen centers in Cascade County and surrounding counties.
- *Transportation.* Montana Deaconess provides free nonemergency transportation to the Medical Center. The transportation service operates 12 hours a day, 5 days a week, and is dispatched through the Medical Center. Through the development of the transportation system, Montana Deaconess has eliminated what it considered to be the primary barrier to the access of health care by the elderly, namely, the inability to get to the hospital or physician's office. This program provides 10,000 transports a year. It has resulted in use of the hospital by more elderly and increased physical therapy, occupational therapy, speech therapy, and emergency department business from all age groups.

Goals

With the advent of the ad hoc advisory committee and the establishment of its Senior Care Program, Montana Deaconess established four goals for the program:

1. The discount portion of the Senior Care Program must be self-funded. This was to be measured by the increase in new Medicare business as the result of implementation of the program.
2. The Medical Center would capitalize on the positive public relations generated from the program.
3. The Medical Center would "lock in" a greater market share of the Medicare business and thereby apply pressure to its major competitor.
4. The program would complement the mission statement of Montana Deaconess, namely, "to take an active part in the promotion of general health in the community; to cooperate and affiliate with persons and organizations having similar purposes; and to establish and maintain a physical and attitudinal environment within which these purposes may be accomplished with the utmost efficiency and economy but without in any way detracting from the quality of the care and service provided."

The realization of these goals is measured in a variety of ways. The first measurement is the total number of members enrolled in the Senior Care Program as a percentage of the total population of Cascade County over age 65. To date, Montana Deaconess has over 70 percent of the eligible population enrolled in the program and has set a realistic goal of 75 percent of the total eligible population becoming enrolled by the end of 1990.

Another measure of the program's success is the number of new members (approximately 15 percent of the total membership) who have not previously been patients at Montana Deaconess. Additionally, approximately 160 members have used services at Montana Deaconess for the first time. This represents an average of slightly more than one new patient per week and, as will be seen in the following section, is a very important measurement in analyzing whether the program is paying for itself and/or generating new revenue for the medical center.

Financing

As noted previously, the program pays for itself. The incremental revenue and margin generated by new Senior Care Program patients at Montana Deaconess have exceeded the cost of discounting cost to the organization. However, it is necessary to allocate resources to the program. These marketing costs are estimated at $5,000 per year. Additionally, there is a cost for the transportation segment of the Senior Care Program, running approximately $50,000 per year. These costs partially arise from a full-time dispatcher, two drivers, and the fees paid to the local taxi company. However, it is felt that these costs are reasonable, because Montana Deaconess has been able to attract an ever-increasing market share of senior citizens.

Perhaps the most important implication of this program is that its organization is flexible and expandable. New segments can be added at any time and with relative ease. Additionally, Montana Deaconess has gathered a very powerful group in Great Falls and Cascade County comprising advocates of the Medical Center on many issues, especially those relating to senior citizens, such as their letters of support for the installation of a magnetic resonance scanner at Montana Deaconess. The Senior Care Program gives the Medical Center a distinct advantage in dealings with the congressional offices and bureaucratic organizations that would not be available under a disorganized or decentralized program.

By initiating the transportation component of the program, Montana Deaconess feels that those elderly individuals who were not accessing health care due to limitations in transportation are now able to be cared for properly, either by their private physicians or at the Medical Center. Additionally, the sliding-scale discount program has also eliminated another barrier to the access of health care by older adults.

Conclusions

Montana Deaconess Medical Center's Senior Care Program has evolved from an initial attempt by a small, organized group of older adults in

Cascade County to increase their political power through a proposed health care plan at Montana Deaconess to a multisegmented program with broad representation from all senior citizen groups. The program consists of an income-based sliding-scale discount on the Medicare deductible and coinsurance payments, education for the elderly in the Medicare program and its ramifications, clinical screenings for various ailments, and a transportation system allowing access to health care by the elderly.

Montana Deaconess, through its Senior Care Program and its ability to expand that program, has positioned itself for the opportunities in the future in developing programs for older adults. Montana Deaconess has developed a program to meet the present needs of the elderly and, through a strategic planning process, is developing the organization to meet the long-range needs of the aging population. Montana Deaconess will continue to develop programs that are accessible, affordable, expandable, and promotable. This is in keeping with Montana Deaconess Medical Center's philosophy–"Excellence with a Personal Touch."

Chapter 14

A Center for Geriatric Care with Case-Management Services

Robert B. Culbertson

Introduction

Morristown Memorial Hospital is a 687-bed health care system located in Morristown, New Jersey, approximately 40 miles from New York City. It includes a 541-bed acute-care division and a 146-bed step-down facility specializing in restorative, rehabilitative, and "short-term long-term" care.

Morristown Memorial is a not-for-profit community teaching hospital affiliated with Columbia University College of Physicians and Surgeons. It serves a middle-income to upper-middle-income suburban population of 426,000, roughly 11 percent of whom are elderly. Morris is among four New Jersey counties with the highest percentage of residents age 75 and over.

Internal/External Environment

With the advent of a large corporate sector, over the years the Hospital service area has experienced significant growth, both in size and income levels. Although there are pockets of low-income elderly in Morris County, the majority are middle income and ineligible for Medicaid or other such programs. Those with chronic needs requiring services beyond the short-term Medicare benefits generally must pay privately for nursing home or home care until their funds are depleted and they become eligible for Medicaid. Most are reluctant to exhaust their funds, however, and will often do without necessary services for as long as possible.

At Morristown Memorial Hospital, Medicare patients comprise 25.1 percent of total admissions and 40.1 percent of total patient days at the acute-care facility. They also account for 73.6 percent of patient days at the skilled nursing and rehabilitation units. Clearly the elderly represent a sizable market for the hospital.

The socioeconomic composition of Morris County makes recruitment of home care and nursing home personnel particularly difficult. This dilemma, coupled with the demands of a growing elderly population that is moving out of acute care more quickly, has driven long-term care costs prohibitively high. Increased mobility of children and dual-career families have resulted in diminished and thus more highly stressed informal supports. These factors have underscored the need for a variety of affordable community support services such as adult day care and respite care.

Planning/Development Process

The evolution of geriatric services at Morristown Memorial Hospital is an excellent example of how optimal planning can become a reality only after the necessary market forces converge. Several independent events coincided over a number of years that led to the development of geriatric services at Morristown Memorial Hospital. First, one of the hospital administrators was interested in expanding hospital services by purchasing Community Medical Center, a small neighboring acute-care hospital, in the mid-1970s. However, this was unacceptable to both hospitals' boards of trustees at that time. Concurrently, the Hospital's assistant vice-president for community services and the assistant to the chairman of the department of medicine perceived mounting unmet service needs of Morris County's elderly, based on the hospital's extensive interactions with community agencies. These three individuals discussed the potential use of the proposed acquisition and identified geriatric services among those that might be appropriate.

In an unrelated but significant development, the New Jersey Department of Health became interested in reducing the oversupply of acute-care beds in Morris County. Consequently they were supportive of the acquisition and its conversion to a step-down facility. When Community Medical Center filed for bankruptcy and a competitor hospital became interested in taking it over, the Morristown Memorial Hospital board approved its purchase in 1978. A feasibility and financial analysis by a consulting firm endorsed the development of skilled nursing and rehabilitation units, and geriatric step-down services were initiated—the culmination of planning influenced by events.

Subsequently, in 1979, the development of a comprehensive geriatric center was endorsed by the Hospital's Long-Range Planning Committee and its board of trustees. Accordingly, an Interagency Planning Committee, chaired by Morristown Memorial Hospital, was established to assess the needs of the community's elderly and to develop a long-term care proposal. State funding of $100,000 was granted in 1980 for capital expenses to develop a comprehensive eldercare center, The Geriatric Living and Learning Center. However, efforts to secure operational funding from government and foundation sources were unsuccessful and development was postponed.

In 1980, the Hospital initiated outreach medical and social services to a neighboring older adult housing complex. Medical services were provided by second-year medical residents under supervision of the assistant to the chairman of the department of internal medicine and the codirector of the residency program. The service was targeted to those who had no family physician and was provided free of charge. It served as a valuable outpatient experience with relatively well elderly for the medical residents. Social work services were provided by graduate social work students. In 1982, a second outreach program was established at Ridge Oak Senior Housing, 8 miles from the Hospital; both programs are still in operation today.

In 1983, the Robert Wood Johnson Foundation (RWJF) issued a request for proposals under its *Hospital Initiatives in Long-Term Care* program, calling for program elements similar to Morristown Memorial's earlier long-term care proposal. A new planning committee was established consisting of key Hospital and community agency personnel. A consensus was reached as to the community's need for eldercare services, and a proposal was submitted. In 1984, the Hospital was awarded a grant by RWJF, and an expanded array of geriatric services was developed under the Center for Geriatric Care.

Because Morristown Memorial Hospital had been under diagnosis-related groups (DRGs) since 1980, the changing nature of health care delivery and its impact on the elderly became apparent fairly early at the Hospital. Accordingly, the need for alternative systems of care and the role of step-down services with decreasing acute-care lengths of stay became fairly well defined. The RWJF funding, received in 1984, enabled the Hospital to develop community care components to broaden its continuum of services for the elderly. Geriatric assessment and case-management programs were seen as crucial toward avoiding inappropriate institutional admissions and maintaining elderly people in their homes.

Upon service development, however, several territorial issues arose. Hospital staff were concerned that these services might duplicate or usurp their role; community agencies claimed they were already doing case management and feared duplication of service and competition for clients. Physicians viewed the geriatric assessment program as competitive and feared the Hospital would steal their patients—not uncommon in areas with an ample supply of physicians and few Medicaid patients.

Additionally, without funds to purchase services, it was difficult to establish credibility and authority with other providers. Morristown

Memorial's funding supports program staff and related costs, not other support services.

Another problem faced in the community is the declining pool of home health aides as requests for service increase. In middle- to upper-middle-income communities, where most people aspire to a college education, there are a limited number of people interested in home care careers, and this same pool is being further drained by working mothers who are hiring them for child care.

Organizational structure issues have also been of concern. While developing the Center for Geriatric Care, the Hospital wrestled with whether it was better to create a new, separate geriatric department or utilize parts of existing units. It was decided that a separate department would create a distinctive geriatric entity whose function would not be clouded by other activities or viewed as belonging to any *one* hospital discipline. Thus, after it was established, the Center for Geriatric Care reported directly to administration, and each discipline (medicine, social work, and nursing) reported to the Center rather than to its respective professional department. This had a number of advantages. The Hospital now had a distinct geriatrics department and the personnel had solely geriatric responsibilities. Also, this structure seemed to dilute interdisciplinary rivalry, with primary allegiance to the Center rather than to the broader disciplines. The Center's administrative and medical directors, formerly from the Hospital departments of social work and internal medicine, relinquished their previous responsibilities and embarked on their new assignments.

Because the Center is located at the step-down facility, over time past ties to the acute division became more distant. Eventually it became apparent that there were some disadvantages to having created a new department removed from the acute-care facility—namely, that the lifeline had been cut, that the Center had become somewhat isolated from the Hospital inpatient setting, and that its previous power base had been eroded. Subsequently the Center has worked to link itself more closely to the inpatient role, reestablish previous connections, and regain old positions of influence. Whereas such an evolution may have been necessary to develop and refine the nature of Morristown Memorial's geriatric program, other institutions considering a similar program should be mindful of the need for visibility, connection, and power positioning within the inpatient mainstream of hospital activity.

Goals

In recognition of the community's growing elderly population and the changing pattern of health care service delivery, Morristown Memorial Hospital established several goals for its geriatric programs. First, the Hospital aimed to develop a competent and caring staff, sensitive to the needs of the elderly and able to provide care of the highest quality to its elderly patients. Education was viewed as a significant vehicle toward this goal, and in 1980 the Hospital hired a geriatric clinical nurse specialist to provide education and consultation with nursing staff. Social work services began extensive in-service training in gerontology, and medical residents were required to serve in the Senior Housing Medical Clinics. A Geriatric Faculty Development Grant was awarded by the state of New Jersey in 1985, and monthly seminars in geriatrics were held for attending physicians, residents, and allied health professionals. Geriatric education for all levels of staff continues to be an ongoing program.

A second goal for the Center for Geriatric Care was to develop a vertically integrated continuum of services that could provide high-quality, cost-effective care for its elderly population, allowing for patients to be moved to the appropriate level of care in a timely, coordinated fashion. Morristown Memorial has developed a variety of step-down services to accomplish this:

- A 50-bed short-term skilled nursing facility (SNF)
- A 28-bed rehabilitation unit
- A geriatric assessment program
- Community case-management service
- In-home and inpatient respite care services
- Outreach clinics
- A Lifeline emergency response system
- Support groups
- Meals on Wheels and weekend meals
- A durable medical equipment for-profit subsidiary

A third goal was to prevent inappropriate hospital and nursing home admissions, thus helping to maintain the elderly in their homes for as long as possible. This goal has been addressed in many ways, particularly by the geriatric assessment and case-management programs. The outpatient geriatric assessment program provides a multidisciplinary evaluation of client and family needs for those elderly having difficulty maintaining their independence. It helps clarify medical diagnoses, ensuring that treatable conditions are identified, and helps develop an appropriate plan of care. Case management coordinates services and ensures continuity of care—in the Hospital and in the community. It ensures that elderly clients' posthospital needs are being met, and it can help avoid unnecessary acute flare-ups of chronic conditions resulting from inadequate home support.

Case Management and Assessment

Morristown Memorial Hospital began providing case-management services in January 1985, through the Center for Geriatric Care.

Since the Center proposal was developed by both hospital and community personnel, entry to its case-management component was designed to be available from both the Hospital and the community. Individuals age 65 and above in the Hospital service area who are identified as "at risk" and in need of planning, coordinating, and monitoring assistance are eligible. Persons are considered at risk if they:

1. Have significant physical impairment that interferes with functioning
2. Have cognitive or behavioral difficulties that interfere with functioning
3. Require home or community-based health or social services to remain in the community
4. Have fragile informal supports that may no longer be able to provide needed services

These criteria were purposely written broadly and were intended to make the service accessible.

Case management is provided by a bachelor's-level case manager, a master's-level social worker, and a master's-level geriatric clinical nurse specialist. Clients eligible for the New Jersey Medicaid Community Care Waiver Program are case managed by the Medicaid office, so that most services are purchased with the client's funds.

Many demonstration (model) community care projects have focused on an indigent population eligible for Medicaid benefits and other such services. These, however, have limited application in the middle- to upper-middle-income community here because there are so few Medicaid-eligible residents. Even if one is eligible for Medicaid, he or she is managed by the Medicaid Community Care Program, so there are no clients who can garner significant publicly sponsored services beyond the short-term Medicare–funded home care services. Furthermore, although many people in the community have some financial resources, they are reluctant to spend these lest they deplete their funds and become impoverished. It is hard to explain to someone that, to become eligible for Medicaid-sponsored home care or nursing home services, he or she must exhaust life savings.

There are four case-management agencies in Morris County, and a case-management committee was established to develop a common definition of case management so as to establish an assignment protocol. The two public case-management agencies are the Morris County Board of Social Services and the Medicaid District Office of Morris County. The two private agencies are at Morristown and the Pequannock Valley Mental Health Center. It was agreed that the case-management agency from which a case originates is designated as the case manager, unless regulatory or funding guidelines mandate a reassignment. In situations not resolved in this manner, the case manager is determined by the case-management committee. Complex care cases can also be brought to this committee for interagency planning and problem resolution. The Center for Geriatric Care is the central access point into the case-management system for Morristown Memorial Hospital patients and provides case management until the client is either enrolled with another provider or is no longer appropriate for case-management services.

Case management extends Hospital services into the community and provides ongoing follow-up, coordination, and monitoring of health care needs for frail elderly clients before admission and after discharge. In many respects, the Center for Geriatric Care model initially resembled a community social services agency that just happened to be located at this site. Primary focus was on assessing the needs of clients in the community and mobilizing and coordinating community services. After a trial period of several months, however, it appeared that hospital discharges could be expedited and lengths of stay shortened if the Center became a resource to which Hospital staff could refer frail elderly with limited posthospital resources for postdischarge follow-up. Physicians, discharge planners, and other staff felt a bit more comfortable knowing that these patients would be monitored after discharge, and some of the pressures they were feeling under the DRG reimbursement system were eased.

Several months later, as a considerable number of clients were enrolled in the case-management service, perhaps its most important role to the Hospital was identified, the role it can play when these clients are admitted to the Hospital as inpatients. As case-management clients they are not new patients to the Morristown Memorial Hospital system *but simply new to the acute-care part of the system.* The case manager has access to voluminous client information that can be communicated to the inpatient staff—home setting, family and other supports, physician, prior level of functioning, even finances, for example. All are data vital to trying to assess, treat, and plan for discharge of a new patient. When the Center could profile a new admission for the acute-care social worker and include a tentative discharge plan—all *before* the social worker had even heard of the patient—proof of success was evident. Now all admission slips are reviewed each day by the case managers, and inpatient staff is notified of admissions of case-managed patients. This has saved time, improved the acute-care staff's understanding of the patient, helped ensure better continuity of care, and contributed to shorter patient stays.

Innovative Services

With the advent of the RWJF-sponsored Center for Geriatric Care, a number of new services were developed:

- Comprehensive Geriatric Assessment Program
- Case Management

- Holiday Guest Program
- Medicare Education, Counseling, and Form Completion Service

Comprehensive Geriatric Assessment Program

The Comprehensive Geriatric Assessment Program is an outpatient consultation service targeted to the frail elderly (and their families) who are having difficulty maintaining their independence and seek clarification of medical diagnoses and help in planning how the older adult can best be cared for at home. It is supplemental to the family physician and is to be viewed similarly to other specialty consultations.

The core interdisciplinary geriatric team (geriatrician, geriatric nurse practitioner, and geriatric social worker) assesses the patient and family needs over a two- to two-and-a-half-hour period. The geriatric nurse makes the initial visit to the home, and social work and physician assessments are conducted at the Center. Medications, nutrition, family interaction, supports, financial resources, and medical condition are evaluated; and laboratory, X-ray, and EKG studies are conducted. Any additional tests are subsequently ordered as needed, and the patient and family return to the Center within one or two weeks for a conference, during which the team's findings and recommendations are thoroughly discussed. It should be noted that this hour-long conference, for which all team members including the physician are present, is highly valued and appreciated by the clients. Their questions are answered in an unrushed forum, and they can consider care-planning suggestions more readily when they are reinforced by the physician. A report outlining findings, recommendations, and a plan of care is sent to the family physician for follow-up, and a copy is given to the patient and family. The majority of referrals have come from care givers, particularly adult children. Only a minimal number of physicians have referred to this service, which many deem competitive or threatening.

Case Management

The case-management service has been described in this chapter in considerable detail and will not be repeated here. The Center has joined the Lifeplans Family Caring Network, a national network of case-management agencies serving purchasers of long-term care insurance; referrals have been received only since January 1990.

Holiday Guest Program

The Holiday Guest Program offers clients an overnight stay in the SNF for those requiring a more extensive respite. The elderly person is registered as a guest rather than admitted as a patient. This precludes a physician's history and physical and extensive departmental documentation requirements, which reduces costs. The guests bring their own medications from home, which are reviewed, stored, and administered by nursing staff. Guests participate in recreational activities, take their meals in the dining room, and have new socialization opportunities while their care giver has a break or goes on vacation. Guests may stay from one night up to two weeks. The fee for patients with Alzheimer's disease may be defrayed by funding from the Alzheimer's Disease Family Support Group of Morris County. Other clients must pay privately. The program provides much-needed overnight respite for highly stressed families and may provide a way for hospitals to fill empty beds, particularly on weekends.

Medicare Education, Counseling, and Form Completion Service

A program to help the elderly and their families understand Medicare, its gaps, supplemental insurance, and claim forms was developed jointly by the Morris County Retired Senior Volunteer Program (RSVP) and the Center for Geriatric Care. A group of volunteers was recruited by RSVP, and training sessions were conducted by local insurance professionals and agency staff. Retired Senior Volunteer Program volunteers staff several community sites and visit people at home to discuss Medicare and help complete claim forms. Not only has this service been helpful to the elderly in the community but has provided a rich experience for the volunteers.

New services being considered include congregate housing, life care, adult day care, specialized units for those with Alzheimer's disease, transportation service to the Hospital, and development of long-term care beds.

Financing

As previously discussed, initial components of the geriatric program were funded by the hospital through existing and new personnel and complemented by medical residents and graduate students in the allied health professions. Step-down facility renovations were funded by a bond issue. Additional elements were funded in a variety of ways, generally combining governmental and foundation funding with internal sources of support. For instance, Lifeline (the emergency response system) was initiated with support from Morristown Memorial Hospital's Women's Association and is maintained through a sliding-scale client fee system.

The weekend meals program is also supported by Morristown Division on Aging and Morristown Memorial Hospital subsidies combined with client fees. The State of New Jersey Department of Higher Education supported the geriatric education program for attending medical staff. The Division of Aging of the New Jersey Department of Community Affairs, in conjunction with the Morris County Department on Aging, helped initiate respite care programs. Additional support for inpatient respite care was received from the Alzheimer's Disease Family Support Group of Morris County. The Edythe and Dean Dowling Foundation provided generous support for the development of an extensive geriatric collection in the Morristown Memorial Hospital library and for education programs for seniors and the community. The Robert Wood Johnson Foundation provided a large grant, which enabled the Hospital to develop its community care component—comprehensive assessment, case management, and outreach programs—and to broaden and refocus its overall geriatric services. Support from the New Jersey Department of Health Gerontology Program, the Rutgers Community Health Foundation, and the Morris County Department of Human Services have helped maintain the program.

The comprehensive assessment service is reimbursed by Medicare and should at least become self-supporting, as it is not a revenue producer for the Hospital. Case-management services were initially provided at no charge, but fee structure experimentation is under way as of this writing. Although no firm results are in, early impressions suggest that it is difficult to ascribe charges for the case-management service and that several charging methods may be required. There appears to be one group of clients who need long-term case management, and they or their families may be willing to pay a fixed monthly fee on an ongoing basis. The larger group, however, appears to require short-term case management, perhaps one to six encounters, and may be charged on an hourly basis or at a package rate. People who have requested the service are more likely to pay than those referred by Hospital staff or other third parties. It is suggested that, whereas some revenue can be generated through a fee-for-service system, it is unlikely that case management can be totally self-supporting. What appears more likely is that the case-management service may be viewed by the Hospital as a loss leader—bringing clients into the Hospital system, directing them to many of its services, and helping them more easily utilize these services. This may enhance the Hospital's reputation as a caring, efficient, and "user-friendly" institution that provides exceptional care to its elderly clients, thus preserving and enhancing market share.

Conclusions

Morristown Memorial Hospital has developed a range of services for the elderly, allowing it to move patients to the most appropriate, least-costly level of care in a timely fashion. It has the core components of a system of care and now needs to add new elements to the continuum and link them together in a new, more cohesive organizational structure. The elderly appear to be the largest future market for hospitals, and it is in Morristown Memorial's interest to develop a caring, efficient, and cost-effective health care system that is sensitive to the needs of these consumers. It is toward this goal that Morristown Memorial Hospital has striven and will continue to strive in its quest to be a center of excellence in care for the older adult.

Chapter 15

A Geriatrics Department at a Major Metropolitan Hospital

Judith L. Howe, Rein Tideiksaar, and Robert N. Butler, M.D.

Introduction

The Mount Sinai Medical Center consists of the Mount Sinai Hospital, one of five large teaching hospitals in the New York City metropolitan area, and the Mount Sinai School of Medicine, one of nine medical schools in the metropolitan area.

The hospital, founded in 1852, now has 112 beds; it had 336,933 inpatient days and 309,252 outpatient visits in 1989. The medical school, established in 1963, has an annual enrollment of 492 medical students and 41 M.D./Ph.D. students. The Mount Sinai Medical Center is affiliated with Beth Israel Medical Center, City Hospital Center at Elmhurst, the Jewish Home and Hospital for Aged, North General Hospital, the Bronx Veterans Administration Medical Center, and Englewood Hospital, all of which are located in the New York City metropolitan area.

The Mount Sinai Hospital's informal catchment area is between East 96th Street and East 129th Street, bordered by Fifth Avenue and the East River. This is a 288-square-block area located on the upper East Side of Manhattan. There were almost 12,000 people age 65 and over in the hospital catchment area in 1980, with almost 40 percent of this population in the age 75–84 category. Eighteen percent of the older population is white, 35 percent Hispanic, and 45 percent black. Forty percent of this older group live alone.

The Gerald and May Ellen Ritter Department of Geriatrics and Adult Development, the first department of geriatrics in a U.S. medical school, was founded at the Mount Sinai Medical Center in 1982.

Goals

The overall goal of the Ritter Department of Geriatrics is to assist contemporary medicine in learning and applying the skills, knowledge, and attitudes that will ease the impact of the demographic revolution described in chapter 2. Specific objectives of the Department of Geriatrics are as follows:

- To develop clinical programs in geriatrics encompassing the care of older adults in the hospital, community, and nursing home settings. The clinical programs are designed to address acute and chronic medical problems, rehabilitative care, and preventive care.
- To develop educational and training programs for medical students, physicians, and other health professionals, as well as older adults themselves.
- To develop basic biomedical, clinical, and health policy research directed toward current topics in geriatrics and gerontology.

During the past seven years the department's impact within the institution has grown substantially, aided by increased awareness among the general population of the growth in the number of older adults. The department now works collaboratively with many departments and programs within the medical center, sharing clinical and research resources and goals. For instance, it works with the Department of Psychiatry in providing psychiatric inpatient and outpatient care to older patients with dementia and depression. The department operates an osteoporosis clinical assessment and treatment program with the Department of Obstetrics, Gynecology, and Reproductive Sciences. Recently the department entered into an agreement with the Department of Medicine enabling all medical house staff to rotate through the geriatrics inpatient unit for one month. This will ensure that all medical residents are exposed to the content and approaches of geriatric medicine, particularly important because an increasing number of patients will be older.

Collaborative programs with Mount Sinai's institutional affiliates have also expanded. Geriatric fellows rotate throughout The Jewish Home and Hospital for Aged and the Bronx Veterans Administration Medical Center. Departmental faculty members also supervise clinical programs in geriatrics at these sites.

Planning/Development Process

The creation of the Department of Geriatrics and Adult Development in 1982 culminated the efforts of the president and dean of the Mount Sinai School of Medicine, Thomas Chalmers, M.D., and key members of the board of trustees. They had been working for several years to create a stronger focus on aging within the medical center, believing that population aging represents a major global public health problem that Dr. Chalmers regarded as second only to the threat of nuclear war. This group saw the training of physicians and other health professionals in the principles and practice of geriatrics as crucial for the care of a rapidly expanding older population.

Original plans called for an institute on gerontology and geriatrics to replace the already existing Division of Geriatrics within the Department of Medicine. However, after consultation it was decided that a freestanding department of geriatrics with clinical, educational, and research components was needed. This arrangement would more adequately meet the needs of the older population, give geriatrics academic presence within the institution, and provide a model for other academic institutions. As a department, there would be a greater claim on the institutional resources needed to make an impact on clinical, educational, and research programs. For instance, a full department in both the medical school and the hospital could have access to hospital beds and curriculum teaching time, whereas an institute could not lay claim to these resources as easily.

The primary barrier to the department's development was the pressure to establish it in a very brief period, whereas under usual circumstances a program with as many components would be developed over many more years. Expectations to develop comprehensive clinical, educational, and research programs may have been unrealistically high on the part of senior management and clinical staff at Mount Sinai because of positive advance publicity prior to the department's establishment. However, necessary resources, such as space and planning staff, were not in place, and key understandings (for example, about bed reallocation) had not been completed with other departments. Institutional barriers have been overcome to a great extent, assisted in part by the recruitment of faculty with geriatric experience and strong external supports from foundations, the media, and key individuals.

Within the institution some resistance has been encountered from physicians, generally internists, who do not understand the rationale for a freestanding clinical department of geriatrics. However, this is not a uniform reaction and has abated over time, in part because of an increasing awareness among physicians about the impact of the older population on health care trends. This has come about for a number of reasons, including the impact of DRGs on practice and successful efforts to educate physicians and other providers about geriatrics. The department has developed several education programs geared to practicing physicians. These include a geriatrics education center in conjunction with Hunter College's Brookdale Center on Aging, one of 30 such centers funded by the federal government, which trains physicians and other health professionals in geriatrics. The New York Statewide Resource Center for Geriatric Education, operated in collaboration with the Health Sciences Center at Syracuse, disseminates information on geriatrics to a wide professional audience. The department also sponsors a review course to prepare physicians for the geriatrics competency examination. These programs have mainstreamed geriatrics and contributed to a greater understanding of the principles and practice of geriatrics among physicians and other health professionals.

Case Management and Assessment

The underlying principle of case management for the Department of Geriatrics is the interdisciplinary team approach. Only through this approach can the fragmentation of care for older adults in the hospital, nursing home, and community settings be avoided. Case management has taken on much greater importance since the institution of DRGs and the need for more timely discharge. The department has developed a range of both inpatient and outpatient services for older adults, with as much continuity of care as possible. For instance, physicians attend to different services and the nursing and social work departments have organized geriatric units to better ensure coordination of care and tracking among clinical components. The outpatient clinic has established a mechanism for alerting physicians if a patient has an unscheduled hospital admission.

Inpatient Geriatric Services

Inpatient geriatric services consist of the Geriatric Evaluation and Treatment Unit, the Geriatric Consultation Service, the Jewish Home and Hospital for Aged and the Bronx Veterans Administration Medical Center, described below:

- *The Geriatric Evaluation and Treatment Unit* is a 16-bed unit designed to assist frail elderly patients (generally 75 years or over) in achieving their highest functional level, using an interdisciplinary approach. In general, these are patients who would be candidates for follow-up in the geriatrics clinic or faculty practice after discharge from the hospital. Patients are referred through attending physicians in the Department of Geriatrics, thus ensuring the appropriateness of patient admissions. In addition, patients not previously known to the department may be evaluated for admission in the emergency room.
- *The Geriatric Consultation Service* assists medical and nonmedical services in evaluating and treating frail elderly patients with multiple medical and functional problems. Patients are referred to the consultation service from Mount Sinai Hospital's emergency room, outpatient clinics, medical and surgical inpatient services, individual attending physicians, and to the Jewish Home and Hospital for Aged.
- *The Jewish Home and Hospital for Aged* is the department's teaching nursing home and operates a rehabilitation unit for the frail elderly. This

program uses a team approach to help patients achieve a level of independence that will enable them to return to the community. Many of the patients, with an average age of 80, have complex medical problems, have experienced prolonged hospital stays, and would be at high risk for permanent institutionalization if rehabilitation services were not available. Referrals are accepted from all components and affiliates of Mount Sinai, as well as a variety of other hospital and community sources within the New York City metropolitan area.

Criteria for admission include a minimum age of 60, cognitive ability to comprehend and follow the rehabilitation program, stable medical condition, and the potential to return to a suitable home environment or more independent life-style in a long-term care institutional setting. The rehabilitation team is made up of a geriatrician, a nurse social worker, a geriatric fellow, a physiatrist, a psychiatrist, and a medical student.

- *The Bronx Veterans Administration Medical Center* operates a 120-bed nursing home that is managed by several departmental faculty members. In addition, special attention is being directed to the care and study of spinal cord injury victims, a population that is living longer than in the past.

Outpatient Geriatric Services

Outpatient services include a number of different programs:

- *The Phyllis and Lee Coffey Outpatient Geriatrics Clinic* provides comprehensive care to the frail elderly who often have multiple interactive problems. The clinic opened in 1983; its mission is to restore and maintain the patient's functional independence in the community. The clinic has a team of professionals trained in geriatric medicine, nursing, social work, neuropsychology, neurology, psychiatry, clinical pharmacology, and physical and occupational therapy. In 1989 the clinic served about 700 patients through approximately 3,500 visits.

  Both primary and/or consultative care is provided, depending on the patient's underlying health problems and whether the patient already has a primary care clinician. The clinic's population is frail, with an average age of 83 and a high incidence of cognitive impairment (acute confusion, organic brain syndrome, depression, and anxiety). Those patients with specific problems, such as urinary incontinence, falling or gait problems, and osteoporosis, are referred to the subspecialty clinics, such as the Falls and Immobility Program.
- *The Falls and Immobility Program* identifies, diagnoses, and treats elderly patients who have fallen or are at risk of falling, in order to prevent further falls. Established criteria for acceptance include community living status, age 60 or older, a history of falls, and a commitment to

participate in ongoing evaluation. The treatment team consists of a geriatrician and a gerontologist/physician's assistant.
- *The Osteoporosis and Metabolic Bone Disease Program* provides screening, diagnosis, and treatment for patients with a variety of metabolic bone diseases. This program is managed in collaboration with the Department of Obstetrics, Gynecology and Reproductive Science.
- *The Urinary Incontinence Program* involves the departments of Geriatrics and Urology, offering a team approach to the assessment and treatment of incontinence.

In association with the Senior Division of the 92nd Street YMCA–YWCA, the Department of Geriatrics sponsors a *Well Elderly Program* at the 92nd Street YMCA–YWCA geared to health promotion and disease prevention for independent elderly living in the community.

- The Ritter Department operates a *faculty private practice,* Geriatric Medicine Associates, which offers both consultation and primary care for a broad range of problems. In addition to specialized geriatric assessments, the private practice emphasizes the integration of all components of a patient's care and refers patients to the Ritter Department's special emphasis programs as appropriate.
- The department participates in several community programs, including the East Harlem Living at Home Program, a multifoundation-funded case-management effort sponsored by the East Harlem Council for Human Services and other agencies. It also participates in patient education and information dissemination programs. For instance, an Alzheimer's disease information coordinator works with community groups to increase awareness of available resources and services.

Financing

The Ritter Department is supported by budgetary, grant, affiliate, faculty private practice, and endowment funds. In addition, seed money was provided for start-up costs such as clinic, office, and laboratory renovations. Although the Department of Geriatrics has a guaranteed budget from both hospital and school sources, it is necessary to continually seek funding from outside agencies, both private and governmental, to maintain current levels of operation. During 1989, grant and affiliate funds exceeded budgetary funds by a ratio of 2 to 1. The department successfully sought funding for four endowed professorships, including the chairman's, a vice-chairman's, and two research professorships.

In addition to major multiyear research projects in the areas of Alzheimer's disease, osteoporosis and metabolic bone disease, gait and falls, and data management, to name a few areas, the department has received funding for several training programs geared to midcareer physicians, academic physician development, and geriatric nurse practitioners. In addition to budgetary and grant funds, faculty and fellows are supported by budgetary agreements with Mount Sinai affiliates.

The department supports 11 fellows in its two-year fellowship program and, in addition to budgetary, grant, and affiliate support, has received private funding for several of these positions. In the beginning the facility lacked stable funding for fellowships. However, fellows in geriatrics are now supported by Medicare (Part A) funds through a federal waiver aimed at stimulating training programs in geriatrics.

Revenues from the department's faculty practice, although relatively small, provide important discretionary funds to the chairman for such activities as research projects, travel, and staff bridging support.

The department also sponsors a unit devoted to policy studies, which has received substantial funding from private foundations and donors. It has directed its attention to health policy issues such as long-term care and productive aging, for example, how to mobilize the continuing productivity of older adults.

Looking into the future, it is clear that the department's fund-raising initiatives must continue with even greater intensity, particularly in the face of reimbursement mechanisms such as Medicare DRGs and substantial cutbacks in National Institutes of Health research funds. This, of course, has an impact on departmental operations because of the considerable staff resources necessary for proposal writing, fund-raising, donor relations, community outreach, and the myriad of activities related to developing outside sources of funding. In light of these considerations, the department recently established four major endowment funds for junior faculty, faculty research, Alzheimer's disease research, and clinical services. To some extent these funds will offset continuing cutbacks in Medicare reimbursements and federal support for research.

Conclusions

The Ritter Department of Geriatrics and Adult Development has developed clinical, educational, and research programs that encompass the community, acute hospital, and nursing home settings. Emphasis is placed on addressing those problems unique to older people, for example, dementia, urinary incontinence, osteoporosis, falls, and immobility, and on teaching preventive, acute, and chronic care as well as rehabilitative care to medical students, physicians, and other health professionals. The department's challenge will become even greater in the years ahead as the population ages in the face of diminishing resources for the provision of adequate health and long-term care.

Chapter 16

A Geriatric Program Serving an Indigent Population

Paula A. Loftis, Maria Garza Reynolds, Craig D. Rubin, M.D., Mark T. Sizemore, and Ron J. Anderson, M.D.

Introduction

Parkland Memorial Hospital is a 750-bed public hospital located in Dallas, Texas. It is the primary teaching hospital for the University of Texas Southwestern Medical Center at Dallas and serves the residents of Dallas County, which includes the city of Dallas and 22 additional communities.

Parkland provides a wide range of primary and tertiary health care services. In 1984, when the Parkland Geriatric Initiative was under development, there were 35,526 admissions, 272,125 outpatient clinic visits, and 153,215 emergency room visits. Approximately 3,000 (rounded) of the patients admitted were over age 65 (see table 16-1), with this number accounting for slightly more than 8 percent of the inpatient admissions and 13 percent of inpatient days. Demographic shifts have brought significant growth into the Dallas and Southwest area, and in the future these percentages should increase. The 1980 census reported that 121,532 people over age 65 reside in Dallas County. An increase to 153,471 is projected for 1990.

The elderly are more likely to have multiple medical problems than are their younger cohorts. Exacerbations of underlying medical problems necessitating hospital admission often occur. For example, the extreme summer temperatures in Dallas have resulted in high morbidity and mortality rates for this population.[1,2] Malnutrition and volume depletion are frequent hospital admission diagnoses.

In addition, a substantial portion of the elderly served in the area have lived and continue to live below the poverty level. The frail elderly who are also poor comprise a special "at-risk" population that is 2.5 times more likely to be unhealthy than the nonpoor. Their needs and service demands are wide ranging and include housing, transportation assistance,

Table 16-1. 1984 Admissions for Patients over Age 65, Parkland Memorial Hospital, Dallas (in percent)

Race	Male	Female	Both Sexes
Black	55	53	54
White	35	36	35
Hispanic	10	9.5	10
Other	1	1.5	1
	43	57	100

N = 2,964.

homemaker help, home-delivered meals, home health care, financial assistance programs, adult day care, nutrition, hospice care, and respite care. The elderly require more *coordinated care,* and a cost-efficient system for providing this care has emerged as a high-priority concern.

Internal/External Environment

Because of the volume of patients and the continual demand for hospital beds, Parkland's main priority is acute care. With Parkland Hospital serving as a teaching hospital for the University of Texas Southwestern Medical Center, the physician staff consists predominantly of interns and residents. As house staff, these physicians constantly rotate through different inpatient and outpatient services, and their tenure at the hospital is limited to their required years of training.

Parkland's extensive outpatient clinic, which attempts to provide long-term follow-up care, is constantly confronted with two major barriers to delivering this care. First, the large volume of patients often makes waiting times longer than desired and physician contact briefer than desired; second, unavoidable gaps in continuity of care are imposed by the rotation of physicians.

Ancillary services exist at Parkland with an extensive staff of social workers who attempt to meet the needs of the patients, nursing personnel who function in positions as discharge planners, and nursing staff trained in patient education. These services, however, often are not fully utilized because of the emphasis placed on acute care. Patients come to Parkland physically ill and once deemed "well" are returned to the community. Communications with the ancillary services may be limited, and frequently no attention is paid to discharge planning.

Unless a physician is sensitive to the social, nursing, and long-term needs of an elderly patient, those needs will not be addressed. Despite the need for physician education in this regard, until recently there had been no formal education of the house staff in the area of geriatrics. Elderly patients were viewed merely as part of the continuum of the population that Parkland serves.

Community organizations in the hospital's service area have contributed to the development of an improved system of long-term care to meet the social and health needs of the elderly. In the forefront has been the Dallas Area Agency on Aging (DAAA), which has as its major responsibility the development of a comprehensive and coordinated delivery system of supportive services for the elderly population. Since 1979, the DAAA has funded the Access Center for the Elderly (ACE), a case-management program for individuals age 60 and over with multiple and/or complex needs. In that capacity ACE has functioned as a catalyst for agencies serving the elderly population to merge in a coordinated effort to provide comprehensive services. Initially sponsored by the Community Council of Greater Dallas, the ACE project is now administered by Parkland with continued DAAA funding. Home health care agencies and other social services agencies also have established links with Parkland.

Over the years, however, communications between Parkland and the community agencies have been less than optimal. Although no area institution is as important to the elderly indigent community as is Parkland, Parkland was in many ways an island. Patients were sent from the community and were often "lost" in the Parkland system. The case managers for ACE found that continuity of care following hospital discharge was not evident for many of their clients and that their efforts to achieve it often were thwarted by "the system." Also, ACE clients were found to continue to use Parkland services as their primary source of entry into the health care system.

In 1983, to improve communications DAAA funded a geriatric case-management program based at Parkland to coordinate the case management and discharge planning for elderly persons with difficult and/or multiple health and social problems. The geriatric case-management program, staffed and managed by Parkland, now works closely together with ACE. Some patients are referred to ACE case managers by social workers in geriatrics for continued coordination of services and follow-up in the community. Conversely, ACE case managers refer those requiring health care to Parkland social workers for assistance in finding their way through the hospital system. Geriatric social workers provide valuable input in developing patient care plans and in providing follow-up to ACE for continued supportive intervention. Perhaps this program more than any other paved the way for what was to become the Geriatric Assessment Team through its reinforcement of community links.

Goals

Serving one of the country's largest indigent populations and operating as the teaching hospital for the University of Texas Southwestern Medical

Center, Parkland represents a community and national model, and these functions are essential to its goals. Parkland's main goal is to provide the highest quality of medical care to the medically indigent population of Dallas County. Working with limited resources and faced with increasing demands placed on these resources, Parkland is exploring cost-efficient ways of delivering this care.

Planning/Development Process

The need for an alternative approach to eldercare was widely acknowledged at Parkland. In 1983, a formal assessment of service gaps to the elderly was conducted with assistance from the Southwest Long-Term Care Gerontology Center at the University of Texas Southwestern Medical Center. Medical records of patients age 65 and older were randomly selected and reviewed to examine utilization patterns, complexity of problems, and thoroughness of discharge plans. Results of the analysis confirmed observations by the ACE case managers:

- Many elderly Parkland patients were found to be long-term and multiple-repeat users of inpatient and outpatient services.
- Many were found to have multiple medical and social problems.
- A number of them had no well-documented discharge plans.

The findings suggested poor continuity of care into the community. A series of feasibility studies addressed reorientation of Parkland's acute-care goals to consider the more comprehensive social and health care needs of the elderly. The community support systems were reexamined, and interest grew in the development of an interdisciplinary approach to the care of the ambulatory older adult patient.

Ironically, at the same time a grant was offered by the Robert Wood Johnson Foundation for the establishment of alternative approaches to the long-term care of the elderly. Parkland Memorial Hospital was chosen as one of the sites to be funded by the grant.

In 1984, preliminary meetings were held to further define this "interdisciplinary approach." Participants included representatives from Parkland Memorial Hospital (social work, nursing, administration), the community (DAAA), the Southwest Long-Term Care Gerontology Center, and the Southwestern Medical School (representatives from internal medicine and psychiatry). During these sessions the links with the community were strengthened, and commitments from individuals to participate in the final project were determined. The final structuring and the mechanics of operation of the Geriatric Assessment Team was formalized.

Implementation of the program met with certain difficulties. First, because the concept of geriatrics was new at the medical school, no physicians were available who had specialized training in the field. The decision was made to recruit internists already familiar with the system who had an interest in and a willingness to become knowledgeable about geriatrics. Second, much debate revolved around the proposed study design of the program and the eventual eligibility criteria. Community representatives wanted to make direct geriatric referrals to the team from its inception. However, because of the agreed-upon study design and the need to collect a data base on each patient, patient eligibility criteria were based on a research protocol.

Geriatric Assessment

In its final structuring the Geriatric Assessment Team at Parkland consists of the following:

- A director/advanced nurse practitioner
- A geriatric clinical nurse specialist
- Nurse clinicians
- A geriatric aide/assistant
- Geriatric social workers
- Internal medicine physicians
- A dietitian
- An education coordinator
- A geropsychiatrist

In an attempt to overcome the impediments to optimal care for the elderly at Parkland, the objectives of the Geriatric Assessment Program were the following:

- To improve the quality and delivery of coordinated long-term care services to the elderly of Dallas County through case management and an interdisciplinary geriatric assessment process
- To provide leadership within the community through the education of hospital staff and students, community health care workers, physicians, and other professionals who provide services to the elderly
- To develop a model program that will best utilize existing resources and create alternative programs to meet the needs of the elderly requiring long-term care
- To establish a research model to provide objective data on interdisciplinary care of the elderly and to provide other geriatric research opportunities

The Geriatric Assessment Team offers continuity in patient care, health maintenance, and promotion measures, in addition to total assessment of the patient's physical and psychosocial status. The team coordinates a wide range of services to enable older adults to remain in the community and at a maximum functional level. The team works with social services organizations, local home health care providers, and visiting nurse associations to enhance the follow-up care. The cooperative relationship, feedback, and assistance provided to the team from these community resources is indispensable.

The team intends that the following benefits will accrue:

- Early detection of problem cases
- Integrated, interdisciplinary approaches to case management and service delivery
- Increased continuity and quality of care
- Creation of a cadre of highly trained geriatric health care providers who will have an impact on the hospital delivery system
- Education of other hospital personnel regarding geriatric health care and optimal utilization of the Geriatric Assessment Team
- A basis for investigating cost-effectiveness of specialized team management and treatment
- An increase in patient compliance and satisfaction
- A willingness and cooperative spirit among community-based providers, health science center educators, and the Parkland staff

The question has been raised of whether a team such as Parkland's might be replicated in other settings. Although Parkland's program is unique in many ways, replication should be feasible. Key steps in the process are, first, recruit team members from within the system. It is of great benefit to work with those familiar with the system's strengths and limitations and those eager to work together to improve that system. Second, develop links with community agencies whose assistance frequently will be needed. If community contacts have been established, strengthen these links through increased communication and feedback. Third, recognize the limitations of the team. It must not be prematurely overextended, or the unique benefits the team offers will be sacrificed.

Accurate patient selection, evaluation, and case management are the keys to successful geriatric assessment.

Patient Selection

Patient selection targets the frail elderly, those whose illnesses, impairments, and social problems reduce their functional ability. Because of their multiple and chronic problems, these vulnerable high-risk patients are candidates for frequent hospitalization and premature institutionalization. To be accepted for geriatric assessment the individuals should be age 70 or older and have evidence of functional impairment. An attempt is made to exclude patients who will not benefit from services, such as terminally ill patients or those who otherwise have no rehabilitation potential.

Referrals are accepted from physicians, other health care professionals, family, and friends. The patients are assessed by the interdisciplinary team. The assessment is based on mental and physical health status, functional abilities, financial/social situation, and medical profile.

Patient Evaluation and Case Management

Geriatric case management is defined here as the coordination of multiple services for older adult clients through a process of assessment, planning, and arranging for and monitoring of services. To accomplish this, the active patient is evaluated by appropriate team members with regard to his or her specified medical, social, and nursing needs. All members of the Geriatric Assessment Team then meet for a formal staffing session during which recommendations are made for the patient's discharge and long-term care. Referrals are made as needed to community services, which include the following:

- Home care and individual support
- Transportation
- Housing
- Community-based mental health services
- Financial assistance
- Informal and family support
- Nutrition and meal services
- Socialization and/or day care
- Nursing home placement if required

Even though some patients are referred to ACE and other outside agencies, they continue to be followed by the assessment team members, who are ultimately responsible for the continued monitoring of needs and coordination of services.

Follow-up in the geriatric clinic, which is staffed by the entire geriatric assessment team, includes:

- A review of the effectiveness of the discharge plan
- A review of the effectiveness of community-based referral services
- A reassessment of health maintenance, physical and psychological
- Immediate telephone follow-up for missed clinic appointments
- Regular rescheduling to the geriatric clinic

Innovative Services

Geriatric assessment at Parkland began with development of the Geriatric Assessment Team. Once data collection was completed, the team was expanded to be open to hospital and community referrals through geriatric outpatient consultation and primary care clinics. The patients most likely to benefit from these geriatric services have full access to them.

Geriatric Assessment Team activities are now concentrated mostly on ambulatory care. The five-year strategic plan for geriatrics at Parkland includes the establishment of a separate geriatric evaluation unit specialized in providing acute inpatient care for elderly patients and educating the house staff in this acute geriatric care. Other activities will focus on the development of an inpatient geriatric consultation service for evaluation of complicated clinical presentations, continued geriatric research, and decentralization of services through a community-oriented primary care system.

The team is now in its infancy. Realizing these long-term goals will require staff expansion and certainly increased financial support.

Financing

In 1984, the Geriatric Assessment Team was initiated by a grant from the Robert Wood Johnson Foundation Program for Hospital Initiatives in Long-Term Care. A total of $650,000 was allotted to fund the team for four years. Parkland Memorial Hospital has made a commitment for continued support from the board of managers to continue the program and fund its operation from regular operating funds and additional grants.

Conclusions

Those experienced in eldercare readily acknowledge the special needs of the elderly. Those in different fields, however, emphasize those needs from their own perspectives. Physicians have their own biases, as do social workers, nurses, and other providers. All of these providers of gerontological services, however, are limited in what they can accomplish independently; therefore all disciplines must recognize their need for each other.

Efforts have been made to make maximum use of the resources of the community and of Parkland Memorial Hospital to provide care for the indigent geriatric population of Dallas County. Funding through the Robert Wood Johnson Foundation permitted initiation of these efforts.

Through a combined interdisciplinary and synergistic approach, the quality of geriatric care has been improved. Efforts will continue to educate the academic and private medical communities to recognize the need for a continuum of care based on case management and geriatrics as a distinct clinical science.

References

1. Hart, G. R., Anderson, R. J., Crumpler, C. P., Shulkin, A., Reed, W. G., and Knochel, J. Epidemic classical heat stroke: clinical characteristics and course of 28 patients. *Medicine* 61:189–97, 1982.
2. Anderson, R. J., Reed, W. G., and Knochel, J. Heatstroke. In: G. H. Stollerman, editor. *Advances in Internal Medicine,* Vol. 28. Chicago: Year Book Medical Publishers, 1983, pp. 115–40.

Chapter 17

A Comprehensive Geriatrics Center Associated with a University

Edward jj Olson and Linda Cutler

Introduction

Sinai Samaritan Medical Center of Milwaukee, Wisconsin, is a two-campus entity operating under the aegis of Aurora Health Care, Inc. It was formed in 1987 with the merger of two large hospitals in Milwaukee, namely, Mount Sinai Medical Center and Good Samaritan Medical Center. Mount Sinai Medical Center was a major medical, teaching, and research facility of 400 beds. It provided primary, secondary, and tertiary care and maintained affiliations with both the Medical College of Wisconsin and the University of Wisconsin Medical School.

More than one million persons reside in Milwaukee and the surrounding metropolitan area. Presently, 12.4 percent of this population is elderly. The older adult population continues to expand, with especially significant growth in the number of frail elderly over 75 years of age. The Geriatrics Institute of Sinai Samaritan attracts patients from throughout southeastern Wisconsin as well as other areas of the state and neighboring states. Because Sinai Samaritan Medical Center is located in and serves the central city, its patients include many individuals living in isolation or poverty, as well as substantial numbers of minority elderly.

The impetus for development of comprehensive geriatric services grew in part from a concern for medical education. Mount Sinai serves as Milwaukee Clinical Campus for the University of Wisconsin Medical School. Recognizing a need for more geriatric training of medical students and residents in internal medicine, the Department of Medicine recruited a trained geriatrician in 1977. Incorporation of this newly recognized specialty into the medical school curriculum was accompanied by efforts to develop a more comprehensive health care program for older adults than was currently available in the Milwaukee area. The community had a history of progressive government and a broad array of health and social services, but no health-related programs targeted specifically for the elderly. As in most communities, the resources that existed were fragmented and complex.

The resulting program, known as the Wisconsin Regional Geriatric Center (WRGC), was started in 1978 with an affiliation between Mount Sinai Medical Center and Family Hospital, a smaller community facility. Like the Mount Sinai Medical Center, Family Hospital was located in the central city on the fringe of the downtown area. Both hospitals had a strong commitment to serving the community and realized the need for meeting the physical, social, and mental health needs of Milwaukee's elderly. Both also perceived the wisdom of deeper market penetration in the area of eldercare. The WRGC was based at Family Hospital and began operation in July 1978, with the geriatrician serving as medical director.

In 1983, the affiliation with the smaller hospital ended, and the program became the Geriatrics Institute of Mount Sinai Medical Center. The Geriatrics Institute, now known as the Geriatrics Institute at the Mount Sinai Campus of Sinai Samaritan Medical Center, provides an integrated continuum of health and social services for older adults and their families. Emphasis is on a multidisciplinary, team approach to care, maintaining independence and avoiding unnecessary institutionalization. The Institute currently is composed of the following major components: the geriatrics outpatient clinic, rehabilitation day hospital, Alzheimer's disease day care programs, community-based wellness clinics, inpatient and outpatient geropsychiatry, specialized clinics (comprehensive geriatric evaluation, dementia, incontinence, and falls prevention), and a care coordination system.

Most patients come to the Institute for primary geriatric care, continue as outpatients, and are seen three or four times a year for their multiple medical and psychosocial problems. Some patients are referred by outside physicians for consultation and then return to their regular physicians for care. The majority of patients coming to the Institute are either self-referred or referred by home care nurses, public health nurses, social workers, or other agencies within the community.

Data maintained by the Geriatrics Institute on 2,043 patients seen over a four-year period provide insight into the complex health-related problems faced by many elderly persons in the area (see figure 17-1). The mean age of the patients was 77 years. Approximately two-thirds were female, and nearly one-half of all patients lived alone. The majority were found to have limited social and financial resources. They suffered from an average of six different medical problems. Problems most commonly seen included gastrointestinal disease, cardiovascular disease, hypertension, arthritis, Alzheimer's disease, and psychiatric problems,

Figure 17-1. Patient Profile, Geriatrics Institute, Milwaukee

Data on 2,043 patients, 7/11/83–10/26/87

Mean age	77 years	Social resources		Mean physical ADL	2.7
Sex		Excellent or good	28.6%	(independent: 4.0)	
Female	68%	Impaired	71.4%	Mean instrumental ADL	2.4
Male	32%	Economic resources		(independent: 3.3)	
Marital status		Excellent or good	35.2%	Services before first visit in prior	
Married	38.2%	Impaired	64.8%	12 months	
Widowed	44.4%	Medical problems	6/pt.	Hospitalized	21%
Single	10.0%	Mean Mini Mental Status		ER	21%
Separated or divorced	7.4%	(Folstein)	22	Nursing home stay	4%
Living arrangements		(Normal: 24–30)		Home care	13.9%
Alone	45.8%	Mood assessment		Day care	3%
With spouse	28.3%	(Yesavage)	27.8%>9	Doctor's office	74.1%
With relatives	15%	(Depression: 10–30)			

usually depression. Approximately 25 percent of the patients suffered chronic dementia.

Goals

The starter program for the Geriatrics Institute, the WRGC, was funded initially as a demonstration project by the United States Administration on Aging (AoA) and the Milwaukee-based Faye McBeath Foundation. Its overriding goal was the enhancement of the quality of life of older adults so that they could maintain their independence and avoid unnecessary institutionalization. This was to be accomplished by providing a comprehensive range of inpatient and outpatient services that focused on the individual medical, psychological, and social needs of the elderly and their family care givers. The result of this effort was the development and demonstration of a coordinated model of care that reflected a multidisciplinary, integrated approach to dealing with functional limitations resulting from chronic health conditions or the deterioration that often accompanies old age.

In addition to the service goals, educational goals focused on the development and implementation of a geriatric teaching service for medical students and resident physicians in internal medicine from the Milwaukee Clinical Campus of the University of Wisconsin Medical School. Educational efforts also were directed at training health and social services professionals in specific coping and caring skills for dealing with the needs of the elderly.

At the completion of the five-year demonstration phase of the WRGC ending in 1983, a more competitive environment for hospitals in Milwaukee contributed to the dissolution of the affiliation with Family Hospital. It had become clear that the two cosponsoring institutions differed on future goals. Family Hospital did not want to continue its support for the teaching and research goals of the WRGC, whereas Mount Sinai decided to develop geriatric services on its campus and refocus its teaching and research efforts. In July 1983, the medical director, administrator, and other personnel moved to Mount Sinai Medical Center to expand and refine the model of care as the Geriatrics Institute.

Also in 1983 a proposal for funding was submitted to the Robert Wood Johnson Foundation (RWJF) *Hospital Initiatives in Long-Term Care* program. The proposal articulated goals, objectives, and implementation strategies in three broad categories. Under "Coordination and Monitoring of Services," the goals included development of a coordinated continuum of geriatric care, which emphasized the implementation of a case coordination system, a quality assurance plan, and a comprehensive data system. "Service Implementation and Delivery" goals covered each of the nine inpatient and outpatient program components. These programs included:

- An outpatient clinic
- An inpatient unit
- Four wellness clinics
- A rehabilitation day hospital
- An Alzheimer's disease day care program
- A geriatric consultation service
- Geropsychiatry inpatient and outpatient services
- Community educational service

Under the heading of "Planning Projects," relationships with community institutions and agencies were discussed, as well as development of an affiliation with a Medicare HMO.

In January 1984, the Institute became one of 25 sites selected by RWJF to demonstrate the effectiveness of comprehensive geriatric services. A total of $650,000 was awarded over the four-year demonstration period. The goals and strategies outlined in the successful proposal continue to represent the Institute's priorities. With minor modification they serve as guidelines for the development of all Institute components.

Planning/Development Process

In the evolution of the Geriatrics Institute, a variety of issues, barriers, and problems arose that are of special interest to those involved in developing comprehensive long-term care programs in hospital settings.

Hospitals are increasingly complex institutions. It is difficult for them to redirect their resources from established line departments to innovative programming. Because of limited resources, new programs have to be perceived either as generating new patients or as catalysts for attracting outside funding support.

Hospital support for the WRGC and the Geriatrics Institute was in part an acknowledgment of the need to tap the older adult market. The AoA and RWJF provided the outside impetus for innovative programming through their national long-term care initiatives. Their planning and implementation monies facilitated the development of experimental geriatric models of care because the funding sources set the framework for the range and scope of service components. The proposals submitted to AoA and RWJF therefore served as statements of policy by the hospitals that they would provide comprehensive geriatric programming for Milwaukee's elderly. Mount Sinai, in fact, designated geriatrics as one of its top corporate priority areas.

Although neither the WRGC nor the Geriatrics Institute was a separately incorporated organization, both Family Hospital and Mount Sinai acknowledged their uniqueness by separating their administrative and programmatic functions from the normal activities of other hospital departments. This organizational independence allowed the programs to recruit new geriatrics-trained professionals, develop protocols that reflected the needs of the elderly, and design clinic space to reflect a warm and inviting environment rather than an impersonal one. In addition, independent budgets fostered flexibility in allocating limited resources.

The difficulties associated with the development of a hospital-based geriatric program cannot be overlooked. During the pilot phase of the WRGC, intraorganizational conflicts arose regarding the complexity of the new system, differing expectations and priorities between staff and other supportive departments, quality of care issues associated with the model, and various territorial questions. Specifically, the social work and therapy departments found it particularly difficult to accommodate the need to revise their staffing patterns and implement new protocols for the frail elderly population seen in the WRGC programs.

Some of these same issues had to be addressed at the Geriatrics Institute. However, because of the acknowledged interest and need for such a program within Mount Sinai Medical Center, traditional red tape and negative attitudes toward the elderly could be addressed in a positive fashion. Sponsoring organizations must be cognizant of the special programmatic needs of the elderly and prepared to support some of the institutional change issues that arise in implementing such a program.

The model that evolved at the Institute also was influenced heavily by the dramatic changes in the health care field that evolved during the 1980s. Changes in Medicare reimbursement for inpatient care and the emphasis on outpatient service instead of acute care served as the catalyst for the adoption of an organizational model similar to a social health maintenance organization (SHMO). With the introduction of diagnosis-related groups by the Health Care Financing Administration (HCFA), hospitals were motivated to reduce the length of stay of their Medicare patients. Accordingly, the introduction of a diversity of outpatient services such as specialty clinics, day care programs, and case-management services by the Institute allowed the Medical Center creative options in diverting their frail elderly to less costly programs. This acknowledgment of the importance of cost-effectiveness and emphasis on social rather than medical interventions were reinforced by preliminary data from the SHMO demonstrations.

Case Management and Assessment

As with most hospital programs, the first step in case management is assessment. The Functional Assessment Inventory (FAI) is used for assessing patients in all Institute programs.[1] Developed originally by Eric Pfeiffer, the instrument has been modified to meet the needs of Institute professionals and, to a lesser extent, the requirements of the RWJF grant. Information from the assessment is entered into the computerized data system to facilitate research, service delivery, coordination, and monitoring efforts.

The assessment is administered by three professionals: a physician, a social worker, and a registered nurse. The physician administers the mental status questionnaire.[2] The social work section includes descriptions and ratings of the patient's social and economic resources, the mood assessment scale,[3] and a number of special questions dealing with behaviors of demented patients. The nurse's section of the assessment includes an evaluation of the patient's physical health, the patient's instrumental and physical activities of daily living (ADL), a physical health needs assessment scale, and a record of the utilization of health services in the prior 12 months. In addition to the FAI assessment, a health history is developed for each patient, and each receives a physical examination from one of the Institute physicians. Basic and specific laboratory work, consultations with subspecialists, and a neuropsychological evaluation of dementia patients also are included as part of the evaluation. The initial time spent on the assessment by the physician is approximately one hour; the nurse/social worker team takes an additional hour to complete its sections.

After the assessment is completed, generally over a two-week period, each patient case is reviewed in a small multidisciplinary conference including the physician, the nurse, and the social worker. Once a week, the most complex of the Institute's new patient cases are presented at a large multidisciplinary conference attended by all staff. After the patient is reviewed at either the mini or major multidisciplinary conference, the patient and/or family returns to the physician for a summary of the complete assessment.

The assessment process identifies a significant number of frail elderly whose chronic diseases, disabilities, or impairments require complex support systems to permit continued independent living. It is for these individuals at risk of institutionalization that a care coordination or case management component has been developed.

Utilizing planning monies provided under the first year of the RWJF grant, the Institute's care coordination model incorporates direct services and brokers community resources to provide comprehensive care for its clients. Persons in need of care coordination are identified through the assessment process described above. The eligibility criteria include scores from the FAI rating scales for physical ADL, instrumental activities of daily living (IADL), and social resources, in addition to the clinical judgment of the assessment team. Care coordination patients must be impaired in any combination of four ADLs and IADLs and be living either alone or with a frail spouse.

After eligibility is determined, a care coordinator is assigned. The care coordinator and the multidisciplinary team identify the problems to be addressed and develop a preliminary service plan. Finalization of the service plan is completed by the care coordinator who initiates services, working with the discharge planning department of the Medical Center when appropriate. The monitoring and evaluation process includes identifying patient progress, level of service utilization, and appropriateness of the care plan. Dialogue with community service providers ensures that care coordinated patients receive appropriate in-home services. (The Institute utilized RWJF purchase-of-service monies to contract directly for community services and thus ensured continuity between the hospital-based health care and community social services systems.) Patient advocates, who are retired older adults, work with the care coordinator to provide companionship through home visits and also provide monitoring and evaluation data for care plan adjustment.

The care coordination model is administered by the care coordination supervisor, who is responsible for system development and care plan implementation. The care coordinators are nurses and social workers from other components of the Institute who maintain small caseloads of clients in addition to their ongoing work responsibilities.

Integration of a care coordination system into an acute-care institution required changes in the internal and external roles traditionally associated with hospitals. The implementation process focused on developing working agreements with prospective community-based resources for clients and orienting hospital personnel to the goals of the care coordination system. After an initial pilot of the program, a data-management system was designed to facilitate both the operation and evaluation of the program. Figure 17-2 provides data on 216 patients enrolled in the care coordination system. In-home nursing and homemaker aides were the most utilized services. Six percent of the patients required high-intensity follow-up of two to three contacts per week, 34 percent received medium-intensity follow-up (two times per month), and the remainder were monitored once a month. As a group, these high-risk patients were more impaired in their social and economic resources, had lower ADL and IADL scores, and were more likely to live alone than other Geriatrics Institute patients.

Innovative Services

The Institute brings together both traditional and new services in an innovative model of comprehensive care. The pilot program included an outpatient clinic, an acute-care unit, and a rehabilitation day hospital. The outpatient clinic initially was set up as the faculty practice of the geriatrician, who was assisted by a nurse and social worker. Currently geriatricians, internists, a psychologist, nurses, social workers, therapists, and a nutritionist provide care. With its comprehensive assessments and

Figure 17-2. Care Coordination System Data, Geriatrics Institute, Milwaukee

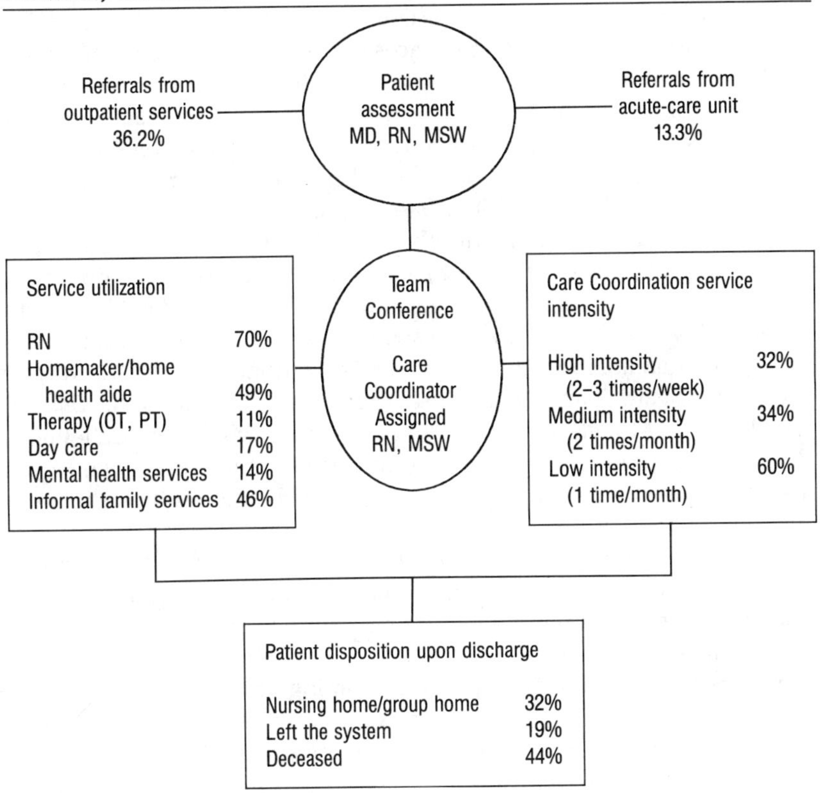

Data on 216 patients, 7/1/85–10/26/87

Mean age	77 years
Sex	
Female	79.3%
Male	20.7%
Marital status	
Married	30.6%
Widowed	52.1%
Single	7.4%
Separated or divorced	9.9%
Living arrangements	
Alone	53.5%
With spouse	22.8%
With relatives	23.7%

Social resources	
Excellent or good	18.3%
Impaired	81.7%
Economic resources	
Excellent or good	17.3%
Impaired	82.7%
Mean Mini Mental Status (Normal: 24–30)	22
Mean PADL	2.54
Mean IADL	2.2

Top 7 medical diagnoses	
Circulatory	39%
Dementia	22%
Depression, anxiety, paranoia	20%
Arthritis	13%
Diabetes	12%
Neoplasms	8%
Respiratory	7%

multidisciplinary conferences, as well as enhanced data system, the outpatient clinic serves as the key entry point to the system. The outpatient clinic provides comprehensive geriatric assessments as well as ongoing primary care and consultative services for more than 1,500 older adults. Each new patient receives a complete geriatric assessment by a physician and nurse and, where appropriate, by a social worker. The clinic also serves as an outpatient teaching site for medical students from the University of Wisconsin School of Medicine, for geriatric fellows, and for resident physicians of Sinai Samaritan.

After evaluating a large number of patients with Alzheimer's disease and dealing with the multiple problems faced by care givers for this illness, specialized services were added to the model. An Alzheimer's Disease Day Care Program was designed to provide socialization, maintain functional abilities, delay institutionalization, and provide respite for families. Participants must meet criteria in the *Diagnostic and Statistical Manual of Mental Disorders, Third Edition* (DSM-III) for Alzheimer's disease, a requirement that facilitates collection of research data. Figure 17-3 provides information on day care participants with Alzheimer's disease.

The Alzheimer's disease program has been remarkably successful. It has generated a great deal of publicity, both nationally and locally, and served as a focal point for emerging community concern. A second community-based day care site opened in 1986. The Sinai Samaritan program has recently expanded its programming to five days a week and has been designated by the Robert Wood Johnson Foundation as one of its dementia care and respite services program sites.

The day care program also includes support group meetings for the family members of day care patients. These meetings provide an opportunity to share mutual problems and anxieties. An eight-hour education series for care givers is offered periodically. As in other Institute components, the involvement of family members and active support of their care-giving efforts are considered to be integral parts of comprehensive long-term care services.

The Wellness Clinic Program also was part of the demonstration project. A geriatrics-trained nurse offers blood pressure monitoring, medication information, health education, and counseling. Currently there are four sites for the Wellness Clinic Program, including one serving predominantly Hispanic elderly.

Other services include inpatient and outpatient geropsychiatry programs to help older adults cope with emotional and social problems that can undermine their health and independence. The Physicians Outreach Consultation Service and Inpatient Team Consultation Service, which was discontinued in 1988, utilized a nurse/social worker team. The team did geriatric assessments at the homes of patients of private physicians and collaborated with the physician to coordinate

Figure 17-3. Alzheimer's Disease Patient Data, Milwaukee

Data on 40 patients with Alzheimer's disease who participated in the 1986 day care programs

Mean age	77 years	Social resources		Mean PADL	2.69/4.0
Sex		Excellent or good	11.8%	Walk long distances	73.7%
Female	73.7%	Impaired	88.2%	Continent urine	79%
Male	26.3%	Economic resources		Mean IADL	1.95/3.3
Widowed	44.%	Excellent or good	11.8%	Prepare food	42%
Living arrangements		Impaired	88.2%	Take Rx	15.8%
Alone	41.2%	Mean Mini Mental Status			
With spouse	35.3%	(Normal: 24–30)	17		
With relatives	23.5%				

appropriate services. The team also provided comprehensive assessments for elderly non-Institute patients in the Medical Center's acute-care units. During 1986–1987, services were provided to 169 patients of 20 physicians throughout the Milwaukee area.

The following case study illustrates how the various Institute components function to provide continuity of care for a patient with multiple medical problems and functional limitations (see figure 17-4).

> A. W., a 73-year-old black woman, widowed and living alone in her own home, was first seen in the outpatient clinic on 2/14/84, having been referred by a public health nurse for increasing weakness, immobility, and isolation. The geriatrician identified the following medical problems: severe degenerative joint disease of hips and shoulders, organic heart disease with angina and congestive heart failure, suspected Parkinson's disease, anemia of chronic disease, hypertension, decreased vision, and a mild left hemiparesis from a previous stroke. The patient was referred for neurological consultation, which confirmed the diagnosis of Parkinson's disease. Medication for the Parkinson's disease resulted in improved mobility. On 5/18/84, the patient started in the rehabilitation day hospital six hours a day, three times per week. Two and one-half months later, the patient was discharged from the rehabilitation day hospital much improved in self-care and motivation. Home care services were maintained, and the patient became active in a church Bible group and a senior center. She was followed up in the outpatient clinic and by telephone contact from the care coordination team for the next year. In 6/85, she was found to have increased congestive heart failure, but she refused hospitalization. One month later, she was hospitalized for six days on the Institute's acute-care geriatric unit for congestive heart failure and angina. Subsequently, she remained relatively well, under the care of her Institute physician and the care coordination team.

The Geriatrics Institute continues to explore new directions for expanding or refining its model of care. Decisions about future directions will be made within a new organizational framework. Building on its metropolitanwide, multihospital foundation, the Institute anticipates the development of satellite sites for services such as geriatric assessment, dementia day care, and rehabilitation programs and/or care coordination. As an example of one type of site, the Institute is providing on-site psychological and geropsychiatric services for residents of a large retirement and nursing home in the metropolitan area.

Although providing comprehensive patient care services, the Geriatrics Institute's mission also includes research. Its research capabilities are greatly enhanced by the medical and psychosocial data collected on

Figure 17-4. Case Study: 73-Year-Old Woman

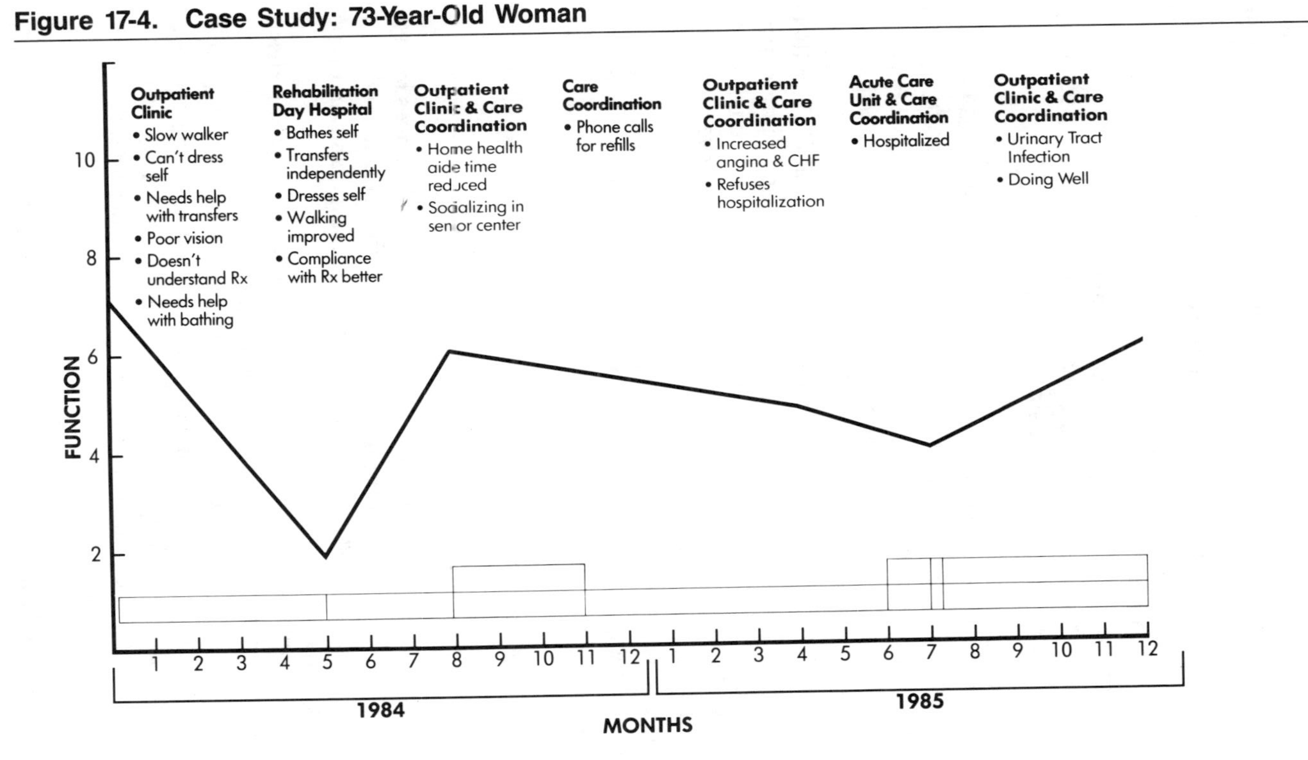

its patient population. The Institute has been involved in research dealing with the following:

- Effects of self-management therapy in patients with Alzheimer's disease
- Burden of care experienced by the care givers of patients with Alzheimer's disease
- Evaluation of the appropriateness of cancer care given to community elderly
- Urinary incontinence
- Development of a prototype dementia patient registry
- Changes in micronutrient requirements in institutionalized elderly
- Patterns of medical care in nursing homes

The Institute continues to fulfill the geriatric education role that contributed to its development. Family practice and internal medicine resident physicians learn to address the medical and psychosocial needs of elderly patients in monthlong geriatric rotations. A geriatric fellowship program was established in 1989. The Institute serves as the clinical site for graduate training of nurses, social workers, and rehabilitation therapists from various local colleges and universities. Continuing education is provided on an ongoing basis for staff and community professionals. In addition, conferences and seminars are given for older adults, their families, and persons who work with the elderly.

The Institute also provides information and technical assistance to hospitals throughout the country seeking to develop or enhance their geriatric services.

Financing

Financing for the Geriatrics Institute is based on a mix of sources including Medicare, Medicaid, third-party insurers, fee-for-service, and grant funds. Funding varies according to the program component and type of service provided.

Patients seen in the Geriatric Outpatient Clinic are billed for physician services and for services by the geriatrics nurse.

Although the main objective of the program is to prevent institutionalization, either in the hospital or in a nursing home, the care of a large group of frail elderly with multiple medical and psychosocial problems inevitably results in an appreciable number of hospitalizations. A substantial inpatient income is generated as a result.

The two Alzheimer's Disease Day Care Programs are not reimbursed by Medicare, Medicaid, or private insurance. The daily charge is $25;

a sliding scale based on financial need is used. The state of Wisconsin recently enacted a program that funds day care services for some patients with Alzheimer's disease. The state also has a Community Options Program that offers financial assistance to patients who otherwise would be candidates for nursing home placement. Administered at the county level, the Community Options Program makes some monies available for day care. With funds available through state, county, private pay, and foundation sources, the Alzheimer's Disease Day Care Programs cover most of their costs. No charges are made for the care-giver support groups that meet in conjunction with the day care programs.

Grants have contributed significantly to the development of innovative services. During the pilot phase of the WRGC, AoA and foundation support totaled $580,000. The four-year $650,000 grant from RWJF supported staff and services needed to provide nonreimbursable geriatric services. The geriatric team consultation service to private physicians' patients and to hospitalized non-Institute patients was funded entirely by RWJF, as was the development of the care coordination system. In addition, the Institute has received approximately $200,000 in local foundation funds during the four-year period. Recently the Institute received a $300,000 grant from RWJF to implement a consortia approach for its dementia care and respite services day care national initiative.

Conclusions

The Geriatrics Institute at the Mount Sinai Campus of Sinai Samaritan Medical Center has become a national model for the delivery of comprehensive health care for the elderly patient. The program is economically viable and provides the Medical Center an opportunity to meet the specialized needs of the elderly as well as generate a substantial number of patients. It has expanded services and implemented new models of care, as well as providing information, education, and training to thousands of older adults, care givers, and the professionals who serve them (figures 17-5 to 17-7). The program also meets the geriatric educational needs of the Milwaukee Clinical Campus for the University of Wisconsin Medical School. The Geriatrics Institute has attracted grant funds, both locally and nationally, which have allowed it to develop innovative programming. The Institute has developed a sophisticated data system that provides a base for research in the areas of Alzheimer's disease, geriatric assessment, and health care delivery. Finally, and most important, the Institute has attracted a group of committed professionals who have worked successfully as a multidisciplinary team to deliver comprehensive health care to the frail elderly of Milwaukee.

Figure 17-5. Expansion of Services, Geriatrics Institute, Milwaukee

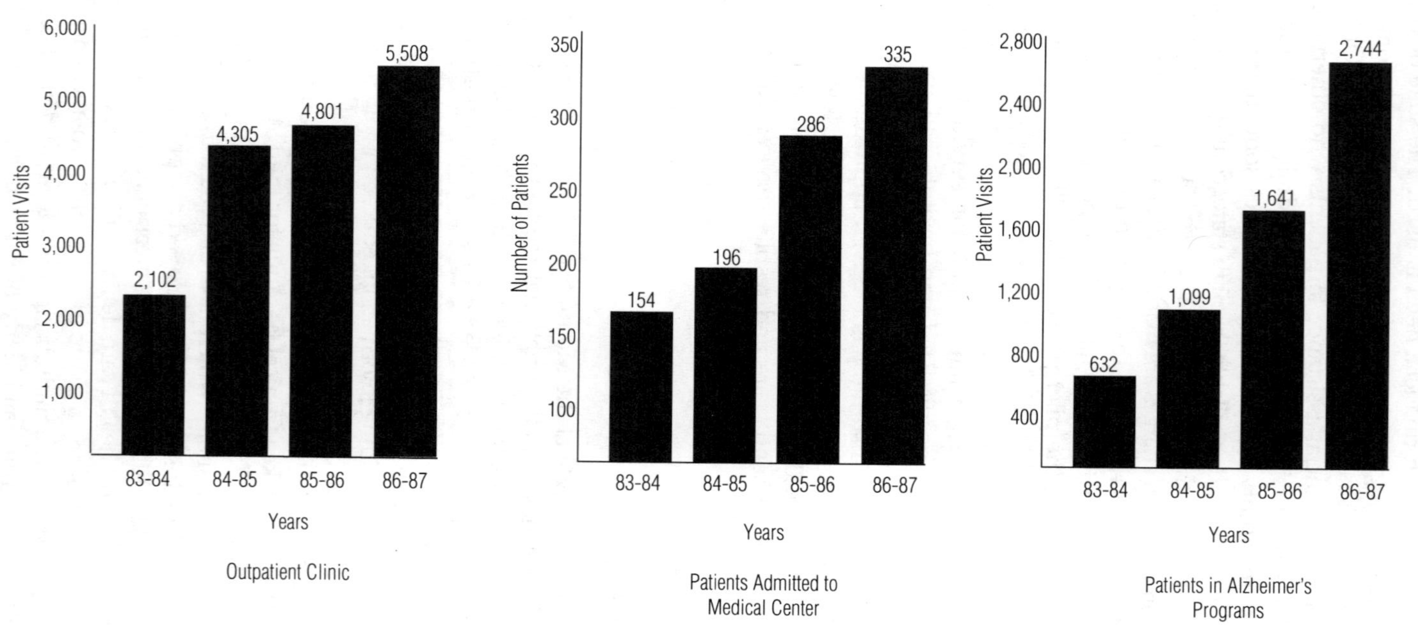

Figure 17-6. Implementation of New Models of Care, Geriatrics Institute, Milwaukee

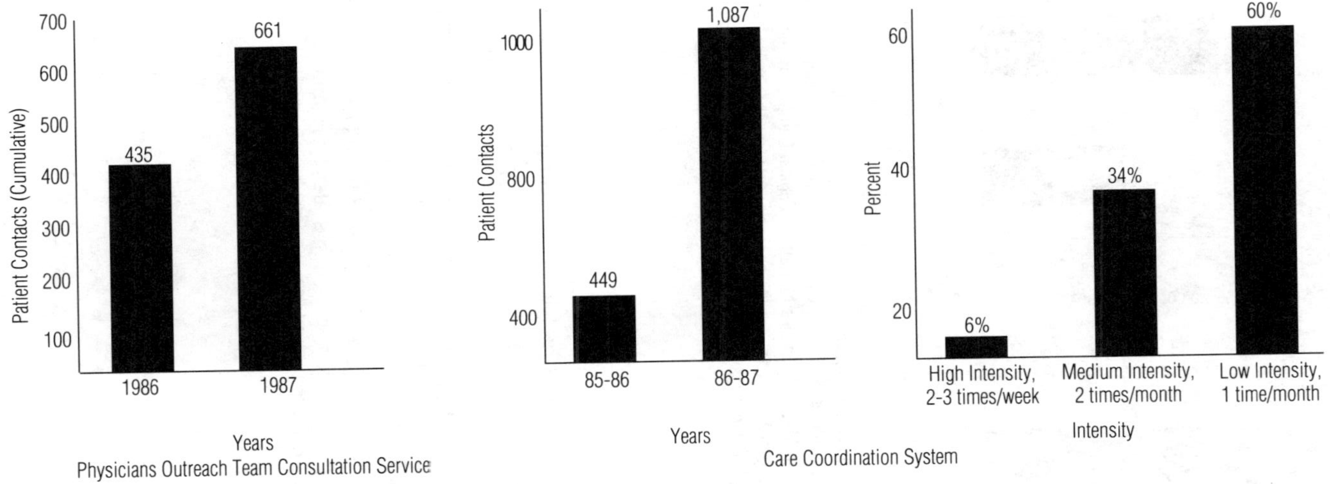

Patient Contacts (Cumulative)
700
600
500
400
300
200
100
435
661
1986
1987
Years
Physicians Outreach Team Consultation Service

Patient Contacts
1000
800
400
449
1,087
85-86
86-87
Years

Percent
60
40
20
6%
34%
60%
High Intensity, 2-3 times/week
Medium Intensity, 2 times/month
Low Intensity, 1 time/month
Intensity
Care Coordination System

Physicians Outreach Team Consultation Service.

In an innovative effort to make multidisciplinary resources available to physicians in private practice, the Institute developed the Physicians Outreach Service. A nurse/social worker team performed geriatric assessments, made recommendations and implemented service for 169 patients of 20 physicians throughout the Milwaukee area. Participating physicians became more familiar with community resources, more able to help patients live independently, and felt the program was a valuable adjunct to their practice.

Care coordination system.

The Care Coordination System manages the care of frail older adults, both inpatients and outpatients, who are at risk of institutionalization. The system includes case finding, care plan development, initiation of services, monitoring and evaluation. It utilizes direct institute services and brokers community resources to provide comprehensive care for institute clients.

Figure 17-7. Expansion of Educational Services, Geriatrics Institute, Milwaukee

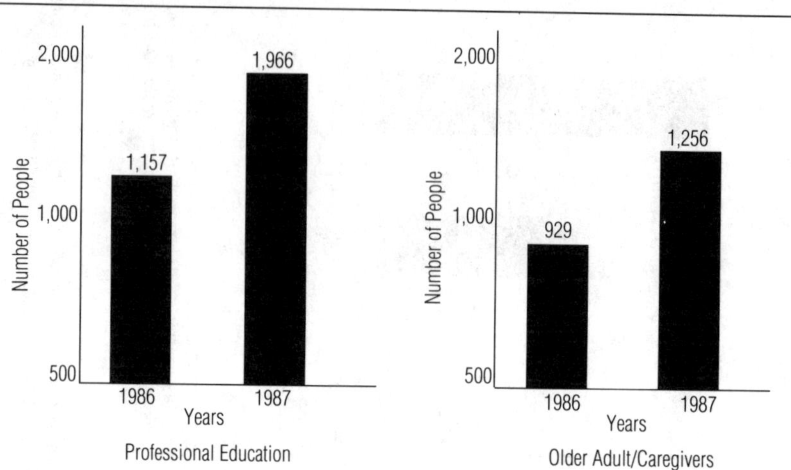

Education.

The Geriatrics Institute conducts educational activities for a wide range of health and social service professionals, emphasizing a multidisciplinary approach to working with older adults. Through the University of Wisconsin Medical School's Milwaukee Clinical Campus, it serves as a resource for training physicians in geriatrics. The institute sponsors extensive health and wellness offerings for older adults as well as educational and support programs for caregivers.

References

1. Pfeiffer, E., Johnson, T. M., and Chiofolo, R. C. Functional assessment of elderly subjects in four service settings. Paper presented at the Annual Scientific Meeting, Gerontological Society of America, San Diego, Nov. 1980.
2. Folstein, M. F., Folstein, S., and McHugh, P. R. Mini-mental state: a practical method for grading the cognitive state of patients for the clinician. *Journal of Psychiatric Research* 12:189, 1975.
3. Yesavage, J. A., Brink, T. L., and Rose, T. L., and others. Development and validation of the geriatric depression screening scale: a preliminary report. *Journal of Psychiatric Research* 17(1):37–49, 1982–1983.

Chapter 18

A Geriatric Assessment and Planning Program

Carolee A. DeVito and William Zubkoff

Introduction

South Shore Hospital and Medical Center (South Shore) is a private, not-for-profit, fully licensed/accredited 178-bed general hospital affiliated with the University of Miami School of Medicine. It is the only hospital and primary health care center for the 3.03-square-mile southernmost tip of the City of Miami Beach island, known as South Beach, and it is located about five miles from the University of Miami Medical Center campus.

South Shore Hospital and Medical Center began its evolution as a model geriatric health center by dubbing its unique location on South Miami Beach, Florida, a "natural geriatric laboratory for the development, implementation and testing of programs in geriatric care." Over the last six years, the needs and opportunities provided by its setting have been matched with wide-ranging program development in long-term care.[1-4] This chapter outlines the strategies and specific methods employed to develop program activities contributing to a meaningful continuum of care for frail older adults in South Shore's service area.

Dade County, Florida, has a relatively high concentration of older adults: about 21 percent of the total population is age 60 or over. Nearly one-third of this elderly population is of Hispanic origin, and about 16 percent are below the poverty level for household income.

The South Beach population can be characterized as an ethnically diverse, poor elderly community in an urban, though geographically isolated, catchment area of the county. At the beginning of the last decade South Beach had approximately 46,000 permanent residents, 60 percent of whom were over age 65. Although current estimates suggest as much as a 10 percent decrease in sheer numbers of elderly, South Beach still has one of the highest concentrations (perhaps the highest) of older persons age 75-plus and age 85-plus, representing 28 percent and 7 percent, respectively, of its total population, or 60 percent and 12 percent of its elderly population. About one-quarter of all South Beach elderly are estimated as being below the poverty level, and over one-half of the elderly live alone.

The development of the Geriatric Assessment and Planning (GAP) Program at South Shore and its various modules has followed a paradigm of community-oriented health care. Thus the GAP Program was founded on the therapeutic objectives of maximizing patient functional health status and patient autonomy, while driven by an assessment of health care needs and evaluated by impact on the health outcomes of a defined community. However, the realities of program implementation have also affected the definition of target populations. Given the reflection of South Beach demographics on the hospital's acute-care services—median patient age of 81 years and 76 percent geriatric—the GAP Program initially targeted more elderly hospital inpatients.

As program modules have been added to the core services, new communities/constituencies have been identified. Following are selected estimates from hospital records from 1986, which provide a profile of the target population:

- Frail
  - About 40 percent are hospitalized more than once a year.
  - The median number of diagnoses per patient admitted is four.
  - Over 10 percent have specific psychoses (for example, are discharged with a psychiatric diagnosis); nearly half are categorized as confused or disoriented.
- Functionally dependent
  - Approximately 25 percent are hearing impaired; 75 percent are vision impaired.
  - Activities of daily living: Katz score at discharge,[5] 26 percent "A," 8 percent "B," 20 percent "C," 6 percent "D," 13 percent "E," 8 percent "F," 20 percent "G."
  - Human help needs at discharge: 17 percent need help to obtain/take medication; 59 percent need help bathing; 34 percent, dressing; 16 percent, using the toilet; 13 percent, transferring (from bed to chair, and so forth); 2 percent, eating; 12 percent, walking; 50 percent, preparing meals; 52 percent, shopping; 50 percent, doing laundry; 52 percent, housecleaning; 25 percent, with transportation.
- Isolated
  - Less than 50 percent of needs identified have formal or informal resources in place prior to the individual's program enrollment.
  - About one-third of the elderly live alone.

- In great need of community-based services
  - –Approximately 53 percent of patients are discharged to their homes; an additional 14 percent are discharged to adult congregate living facilities (ACLFs).
  - –Community-based services are recommended for over 60 percent of patients at discharge.

The demographics of Dade County and, specifically, South Beach, provided the backdrop for defining appropriate directions for the medical center's development through the 1980s. In fact, a number of studies had targeted specific needs and service gaps, such as the following:[6,7]

- A 1979 University of Miami study showed that nearly all of the elderly residents living in South Beach had at least one chronic illness, and the overwhelming majority had multiple illnesses requiring daily medication. The factors above were combined with knowledge of the number of elderly living alone to help support reports from physicians and community-based agencies that mental health problems were particularly pronounced.
- Significant unmet health needs among the elderly were documented (nursing home beds, ACLF beds, and so forth), and South Beach was designated a medically underserved area (MUA). South Shore is the only hospital on South Beach; the next closest is located approximately 40 blocks north.
- Of particular note were problems regarding primary care. Most physicians held very limited service hours in South Beach and maintained offices in other areas. Estimates showed that only about 22 percent accepted Medicare assignment and not even one accepted Medicaid. Unmet needs for primary care physicians were estimated at about 26,000 encounters per year or about 4 to 6 full-time equivalents.
- A summary report, concentrating almost exclusively on the elderly population, was prepared by the Health Systems Agency in 1976, documenting health care services and health care problems in South Beach, including:
  - –Multiple health problems among the elderly, involving the need for multiple clinical interventions
  - –Insufficient home care and homemaker services, unnecessarily hastening institutionalization
  - –Extremely limited alternatives to institutionalization
  - –Prohibitively expensive existing health services, even when partially subsidized by public assistance

Dozens of different social services agencies, including county, state, federal, and nonprofit groups, were servicing the residents of South Beach. However, the programs designed to benefit the elderly low-income population failed to approach the magnitude of need on South Beach. Furthermore, the overlaps among programs and duplication of efforts impaired efficient provision of service to those eligible.

These problems were restated often throughout the late 1970s and early 1980s with widespread agreement among agencies and providers that the South Beach elderly suffered from extensive and ever-increasing unmet needs in the area of health services as well as from problems with housing, income maintenance, and lack of counseling, legal services, and financial assistance.

Clearly, sound methods were needed to guide frail older adults through the medical and social services maze. But the process of creating and implementing new services and initiatives was limited by service delivery capacity, and scarce resources (to fund and/or encourage development of expanded capacity) were becoming scarcer. With so many in need, creative mechanisms to reprioritize or target services from at-capacity programs would be insufficient. Given the magnitude of the problem of meeting long-term care needs of the frail elderly, locally and nationally, and obvious demographic trends likely to result in greater needs, unique solutions or programs directed at select populations that could not be expanded would prove trivial.

The problems of providing a continuum of long-term care services to the South Beach community were described as "largely the same for South Beach as for other communities" but existing in a poignant and blatant form due to "absolute numbers of elderly, widespread economic deprivation, and geographic isolation."[8] Meaningful solutions would have to accommodate three assumptions:

1. The need for changes in the approach to usual and customary care for most frail elderly
2. The need for system coordination as well as service development with targeted growth at obvious gaps in the long-term care continuum
3. The need for large-scale resource development/expansion of service delivery capacity to approach the optimal need/use match

The feasibility of implementing a geriatrics program development strategy was established from within both South Shore Hospital and Medical Center and the larger health care community. At the beginning of this decade, as a relatively young institution (founded in 1968), South Shore Hospital and Medical Center had established itself as a credible, typical provider. It was operating as a full-service community hospital (with the exception of obstetrics and pediatrics).

Dade County, with its more than 40 hospitals, and Miami Beach, with three other large hospitals, provided less than a nurturing environment for typical expansion and little or no protection of a "natural" catchment area. The 1980s began with falling hospital occupancy rates countywide, fierce competition for Medicare inpatients, rapid development of health maintenance organizations targeted at the elderly, the institution of prospective payment systems, and extensive overlap of attending medical staffs at the area hospitals. However, the growth of hospital competitors seemed to be targeted at somewhat different constituencies and obviously variant technologies. Meanwhile, numerous potential partners shared perspectives likely to facilitate South Shore Hospital's transition to a model geriatric health care center:

- The University of Miami School of Medicine clinical activities and teaching programs are based largely at Jackson Memorial Hospital, a 1,350-bed general hospital operated by a nonprofit corporation for the Metropolitan Dade County government. The desire of specific departments to increase opportunities to implement community-oriented health care (especially community-oriented primary care) and continuity models, a search for community-based practice sites, and the dean's vision of collaboration with community hospitals set the stage for planning.[9]
- The University of Miami had relatively little health services research and development activity, and virtually none directed at geriatrics. However, individual faculty members from the School of Medicine and clinical chiefs from the neighboring Veterans Administration Medical Center (VAMC) viewed geriatric program development as a top priority. A number of ideas for training programs or innovative clinical services had failed to materialize, partly attributable to the constraints of large tertiary care centers, start-up funds, and space.
- Long-term care service providers with responsibility or interest in the South Beach Community were well aware of obvious service gaps, difficulties in coordinating services, and long waiting lists for health, social, and personal care services. Numerous local government-sponsored task forces, community agency networks, and areawide committees existed to highlight problems and outline recommendations. Few anticipated changes or solutions necessary to satisfy the unmet needs of the frail elderly, but virtually all matched their skepticism with enthusiastic support for development of any program or program component likely to make an incremental change.
- In addition to local support, dissemination of demographic information about the South Shore Hospital and Medical Center constituency and the South Beach community attracted attention from researchers and health system analysts as a unique site for long-term care program development and evaluation. Colleagues from Dartmouth Medical School and the Burke Rehabilitation Center (White Plains, New York) were among the first to propose specific projects. In recent years the Centers for Disease Control, in cooperation with the Dade County Public Health Unit, have implemented population-based studies on South Beach.

Goals

The long-term goals of South Shore Hospital and Medical Center involve the continued development as a model community health care center in the natural geriatric laboratory of South Miami Beach, pursuing the appropriate mix of patient care, education, research, and community services.[10] As an evolving model site for the development and dissemination of innovations in the long-term care service delivery continuum, the medical center has targeted the systematic identification of health care problems and the cost-effective matching of needs with resources and services as its top priority. Additionally, the goals include a commitment to monitoring and evaluation of program interventions and prioritization of programs focused on maximizing independent living among the frail elderly.

The organization's program objectives have three major themes:

1. Development, testing, and dissemination of relevant innovations
2. Initiation and participation in large-scale service expansion to the target population
3. Recognition as a center of excellence for specific services

The operational challenge has focused on identifying the appropriate role for an acute-care hospital in the long-term care continuum, or the development of a continuum of care for the elderly. The ideal outcome for investments in program development would yield credibility both locally and nationally as well as long-term institutional viability. This includes expanding the definition of target populations/constituencies by becoming a significant referral center, sustaining the ability to respond to changes in demography (for example, community needs), and empowering the institution to create new service capabilities.

The Development Process

A deliberate philosophy and set of strategies have driven the developmental process to date. One tenet has been to recognize and promote the short-term general hospital as an important vehicle in the development of a continuum of long-term care services. The inpatient stay provides the opportunity to address the very long-term needs of frail elderly individuals at critical points in time and brings multiple professional resources literally to the bedside. Instead of facing a question of whether long-term care decisions should be made at discharge, each discharge decision that is made has long-term impact. With large numbers of rehospitalizations among the elderly and a concern for the incentives of prospective payment as well as for community image, hospitals are receptive to and are also appropriate vehicles to promote rational long-term care.

The development process incorporated strategies ranging from sponsorship to cosponsorship, from "hosting" to facilitating/catalyzing of program components. For any program component, the role of organizational affiliates generally increases both program credibility and constituencies.

A general assumption of a "win-win" mode was incorporated to prevent wasting scarce developmental resources on competition with potential allies. Short-term competitiveness was substituted with a belief that in the long run, affiliations among organizations would increase constituencies as well as the likelihood of program expansion. Certainly once affiliations are established, the entire consortium of participants has increased access to developmental funds (for example, grants and contracts) that otherwise may have been targeted at selected organizational types.

The actual steps in the developmental process to date can be outlined as follows:

- In 1981, a technical consultants advisory committee was established to guide the development of the geriatric program to a state-of-the-art level. This committee included expertise in health care systems/long-term health education, volunteerism, information management, and long-term care financing and marketing, as well as clinical geriatrics.
- In 1981, South Shore implemented a National Center for Health Services Research generic drug evaluation contract.
- In 1982, the Geriatric Community Resources Steering Committee was established, portraying the vast spectrum of local advisory and working relationships associated with the hospital's goals and mission for eldercare. The duration and intensity of the individual relationships spanned from years of comembership on task-force committees to years of interaction through individual patient placement. The members are all influential representatives of significant agencies affecting the South Beach community. Their agencies range from agencies within the City of Miami Beach to agencies of Dade County, the State of Florida, and private philanthropic sponsorship. They represent a full spectrum of services (nutrition, housing, day care, ambulatory care, and guardianship) and provide adequate political representation to facilitate activities.
- In 1982, under the leadership of the Department of Family Medicine and Community Health, affiliation between the University of Miami School of Medicine and South Shore Hospital and Medical Center was formalized. The university's Department of Family Medicine and Community Health assumed responsibility for planning, evaluation, and research at the South Shore site. Through this responsibility, a close working relationship developed among the Department of Family

Medicine and Community Health, South Shore Hospital and Medical Center, VAMC, and community service providers. A wide variety of collaborative program and project efforts resulted.

- In 1982, development of the first geriatric fellowship-physician training program in Florida took place, jointly sponsored with the University of Miami School of Medicine and the Miami VAMC.
- In 1982, South Shore implemented an Administration on Aging Grant subcontract with Dartmouth Medical School's Self-Care for Seniors Program Evaluation, obtained an Arthur Vining Davis Foundation grant to disseminate the program throughout community sites, and subsequently developed the Caregiver Training Program.
- In 1983, the South Shore/University of Miami efforts to develop a long-term care continuum were labeled the GAP Program. The original conceptualization of the GAP program components was directed by a consortium including South Shore Hospital and Medical Center, the University of Miami School of Medicine, the Geriatric Community Resources Steering Committee, and the Miami Beach Hebrew Home for the Aged. The program included a broad range of patient care services, the integrated patient information system, professional education programs, geriatric outreach education programs, and program evaluation/research components. The program goal for the consortium was stated explicitly as tailoring services to needs rather than to reimbursement; as a fully integrated, case-managed, health and personal care service system with an enrolled population, central care provider, and realistic financing.
- In 1984, development of one of only two community hospital-based geriatric medical psychiatric units in South Florida took place.
- In 1984, extensive interviews and site visits were conducted with key community-based service providers to establish the character and magnitude of services, the availability and accessibility of patient information, the willingness to share information, and the range of possible interactions. A physician survey informed clinicians of the hospital's goals and assessed the extent of collaboration or resistance that could be expected.
- In 1985, the information requirements of the developing model discharge planning program required the integration of functional health status assessment into the usual care processes, the establishment of an integrated patient information system to facilitate inpatient care, and linkage to community-based services as well as tracking of need and use for evaluation purposes.
- In 1985, specialized nursing in-service education/staff development focused on caring for the elderly
- In 1985, community-oriented continuing medical education and the "Topics in the Care of Older Persons" in-service education series were introduced.

The GAP program development can be described as three distinct phases from 1983 to the present, as follows:

- *Phase I: Development. Setting the foundations of systematic and comprehensive functional health status assessment.* The technical assistance and resources of this phase were enhanced by the selection of South Shore Hospital and Medical Center as one of three national sites in a Kellogg Foundation–supported program "to develop assessment technology in acute care hospitals serving the elderly" under supervision of the Burke Rehabilitation Center in New York.
- *Phase II: Cooperation/Coordination. Establishing mechanisms for the core of GAP program activities.* Specific organizational arrangements and tasks have been implemented to mainstream the core program throughout the South Shore Hospital/University of Miami consortium of providers, focusing on the inpatient stay as an opportunity to initiate and institute the most appropriate long-term care arrangements. These tasks can be summarized as requirements to achieve the following results:
  - Integrate the comprehensive assessment system
  - Provide explicit mechanisms to ensure linkage of patients through posthospital service providers
  - Provide education and training for primary care givers
  - Provide patient education and service utilization information
  - Reassess patients until community-based services are no longer indicated
  - Provide patient educational and administrative seminars for in-house and community providers

  Additionally, patient assessments and utilization data are analyzed to identify major service gaps and explore mechanisms for the consortium to develop needed services. Substantial funding for phase II development resulted from the selection of South Shore as one of 24 hospitals in the nation, and the only site in Florida, as a grantee in the Robert Wood Johnson Foundation *Hospital Initiatives in Long-Term Care* program. Numerous other activities are associated with the core and were developed with varying degrees of direct sponsorship by the hospital. They will be described later in the chapter.
- *Phase III: Collaboration. Identifying mechanisms to mobilize unrecognized potential resources.* This "community action phase" of development is unfolding as a transition and expansion from the core of GAP program activities. Defined as private sector–public sector collaboration, phase III program plans suggest that there are likely solutions possible at an aggregate level within the community that are not feasible on an individual care plan level. Mechanisms to activate the private sector–public sector toward local ingenuity recognize that the problems associated with the elderly becoming institutionalized are of interest

to the varying forces within the community. The community action phase promotes collaborative efforts that can be typified by motivated private business ideas (for example, unique housing arrangements promoted by private developers/owners) matched to facilitating public officials (for example, zoning issues, tax issues, and so forth) while realizing the hidden resources of the elderly (for example, organized volunteer efforts). Four initiatives have been identified:

1. Volunteer resources development
2. Preferred housing initiatives
3. Community awareness, education, and training
4. Service enhancement and expansion

Specific program components that have been partially or fully implemented to date are described later.

Each step of the GAP program development was supported ideologically and financially by the Medical Center consortium at about a 3:1 ratio to developmental grants. The charge at each step was to produce a meaningful program of services, monitoring, and financial arrangements that would persist under usual circumstances (for example, not grant or waiver-dependent) and would be self-supporting at the close of each grant period.

Innovative Services

This section describes the program components of the GAP Program, phases I and II, as follows: case management and assessment, related geriatric assessment and planning program activities, related community-oriented programs and activities, expanded community and professional relationships, and associated geriatric research.

Case Management and Assessment

The goals of both phase I and phase II included changing the care process by mainstreaming the technology of functional assessment and monitoring into a usual part of the hospital responsibility, and creating mechanisms to effectively "pass the baton" of care among community-based providers. The role of the hospital at postdischarge varies, depending on the agency responsible for postdischarge care. Ongoing service is provided by careful monitoring through the hospital's data base and by targeting staff responsibilities for patients categorized as "high risk" for dependence. The assumption guiding the program development is that the ability of frail older adults to live independently is enhanced by carefully and continually matching needs to services. The South Shore service coordination model is offered to all discharged patients in need (regardless of ability to pay), whereas services are provided largely by the multitude of available community-based agencies.

The basic program can be described as intake and assessment, linkage to needed services, monitoring the need–service utilization match, and reassessment. Specifically, the program enrolls South Shore Hospital inpatients and then through the case-management process:

- Integrates the comprehensive patient assessment system with the goal of early identification of those patients likely to need posthospital services and a continuing care plan
- Provides explicit mechanisms that ensure linkage of patients through posthospital service providers with specified and routine information sharing between the hospital and community-based service providers, confirmation of linkage, documentation of services provided, and notification of termination of patient care services
- Provides education and training for primary care givers of patients (as a hospital-sponsored referral service) prior to discharge or immediately following discharge
- Reassesses patients through six months postdischarge from community-based services with recommendations for physician visits (to their own physicians, if possible) and other services as appropriate
- Provides periodic educational and administrative seminars for community-based service providers and in-hospital staff to identify problems associated with linking patients to community services and to detail strategies to overcome them
- Analyzes patient discharge data, with regard to posthospital service needs as well as service availability, to identify major service gaps and explore ways in which South Shore Hospital and its affiliates can provide leadership in developing these services

The actual steps in the program begin with a comprehensive assessment at admission. In fact, the assessment process and the documentation provide the ability to categorize patients, with regard to likely posthospitalization needs, early in the stay. (Obviously, the actual plan is modified throughout the stay as assessment continues up to the time of discharge.) Patients are categorized with regard to level of dependency and availability of informal support (for those for whom noninstitutional community living is indicated). The GAP Program progresses as follows:

- Multidisciplinary discharge planning rounds are conducted approximately two days after admission. Patients who are likely to need continuing care are identified and enrolled.
- Care plans and preliminary discharge plans are detailed. Physician and patient (and family, if indicated) approvals are provided. Patients are referred to the appropriate community-based agency or agencies.

Family members and friends are referred to the Caregiver Training Program as indicated.

- Patients are discharged with discharge summaries and appropriate instruction. Initiation of services is confirmed, or the reasons for nondelivery are obtained. Patients' data are entered into the information system with appropriate "call-up" reminders so that staff can verify the initiation of planned services and/or the need for follow-up assessment and planning.
- Immediately after discharge, follow-ups are conducted on patients who are discharged in the following categories:
  - Confused and living alone
  - Against medical advice
  - Rounds not conducted
  - Dependent persons who go home alone
  - Dependent persons who go to ACLFs
- Notice of termination of services to patients are received from agencies with utilization summaries and reasons for terminations. Patient information is updated, and three- and six-month "call-up" reminders are entered.
- Arrangements are made for three- and six-month follow-ups by telephone/home visit. As a result of contact, further referrals may be made to a variety of sources in the community (for example, physician, community agencies).

Follow-up and tracking for the enrollees includes categorizing patients using activities of daily living and instrumental activities of daily living information by a composite score, as well as according to other key variables such as age, sex, marital status, household composition, insurance coverage, mental status, and past hospitalization experience (for patients and family members). Syntheses of these data are used both to summarize program activities and as a formative evaluation tool (for feedback to the assessment and planning staff) with which to review and modify program activities.

Related Geriatric Assessment and Planning Program Activities

Numerous programs and activities support the core of the GAP Program. The following list highlights some aspects of phases I, II, and III program expansion:

- Development of the Integrated Patient Information System, linking inpatient records with discharge planning and long-term care services
- Development and expansion of the Clinical Geriatric Fellowship to include the Jackson Memorial Hospital site

- Establishment of the Family Practice Residency Rotation at South Shore Hospital and Medical Center, for secondand third-year residents
- Establishment of the "Topics in the Care of Older Persons" continuing education series
- Expansion of the Self-Care for Seniors education program for well elderly and the Caregiver Training Program
- Establishment of care giver support groups, the Pacemaker Club for cardiac patients, and the Alzheimer's support group
- Establishment of the hospitalwide Art of Care Program that provides patient advocacy and focuses on processes of care likely to enhance patient satisfaction
- Training, placement, and supervision of senior companion volunteers providing personal care services to frail elderly under a Community Action Agency ACTION grant
- Location of a faculty practice site for the Department of Family Medicine and Community Health in the hospital's office tower, providing an ambulatory care site for patient care as well as residency and fellow training

Related Community-Oriented Programs and Activities

Although not specifically linked to the core GAP Program, related community programs share the common goal of maximizing the functional ability of the frail elderly and avoiding premature institutionalization. They include the following:

- Establishment of the VA Adult Day Health Center (one of four demonstration programs across the nation) on the South Shore Hospital and Medical Center campus under a lease arrangement
- Establishment of a Lifeline Program (emergency alert system) under a barter arrangement whereby the VA provides equipment and South Shore Hospital and Medical Center provides switchboard/monitoring coverage to a combined veteran–civilian constituency
- Shared assessment technology and referral capabilities among the South Shore Hospital and Medical Center programs and the 4C ("Foresee") Continuing Community Care Program of Jackson Memorial Hospital's Family Practice Service

Community activities also focus on volunteers. Volunteer efforts enhance the core of GAP program activities such that lower-priority patients (not just the highest-risk patients) can be monitored more closely. Volunteer efforts also facilitate the development of new/expanded services including respite, companionship, homemaker, personal care, home maintenance/repair, life management, day care, transportation, and monitoring.

Two models of volunteerism are in place. The first is represented by a Community Action Agency (CAA) ACTION grant awarded for the GAP Program site. Under this program, 16 low-income volunteers from the established Senior Companion Program are based at the hospital and perform tasks assigned by the GAP Program community health coordinator. These services expand the monitoring capability and provide homemaker/personal care services to clients on waiting lists or those ineligible because of financial reasons. Training of these volunteers is conducted jointly by the CAA and South Shore, and explicit monitoring and data collection facilitate the evaluation of all sites in the country in this ACTION grant program. Stipends are provided to the volunteers.

The second and more extensive model of volunteerism is a service credit model. The service credit concept allows resource expansion by creating a new currency, called *credits,* associated with volunteer activity.

The Greater Miami Service Credit Consortium was formed in 1986, representing a broad spectrum of organizations from the triethnic Miami community. Under South Shore Hospital and Medical Center sponsorship, a working-rule group was formed for immediate implementation of the service credit concept. In 1987, South Shore Hospital and Medical Center was awarded a three-year demonstration grant from the Robert Wood Johnson Foundation to lead the program at the hospital and expand to other sites including the Little Havana Activity Centers, Covenant Palms (Urban League housing for the elderly), and Hospice of Greater Miami. The program is designed to help frail older individuals avoid medical crises or institutionalization and live as independently as possible by matching needs with in-home services.

The program uses trained older volunteers who earn credits (one hour of services equals one hour of credit) by providing specified services (companionship, light housekeeping, transportation, respite, accompaniment on errands, telephone reassurance, linkage or referral to formal services) to frail elderly living at home. The hospital provides program administration, training, and record keeping for over 30 sites throughout Dade County. Local supervision is enhanced by 13 VISTA volunteers donated by the Little Havana centers. Currently over 600 volunteers (average age, 67) provide an average of 8,000 hours of service per month; over 1,300 recipients (average age, 80) are served in a one-year period.

Expanded Community and Professional Relationships

Various activities and relationships between the community and South Shore have unfolded. Although specific program capabilities are not directly enhanced, these activities and relationships provide networking likely to enhance future opportunities in several areas. Examples include:

- Participation and membership on the Guardianship Program (court-designated guardians for incompetent elderly) of the Dade County board of directors and the State of Florida Long-Term Care Ombudsman Committee
- Membership on the Miami Beach Health Advisory Board, the Gray Panthers of South Dade, the Steering Committee of the Alzheimer's Disease and Related Disorders Association, and the Southeast Florida Patient Education Association
- Participation in the Miami Coalition to Care for the Homeless
- Participation and active membership on several long-term care committees: Dade County Association of Service Providers for the Elderly, Agencies Concerned for the Elderly, Miami Beach Jewish Community Center Senior Center Board, and the Dade County Clearing House Consortium
- Provision of office space and meeting rooms to community organizations such as Jewish Family Services, Senior Ride, and the Miami Beach Development Corporation
- Cohost of the annual meeting of the North American Primary Care Research Group (Community-Oriented Health Care–A Brave New World)

Associated Geriatric Research

In addition to assuming responsibilities for the planning and evaluation department, the University of Miami's Department of Family Medicine and Community Health has relocated its health services research offices to the South Shore campus. A variety of geriatric health services research activities are directed through this office, including:

- Site coordination for the Seattle-based evaluation of the VA Adult Day Health Center.
- Research direction for the Study to Assess Falls among the Elderly (SAFE), a five-year epidemiological study of falls and burns among the South Beach elderly under a Centers for Disease Control/Dade County Public Health Unit cooperative agreement. This includes establishment of an ongoing surveillance system, a demographic survey (minicensus), a case-control study, and program intervention/evaluation.

Continuity of Care Programming

Two new programs have been implemented:

- The not-for-profit community health center for South Beach relocated to the South Shore Hospital and Medical Center campus in 1988. In addition to significant physical plant improvements and renovations, this relocation brought with it expanded primary care capabilities and a source of referrals to (and from) the GAP Program. Further, the hospital has opened a 24-hour urgent care center, greatly increasing access to service for the community health center patients.

- The University of Miami Comprehensive Plan and Rehabilitation Center, directed by the department of neurosurgery, has assumed responsibility for the hospital's rehabilitative services.

Via reimbursable outpatient services, the community health center seeks to restore and sustain maximal physical functioning with specific training and adaptation to usual activities and independent living.

Financing

The financing of each activity or program component described in this chapter posed unique challenges. The accomplishments were largely a result of commitment of top management to support a core staff, with planning capability to seek out and develop important long-term care activities. Although many of the activities described were funded by grant dollars, a general theme of self-support was evident. Program activities were prioritized to be consistent with the overall mission of the institution and, following investment in their development, to enhance services and thereby attract referral providers and patients to the hospital. Collaboration with the university and other community organizations was founded on a theme of "win-win" situations, as well as sharing resources and benefits (such as an increase in constituents) in a mutually beneficial manner. All resource investment required endorsement at the board level and collaboration at the necessary administrative level via clear directives from officers of the chief executive officer and chief operating officer.

Conclusions

The foundation of systematic assessment and service coordination has guided the core program and development of elderly services at South Shore in order to approach a continuum of long-term care services for the hospital's constituency. The hospital stay is viewed as an opportunity to affect long-term care needs, including those at postdischarge, and innovations are mainstreamed into the usual care of older adults.

Although hospitals may be viewed as complex organizations representing hard-to-move bureaucratic structures, South Shore Hospital has demonstrated commitment and actions toward the development of a long-term care continuum. The challenges of future development are formidable, and widespread modes of caring for frail elderly are likely to remain, at least in part, dependent on the adequacy or inadequacy of support from the public sector. But numerous opportunities to approach an optimal continuum of long-term care exist for the hospital committed to principles of community-oriented health care.

References

1. DeVito, C. A., and Zubkoff, W. South Shore Hospital and Medical Center: A comprehensive care provider. In: *Comprehensive Care for the Elderly Hospital Case Studies.* Chicago: Hospital Research and Educational Trust, 1986, pp. 13–20.
2. DeVito, C. A., and Zubkoff, W. Community resources for post-hospital needs: geriatric assessment and planning program. *Topics in Geriatric Rehabilitation* 1(2):70–76, 1986.
3. DeVito, C. A., and Zubkoff, W. The role of the acute care hospital in long-term care: a model program on South Miami Beach. *Journal of the Florida Medical Association* 72(4):258–62, Apr. 1975.
4. DeVito, C. A., Carmichael, L. P., and Zubkoff, W. Toward community-oriented care: the role of the community hospital. In: P. A. Nutting, editor. *Community-Oriented Primary Care: From Principle to Practice.* DHHS publication No. HRS-A-PE 86-1. Washington, DC: U.S. Government Printing Office. In press.
5. Katz, S., and Akpom, C. A measure of primary socio-biological functions. *International Journal of Health Services* 6(3):495–507, 1976. (For bathing, dressing, transferring, toileting, eating/feeding, bowel and bladder continence: A = performance without assistance in any of the functions; B = needs assistance with one function; C = needs assistance with two functions; D through G = needs assistance with three, four, five, or six functions, respectively.
6. Clients Served and Services provided—1980–81. Report by Douglas Gardens Community Mental Health Center of Miami Beach, 1981.
7. Analysis of At-Risk Population in the City of Miami Beach. Report by City of Miami Beach, July 1982.
8. Zubkoff, W., DeVito, C. A., and Carmichael, L. P. South Shore Hospital and Medical Center—a natural laboratory for programs in geriatric care. In: S. J. Brody and N. A. Persily, editors. *Hospitals and the Aged: The New Old Market.* Rockville, MD: Aspen Publications, 1984, pp. 255–63.
9. Fogel, B. J., and Zubkoff, W. A model for medical school and community hospital cooperation. *Journal of the Florida Medical Association* 70(3):203, Mar. 1983.
10. South Shore Hospital and Medical Center Mission Statement, Fall 1982.

Chapter 19

Programs for the Elderly at a Rural Medical Center

JoAnna DeMeyer

Introduction

Since its founding in 1901, St. Luke's of Boise, Idaho, has evolved into a regional medical center offering a wide variety of sophisticated medical services to an immediate county of 200,000 people, as well as a large, sparsely populated secondary service area of approximately 368,000 people. The tertiary service area of St. Luke's Regional Medical Center includes southwestern Idaho, northwestern Nevada, and southeastern Oregon, with a population of approximately 550,000. Although Boise is the largest city in Idaho, with a population of approximately 127,000, it is geographically isolated from any other metropolitan area. The closest metropolitan area is Salt Lake City, Utah, 350 miles southeast. The state of Idaho, as well as the service area, is very rural. Approximately 15 percent of Idaho residents are over age 60, and 10 percent of the over-60 population in Idaho reside in Ada County where Boise is located.

St. Luke's provides a wide range of services, including obstetrics, neonatal care, pediatrics, cardiovascular services, and oncology. St. Luke's has several outpatient services, including the Mountain States Tumor Institute, the Breast Cancer Detection Center, the Mountain States Surgery Center, outpatient rehabilitation, home care services, patient and family education, and health promotion programs.

Emphasis on programs for the elderly began in 1980 when St. Luke's Regional Medical Center's board of trustees developed the Medical Center's strategic plan, which included the following objective: "[To] develop a plan for a full-service spectrum of senior citizen programs for meeting health and human support needs."

This chapter describes the process and activities of this rural medical center in initiating and developing services and programs to better meet the health care needs of the elderly. The three overall goals were:

- To demonstrate that a rural community hospital, utilizing a private medical practice model, could provide a broad spectrum of cost-effective health care services to the elderly
- To reduce the use of costly hospital and nursing home services by the elderly by helping them maintain independence and retain functional abilities
- To improve the capabilities of both medical and hospital staff to care for the elderly in all areas of the hospital

Internal/External Environment

Within St. Luke's regional service area, the problems of meeting the health care needs of the elderly are largely the same as throughout the country. In addition to the area's increased aging population, a rising number of elderly—particularly those over age 75—have increasing health problems and decreasing resources for addressing those problems. The onset of diagnosis-related groups (DRGs) has shortened an already-short average length of stay for those 65 and over, from 7 days in 1983 to 6.3 days in 1989, allowing little time to prepare a frail elderly person for the return home and for the recovery period. The short hospital stay has resulted in more short stays in nursing homes for recuperation before a return home. Services to facilitate this transition may or may not have been available to each patient, and those that were available were poorly coordinated, resulting in service duplication and inflated costs to the client and/or the family. Also, an issue resulting from some short hospital stays has been rehospitalization among the elderly.

The Boise community has a strong commitment to care of the elderly. This is evidenced by a dynamic senior citizen center, by Boise State University's establishment of studies on aging, by a well-received Growing Younger Program through Healthwise (a not-for-profit health promotion organization), and by an affiliation between the Boise Veterans Administration Medical Center and the University of Washington School of Medicine. This affiliation provides training to interns and medical students in gerontology, as well as support for research in gerontology.

The health care community includes three hospitals: St. Luke's Regional Medical Center (community), St. Alphonsus Medical Center (Catholic), and the Veterans Administration Medical Center. Approximately 333 physicians in the community have hospital privileges.

In 1985, 20 percent of St. Luke's total hospital admissions were over age 65 and used 30 percent of the total hospital days, representing an increase of approximately 6 percent over 1982. In 1989, 22.2 percent of the same age group used 32.7 percent of the hospital days; 9.7 percent of these admissions were age 75 or older and used 14.4 percent of the hospital days.

Several sources of information were used when St. Luke's planned its programs for the elderly. In the *1982–87 Health Systems Plan for Idaho,* the Idaho Health Systems Agency (private, not-for-profit) stated three major concerns:

1. The need for a readily identifiable source of information about existing health services
2. Increased accessibility to existing services
3. Renewed efforts and concern by the region's health planning agencies, health services providers, and local governments to seek ways to strengthen, expand, and establish the health services needed for a comprehensive health services delivery system

It should also be noted that readily identifiable sources of health services information and increased accessibility to health care were especially important for the elderly as their health status changed because of chronic disease and disability.

In 1980, the Ada County Medical Society completed a telephone survey regarding the socioeconomic mix of patients served. These data were utilized in conjunction with a study of St. Luke's Regional Medical Center's statistics. To assist assessment of the environment, St. Luke's also completed a community survey of eldercare resources.

In 1984, St. Luke's was awarded a Robert Wood Johnson Foundation (RWJF) grant, *Hospital Initiatives in Long-Term Care.* One of the first activities made possible by the grant was an internal survey of St. Luke's employee needs and interests with regard to the elderly. The survey included a needs assessment and a facts on aging quiz. Respondents were placed in four categories according to their contact with the elderly: clinical nursing, clinical nonnursing, nonclinical/contact, and nonclinical/no contact. The nonclinical/contact group included people in the business office or admitting; the nonclinical/no contact group included those in areas such as accounting or personnel. The majority of the clinical nursing and clinical nonnursing respondents expressed greatest interest in programs regarding cerebrovascular problems, confusion, nutrition, drugs, and functional assessment. Those in the nonclinical/no contact and nonclinical/contact groups expressed greatest interest in information on preparing for retirement and aging, myths and realities about aging, problems relating to aging parents, health care resources for the elderly, nutrition, and exercise and recreation for the elderly. The majority of all respondents, then, did express interest in the elderly.

The survey also included an interest survey of St. Luke's private-practice physicians. The physician survey identified greatest interest in four general topics and four disease-specific topics. The general topics were normal versus abnormal aging, pathology and pathophysiology of disease relevant to the aging process, preventive medicine for the elderly, and financial issues relating to eldercare planning. The disease-specific topics were osteoporosis, dementia, osteoarthritis, and coping with death and dying. The employee and physician survey data were used extensively to plan and develop St. Luke's programs for older adults.

Educational programs were interwoven throughout as specific services or programs were developed. The needs assessment was repeated annually for the first three years of these endeavors. Educational activities were designed and implemented to relate directly to survey findings. The surveys guided educational endeavors to five categories of activities:

1. Circulation of articles and information to all departments about topics and issues on aging
2. Internal community plan for keeping all medical center staff informed of new or developing programs for the elderly
3. Specialized programs utilizing consultants for either program design and/or program presentation
4. Physician continuing education programs utilizing consultants for physician-specific presentations and increasing materials included about the elderly in all appropriate physician continuing education programs
5. Community programs for the elderly and health professionals

A process was developed for the most effective utilization of consultants. This process included planning consultant visits to coordinate with community agencies; to coordinate with Boise State University; to arrange presentations to staff, at community health night, and to medical staff; as well as to make clinical rounds and/or attend meetings with specific groups or staff (see figure 19-1).

Figure 19-1. Process for Utilizing Consultants

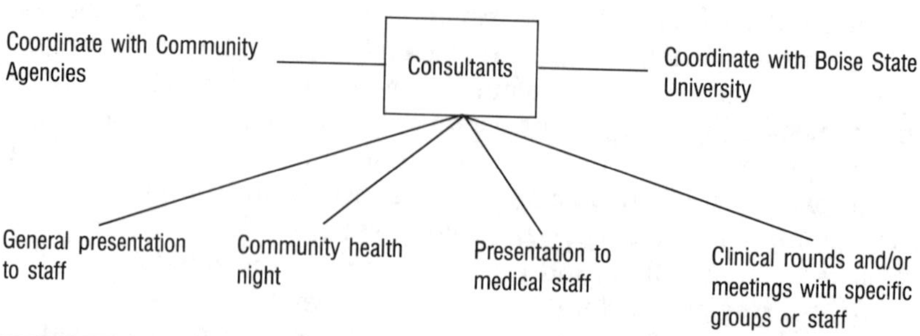

A significant environmental factor was physician reluctance to consider geriatric programs a viable concept. Although the president, the president-elect, and the past president of the medical staff were involved in the very first discussion of concepts and planning, a "wait and see" attitude prevailed. Physician reluctance seemed attributable to a variety of factors. First, the physicians as a group initially appeared not to recognize geriatrics as a specialty. Second, the programs/services for the elderly were new to this physician group. Also, physicians seemed to fear losing these patients from their practices.

Twelve physicians were members of three task forces formed to guide and implement objectives of the RWJF grant. These physicians were essential and crucial in designing the service management system and influenced other physicians' referrals to the service management system.

Expanded involvement of St. Luke's staff, particularly geriatrics-trained staff, with community groups provided information on service needs, areas of interests, gaps in service, support needed, and assistance in developing geriatric services.

In summary, the environment for developing geriatric services at St. Luke's was characterized by a community with a strong interest in older adults and their needs, a medical center with stated planning goals for meeting those needs, a medical staff with no geriatricians on staff or in the nearby community (except at the Veterans Administration Medical Center), and a medical staff with unsolidified goals regarding the elderly.

Goals

St. Luke's identified the many benefits the Medical Center could gain by promoting a comprehensive and coordinated system of care for the elderly. These benefits included a positive, knowledgeable environment in which Medical Center employees could provide services to the elderly, increased patient referrals (resulting from high-quality services and increased community awareness), and decreased duplication of costly services, thus making health care services more convenient for patients and physicians.

The Medical Center's specific goals for geriatric services were:

- To offer those 65 years and older (and their families) access to a system that provides a comprehensive, coordinated continuum of care
- To increase knowledge about special health and social services care of older adults and their families in order to enhance the quality, coordination, and cost effectiveness of care
- To establish and maintain cost-effective programs that contribute to the viability of the Medical Center

- To formalize, organize, and coordinate the activities by creating appropriate organizational structures

Early in 1983, St. Luke's responded to the RWJF request for a proposal on Hospital Initiatives in Long-Term Care. During that same year, SeniorLife Services was designated as a St. Luke's department, and a department director was hired. In January 1984, St. Luke's was awarded the four-year RWJF grant. St. Luke's had already provided some services to elderly persons, but the funding offered an opportunity to expand and develop new programs and demonstrate a model for other similar community hospitals.

The specific objectives of the RWJF grant proposal were:

- To organize a geriatric assessment team to provide consultative services to participating private practice physicians and to assist in assessment, case-finding, placement, monitoring, and follow-up services
- To design and implement a centralized data system for storage and retrieval of data relevant to the health care needs of a selected group of elderly patients and community resources to meet those needs (including development of a community resources directory)
- To design and implement an educational program utilizing modules and teaching aids, to sensitize care givers to the needs of the selected elderly, and to educate care givers to meet those needs

Planning/Development Process

The planning/development process for geriatric services at St. Luke's included St. Luke's Regional Medical Center's board of trustees establishing overall goals for strategic planning and receiving planned feedback on progress and accomplishments. The process included a community advisory committee with representatives of the elderly population segment, as well as representatives from selected community organizations and associations.

In 1984, a steering committee was established within the Medical Center that included the vice-president of patient care services and the chairpersons of the three task forces charged with implementing the objectives. The three task forces were the educational programs team, geriatric assessment team, and centralized data team. Task force memberships included physicians and multidisciplinary representatives from St. Luke's. The overall Medical Center coordinating committee included the president, the executive vice-president, the vice-president of finance, and the vice-president of patient care services. This committee strategy ensured communication with and feedback to medical staff and the board of trustees as well as communication with the multiple Medical Center departments.

A significant aspect of the development process was the need to continually identify motivational strategies to encourage interest and involvement of needed key players—physicians and nursing staff.

Physician involvement was questionable because, as determined at the time, physicians as a whole were ambivalent about whether geriatrics was a "true" specialty. Thus they were doubtful whether a geriatric assessment team, special services, and educational programs were needed. At that time none of the resident internists had a specific geriatric requirement to fulfill, and there were no geriatricians in the community except at the Veterans Administration Medical Center.

Some physicians also indicated they had "grown older" with their patients and knew their needs. Others felt that unless the assessment team would "determine new diagnoses," there was no reason to refer to the team.

Changing these perceptions was a slow and difficult process. It took time before some physicians referred to the assessment team and were willing to say the team had been helpful. (The geriatric assessment team includes a geriatrician, a geriatric nurse specialist, and a social worker.) These physician "pioneers" stated the team had saved them office time through reduced phone calls from patients and families, identified team-coordinated services and new services and resources, helped with social problems among patients and identified other health problems (such as depression), provided information on drugs prescribed by other physicians, and identified environmental issues, and so forth.

A majority of the professional nursing staff had associate's-degree backgrounds and some knowledge of functional assessment and service management. Even so, they also were doubtful that geriatrics should be a service area with a special knowledge base and care needs. Getting them to attend educational programs was a challenge, but once they became involved, behaviors began to change. For both groups, physicians and nurses, motivational strategies were important, such as teaching and demonstrating how educational programs, the geriatric assessment team, and the *Directory of Community Resources for the Elderly* could be helpful to them.

Case Management and Assessment

To work most effectively in a rural community medical center environment that utilizes private-practice physicians, a service management philosophy (case management) was developed. The philosophy is founded on meeting the needs of elderly or chronically diseased persons while ensuring their maximum independence and functional ability and avoiding unnecessary and costly hospital and nursing home services. To implement this philosophy, geriatric assessment activities and centralized, computerized data-system activities were interwoven with care-giver and client educational endeavors, and with the development of the *Directory of Community Resources for the Elderly.*

At St. Luke's the term *service management* rather than *case management* is used. This is due to physicians who commented that it was they who reviewed and managed "cases," whereas the team really managed "services." Thus physicians on one RWJF task force advised use of the term *service management* to gain greater acceptance and more referrals by physicians. The term was felt to be clarifying and helpful in continued endeavors to gain physician involvement.

Referrals for the geriatric assessment team and service management are received from physicians, the home care and discharge planning staffs, and from families. Referrals are accepted for inpatients and outpatients. Once a referral is requested, an order is obtained from the client's physician. The assessment consultation is completed, and the client's follow-up plan of care is coordinated with discharge planning, the geriatric assessment team, and the client/family at the time of discharge. The registered nurse or the social worker for the patient's geriatric assessment team is designated as the service manager. Service management is initiated following the client's discharge (inpatient assessment) or after the initial outpatient visit (outpatient assessment). Clients are followed with at least monthly telephone contact and reassessment visits at three-month intervals.

Patient entry criteria for referrals state that the geriatric assessment team can best assist with those patients who are 65 years of age or over and who have one or more of the following characteristics: a history of falls; difficulty walking; sphincter incontinence; confusion; or medical problems significantly influenced by aging (for example, diabetes and hypothyroidism), those needing presurgical assessment, those involving multiple medications, and so forth.

The geriatric assessment team completes the initial intake monitoring, including comprehensive assessment of medical status, functional status, service needs, and available resources. The team consults appropriate ancillary services, family members, direct care nurses, and discharge planners in formulating its recommendations, which it then shares with the private-practice physician. At this point the patient becomes a part of service management, which includes the following elements:

- *Service manager.* A clinical nurse specialist or social worker is designated to coordinate reassessment, services, and data collection.
- *Service management.* This process includes no less than a monthly telephone call and home visits at three-month intervals. Home care nurses and/or discharge planners may assist with collection of data and reassessment as deemed appropriate by the service manager. The client

data are computerized, and copies are provided for the physician's review and office file.

- *Service tracking.* Patients who no longer require home visits are transferred to service tracking, which entails monthly telephone calls only, replacing service management for those patients whose services are being managed adequately by another provider or those no longer in need of service management. Should conditions change, patients will be returned to the service management status.

The computerized management information system was designed to provide for the storage and retrieval of patient data collected by the team during assessment and reassessment intervals. Computerized outpatient summaries are generated for service managers and the referring physicians following the initial assessment and after reassessment visits. These summaries provide baseline data regarding functional status, environmental factors, and resources currently utilized. These data also are used for planning and case utilization monitoring as part of the service management process. Another feature of the management information system is the computerization of a *Directory of Community Resources for the Elderly,* a valuable resource.

Thus service management functions include:

- Validation of initial assessment data and care plan postdischarge
- Monitoring of health status and service utilization
- Service referral and/or procurement
- Advocacy for patient and family
- Coordination of information flow
- Support and education for care giver
- Ongoing reassessment and revised care plan as appropriate

Service management benefits to the patient/family have included a connection following discharge between hospital personnel/services and the patient/family to identify problems, specify action to be taken in a timely manner, and have one person with whom to network and coordinate all services. Service management benefits the primary physician by saving time (in particular phone calls from the patient or family), by relieving the physician from assessing and referring clients regarding social issues better handled by the service manager, and by providing client information that otherwise would not be available. The benefit to the Medical Center has been the development and maintenance of linkages with community agencies, thus avoiding duplication of services and increasing the referral base.

The identification by the community of St. Luke's/Boise as being interested in, caring about, and providing specific programs for older adults has resulted in increased numbers of elderly utilizing the Medical

Center's services. The service management program has demonstrated that program participants have been able to stay in their own homes longer, in some cases until their deaths. Clients or families also have indicated they felt the program enabled them to utilize available services more effectively, many of which they were not previously aware of or where previously there was duplication. Clients also were able to use services in the home rather than be admitted to a hospital or nursing home. Although it is difficult to identify specific dollars saved, these observations indicate more effective utilization of dollars for services as viewed by the client or family and some savings of public and private dollars.

Innovative Services

A variety of services are offered and/or managed by SeniorLife, programs and services developed with the input from senior citizen groups, the grant community advisory committee, staff, and physician groups. Although new programs were being developed, existing services and programs placed increased emphasis in meeting the needs of older adults.

One senior citizen group identified the need for a foot clinic, which it felt should be offered in the senior center. In 1985, St. Luke's started providing these clinics on-site in the senior center once a month with the center handling its own appointment calendar. St. Luke's clinic staff (an aide and a registered nurse) have referred elderly patients to the staff podiatrist, the internist, and the nutritionist. The clinics are well attended and are provided for a small fee or, where necessary, no fee.

In 1984, the *Directory of Community Resources* was developed utilizing a computer system that provides for quick and inexpensive updates. *The Directory* is designed to be used by the elderly, physicians, and care givers, as well as health professionals. It is a resource of services available in the community. *The Directory* is provided at a $10 cost and is free to those unable to pay.

The insurance assistance program was also need identified by the community advisory committee and senior citizen groups. St. Luke's provided the service in 1985 with well-publicized specific hours in an easily accessible area. Soon, however, the hours were expanded, because not only the elderly but other patients as well used the service. No fee is charged for this service.

Geriatric assessment was provided through a detailed health assessment by a physician, registered nurse, and social worker. The geriatric assessment team completed a comprehensive assessment of medical status, functional status, service needs, and available community resources. Recommendations from the team were shared with the patients' private physicians orally and through a printout of the computerized patient assessment data, which was sent to the physicians' offices. Following the initial assessment, the patients are enrolled in the service management program where the clinical nurse specialist or social worker becomes the patient's family service manager to coordinate patient's reassessment and data collection.

The SeniorLife Passport Program was developed in 1987 in response requests from older adults for simplified billing and admitting. The program offers a credit card–like "passport" that when presented at the Medical Center provides access to data needed for express admission. The program also provides for simplified billing as well as many educational and health promotion programs. There is no charge for this program. Other programs and services offered by the medical center are included in table 19-1.

Financing

The geriatric/seniors programs began with support by the St. Luke's Regional Medical Center's board of trustees for the 1980 strategic plan goal, which identified the need for a plan to develop a full spectrum of services for the elderly. The board's initial statement provided resources for developing the plan and supported working with selected department directors and a College of Health Science representative from Boise State University to develop a grant application for the RWJF *Hospital Initiatives in Long-Term Care* program. The grant awarded $495,000 to St. Luke's over a four-year period (1984–1987). It included a commitment that those activities and services demonstrated to be effective would be continued by St. Luke's.

SeniorLife programs, developed during the grant and continued after the end of the grant, are financed in a variety of ways. Payment by Medicare and private insurers is utilized where available. Many senior services or programs are not covered by insurers. Thus educational programs and health maintenance programs (such as foot care) are offered free or at cost. St. Luke's has continued to refine and develop programs and services for seniors. The St. Luke's board of trustees has designated SeniorLife as one of the Medical Center's "centers of excellence."

Conclusions

St. Luke's Regional Medical Center has developed a strategic plan for and progressed significantly toward a "full-service spectrum of senior citizen programs for meeting health and human support needs." These accomplishments have been made with the assistance of a Robert Wood Johnson Foundation grant and the support of the local community. The

Table 19-1. SeniorLife Programs, St. Luke's Regional Medical Center, Boise, Idaho

Program	Provided by	Description	Cost to Client
Geriatric Assessment	SeniorLife	Consultation service; referral from team physician required	None
Staff Education	SeniorLife	Conferences, written materials, Attitudes and Behaviors Workshop, consultant presentations	None
Senior Education	SeniorLife	1. Community seminars 2. Growing Younger/Growing Wiser Programs 3. Senior Health Fair 4. Senior Sit-Ups Program	1. None 2. $15/person, $25/couple 3. None 4. $10/6 weeks
Community Education	SeniorLife	Variety of workshops for professionals and/or lay care givers	Cost varies
Directory of Community Resources for the Elderly	SeniorLife	Hard-copy directory listing detailed information/resources specifically for the elderly in Boise	$10 (if unable to pay, no charge)
Insurance Assistance Program	SeniorLife	Assistance for the elderly and/or families to complete insurance forms and file claims	None
Foot Clinic	SeniorLife	Monthly assessment of foot care referrals for the elderly	$10 (if unable to pay, no charge)
Carrier Alert	SeniorLife	Cooperative program with service/letter carriers to look for mail accumulation at homes of the elderly	None
Home Care Services	Home Care	Nursing, social work, rehabilitation, and aide services for Medicare and private-pay patients	Based on service provided
Phone Care	Home Care	Phone units to alert designated persons of problems and need for help	$10/month (if unable to pay, no charge)
Discharge Planning/ Social Services	Discharge Planning/ Social Services	Assistance for client/family with placement and social services	None
Senior Meal Discount	Dietary	20% discount on meals for senior citizens	20% less than listed price
Blood Pressure Screening	Emergency Department	Blood pressure reading on walk-in basis	None
Physician Referral Service	Medical Staff Office	Assistance and information for the elderly regarding physicians available	None, referral
SeniorLife Passport	SeniorLife/ Admitting	Multiple departments collaborate to provide program for senior members, cards for express admitting, simplified billing, and so forth	None

basis has been that the concept of a continuum of care is a natural framework for geriatric services and programs. St. Luke's envisions a coordinated range of services that includes health promotion, health counseling and education, mental health counseling, acute inpatient care, ambulatory/outpatient care, home care, and information and referral to other community services.

St. Luke's believes the continuum of care, emphasizing access to an array of services for older adults, will enable the Medical Center to respond to and anticipate challenges to the ever-changing health care environment.

Chapter 20

A Gerontology Center Serving People over Age 75

Eugene Dawson, Jr.

Introduction

The general service area of Swedish Medical Center stretches out over the expanding southern metropolitan area of Denver, Colorado, and has an estimated population of 450,000 to 465,000 persons. Even though the bulk of this service area includes new suburbs with a majority of young families, Swedish itself is situated in the heart of an older suburb, Englewood, which is adjacent to the southern portion of Denver. Another older area located farther south, Littleton, and the south central portion of Denver are all in Swedish's immediate service area. Furthermore these areas contain many census tracts with extremely high percentages of people 65 years of age and older. The older adults in these areas represent anywhere from 9 to 25 percent of the neighborhood populations. Approximately 45 percent of those 65 and older are over 75 years of age. This older group is nevertheless a vastly diverse group that spans the socioeconomic spectrum from people with very low incomes to homeowners with comfortable retirement incomes. It was for this group that Swedish established the Gerontology Program in 1976 and opened the Swedish Gerontology Center in 1984.

Internal/External Environment

The Swedish Medical Center Board of Trustees' support for long-term care services dates back to 1975, when it established a task force to examine the needs of the aging population and to look at the hospital's role in meeting those needs. In 1976, that study culminated in the board's affirmation of its commitment to the hospital's role in serving the elderly community and the establishment of Swedish Gerontology Health Resources, Inc. (SGHR). Legal and administrative responsibilities over all gerontological activities at Swedish have been maintained by SGHR.

Swedish's commitment also extends to congregate housing needs of the elderly. In October 1986, the Corona Cooperative—a $26 million 227-unit facility—was officially opened. With 18 different floor plans, from 900 square feet to 1,700 square feet, it represented the only hospital-sponsored cooperative in America. The facilities and programs at Swedish Medical Center, as well as on-site medical and social services consultants, are available to Swedish Corona residents. An emergency system can summon help within minutes. As a cooperative, the entire project is governed by the residents, each of whom shares ownership.

Those age 75 and older constitute the major target population to be served by the Swedish Gerontology Center, an affiliate of Swedish Medical Center. The Center is designated to serve an older population at risk of being institutionalized, or the frail elderly. These individuals tend to be more socially isolated, have few support systems, and have one or two chronic illnesses. A sizable minority of the population served by the Center are diagnosed as having Alzheimer's disease, or severe memory loss. Others served in the Center are dealing with various common frailties associated with advanced age. In 1985, an "Aging Services Impact and Needs Assessment," sponsored by the Denver Regional Council of Governments, Aging Services Division, found that 44 percent of this older population had "health" as their major concern in life. The problems of these older adults resulted from specific illnesses that were incapacitating, severely limited the ability to care for oneself, or were very painful. Other problems included alcoholism, insufficient health care benefits, and difficulties in obtaining health care.

Swedish has a large number of special programs to serve the community. The programs that distinguish Swedish from its competitors are:

- Corporate health management
- Day care for relatives of employees
- Hospital satellite program
- Lifegain
- E.M.S. system involvement
- Comprehensive neuro/neurorehabilitation program
- Health matters
- Comprehensive women's health services
- Employee assistance programs

Other programs partially distinguish Swedish, although both hospital and nonhospital competitors market similar services. Such programs include a breast center, a sports medicine center, a community wellness (former service) center, and seniors programs.

Late in the fourth quarter of 1986, the Colorado Health Data Commission released a report on important data concerning the 17 hospitals in the Denver area. These data indicated that, even with a 5 percent average rate increase, Swedish was a low-cost provider of health care services in what is considered one of the most competitive hospital market areas in the country.

Swedish is investigating or preparing to launch a number of programs that will be used in increasing the access and visibility of the hospital: helicopter/air transport, physician referral program (has been implemented), communications information center, and access card (VIP)-type program.

In the aging field, three other Denver-based hospitals have aggressively sought the older adult market. In all three the emphasis has been on the establishment of senior clinics throughout the city. Swedish has countered by supporting the development of health maintenance organizations (HMOs) for older adults and in the development of a "centers of excellence" concept by concentrating on a few activities and doing what is perceived as most sensible from a market share or volume position.

Fifteen adult day care programs currently are operating in the Denver metropolitan area. Only one hospital other than Swedish serves as a sponsor for day care activities. Swedish's day care programs are comparable in size to other existing day care programs. The Swedish program, small by design (seven to nine participants), is considered by professionals to be the exemplary program within the state. The Swedish Alzheimer's Day Care Program, one of two day care programs in the Gerontology Center, is the longest-standing program of its kind in the state of Colorado. Other such programs throughout the state, with the exception of one, are located within skilled nursing facilities (SNFs).

Goals

The Swedish Medical Center Mission Statement reads as follows:

> To identify community needs, act as an advocate for the community, and provide a continuum of health care and other social services necessary to meet the needs of the Denver Metropolitan Area and immediate hospital service area, and any other communities that Swedish can effectively assist.

The mission statement of the Swedish Gerontology Center is as follows:

The Swedish Gerontology Center, sponsored by Swedish Health Systems, is dedicated to promoting the health and well-being of seniors through a wide range of services that enhance their ability to live actively and independently in the community.

The management structure of Swedish is shown in figure 20-1.

Figure 20-1. Management Structure of Swedish Medical Center, Englewood, Colorado

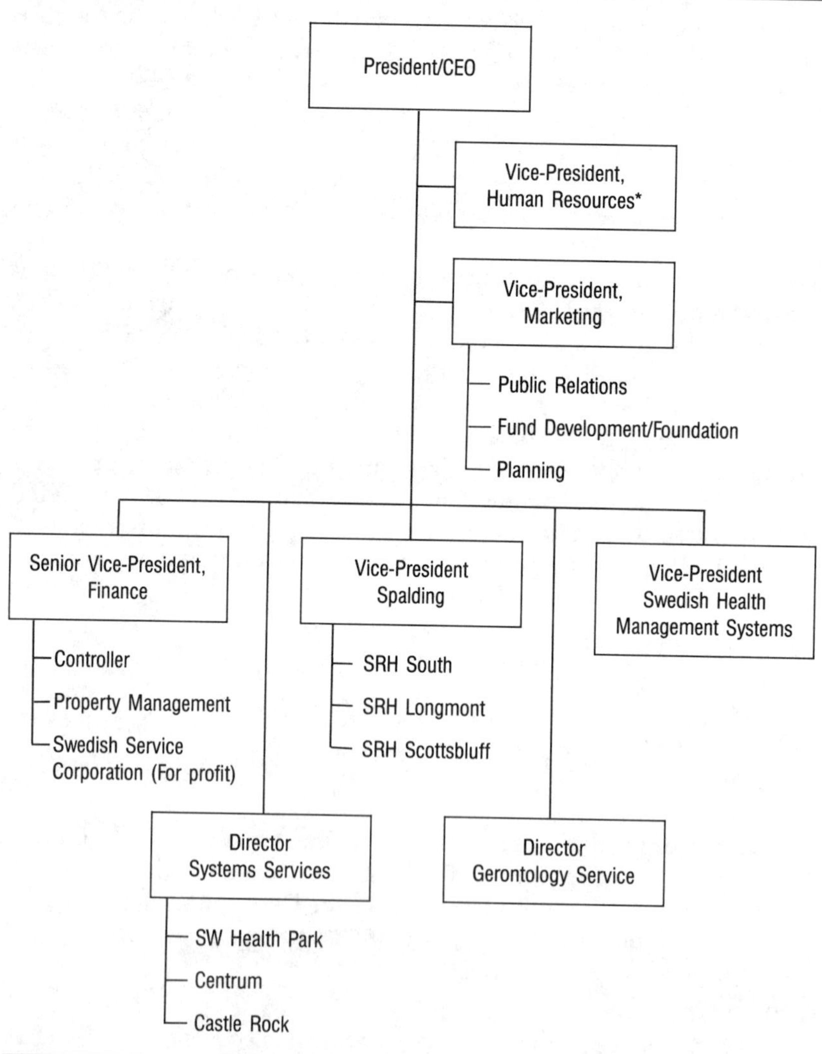

*Also reports to Senior Vice-President, Administration.

Planning/Development Process

The development process of geriatric services at Swedish began with Clarkson Corners, the gerontological program started in 1976, and with the development of the aging services committee in 1986. Gerontology at Swedish originated at a location on Clarkson Street in Englewood on the main campus of Swedish Medical Center. The program consequently called "Clarkson Corners" began as a clinic under the direction of a physician from the medical center. The clinic's purpose was to serve older adults, and it had provisions with the assistance of the Swedish Medical Center Foundation to serve the medically indigent. Funding problems and concerns voiced by other physicians that patients were being directed from their practices to the clinic resulted in the program being developed more along the lines of a "social model" as opposed to a "medical model."

Clarkson Corners

Clarkson Corners evolved into two major areas of emphasis. One, on Alzheimer's day care, was referred to as the Adult Specialized Activities Program. It consisted of a small group who were at risk for institutionalization. They met in a specially designed room on Mondays, Wednesdays, and Fridays from 9:00 a.m. to 1:30 p.m. The other program, referred to as Clarkson Corners, met on Monday and Thursday at noon. The emphasis included good food, socialization, and topics pertaining primarily to health promotion. The social worker in charge of the program provided limited case management and referred persons to appropriate resources when the need arose.

Another program, Outreach to Syracuse Plaza, a subsidized, federally sponsored high-rise for low-income elderly, began in 1982 and represented an important component of the total program. A Syracuse Club of 10 to 50 older persons was developed. Each person paid $10 dues four times a year plus the cost of the meal that was brought over to the residence from the dietary department at Swedish. Again the program emphasis approximated what was being done at Clarkson Corners, except the program was semimonthly as opposed to weekly. During the "off weeks," health screening occurred as did trips and various social activities. The high-rise was in a socially isolated area of southeast Denver, and Swedish's contribution occurred because other agencies, private and public, had not responded to the various needs manifest within that environment. The move and creation of the Gerontology Center, located in Englewood two miles south of the main hospital campus, necessitated the discontinuation of the Syracuse Club. Considerable effort was taken by Center staff to link residents with other resources in the community.

Several considerations went into Clarkson Corners becoming Swedish Gerontology Center. One consideration centered on the larger institutional need to have the structure that housed the Clarkson Corners program be converted into an ambulatory outpatient surgical unit for the hospital. A second consideration focused on the planning effort to reach out to those "more at risk of being institutionalized"–the older population residing south of the main hospital campus in the older suburb of Englewood (identified by demographics to be a sizable number). Clarkson Corners had served a very useful purpose when there were no senior centers in Englewood and few, if any, senior organizations. But in recent years a very impressive senior center–8,500 members–known as Malley Center had been developed. Numerous other specialized programs for the elderly were being developed, and it made little sense for a hospital-sponsored program to be competing for the same clientele already being served by other groups within the city. The mission of serving the more frail and forestalling institutionalization while promoting wellness appeared to be a more logical course of action.

Finally, an attractive former school in a residential park two miles south of the hospital became available for the housing of the Center. A lease was arranged for $25,000 a year, paid to Englewood Public Schools. Major improvements were made to make the building "barrier-free" and conducive to serving the more impaired older adult.

Not all residents in the community or agencies in the area were pleased to see Swedish penetrate their community with a gerontology center. Accusations were made that Swedish was planning to build a high-rise in the park; bring "dangerous, demented older persons" into the neighborhood; and misuse the school building where residents had sent their children. Even numbers of older adults from Clarkson Corners were resentful of the change. The thought of leaving familiar territory and going to a schoolhouse was repugnant. There was bickering over the increase in dues for the Community Circle Program (formerly Clarkson Corners), an increase instituted to cover some of the expenses associated with the move and remodeling of the Gerontology Center. The city council was notified of these matters and letters were written to the editor of the local newspaper. Some dissidents boycotted the program and even tried to encourage others to leave. The good motives of Swedish were impugned. What was being done for noble reasons was being seen by some as taking advantage of a neighborhood, lowering property values, "ripping off" the loyal elderly of Clarkson Corners, and so forth.

Several strategies were employed to counter the negative feelings centered primarily at the Thursday Community Circle, a wellness program that succeeded Clarkson Corners. Concessions were made on the charges for the Thursday program to keep them more in line with what persons paid in their former location. Numerous small group meetings were held with new and former members to discuss why the Center was established and why the mission of gerontology was being modified. These meetings had taken place several months before the move, yet the impact of the change accelerated the need for more interpretation and discussion.

A new advisory council of area elderly was established, because former members had boycotted the move. The council assisted in program planning and in giving a new name to the program—first called Duncan Corners and later changed to Community Circle. A "circle" theme was later developed at the Center, focusing on the theme of the expanded family circle with components of Friendship Circle (day program) and Inner Circle (Alzheimer's day care program). Gradually the new mission and rationale for the Center began to sink in; new people joined the Community Circle and former members, most of whom were not considered frail, went elsewhere. It was a painful rebirthing process for those associated with the program.

The strategy of dealing with the immediate neighborhood took several forms. Open houses were held for residents and professionals in the area. Neighbors adjacent to the Center were hired as staff persons, which proved a very useful concept because of their ready availability, their assistance in recruiting volunteers, and their promotional efforts on behalf of the Center. Neighbors also keep an eye on the facility because hospital security is not available due to the distance from the main campus. Major media coverage concerning the leadership role that Swedish was assuming in adult day care programs and wellness also resulted in an awareness of this important neighborhood resource. In addition, the director visited with local churches, service clubs, city officials, and professional organizations concerning the mission of the Center. After about two years, the concept and intentions of the Center finally began to gain acceptance by the general public.

Another strategy of promoting public acceptance and support for the Center has been the development of a center advisory council. This council consists of 25 professionals, family members, and businesspersons who advise the center director on professional practice issues, assist in resource development, and participate in the public relations and promotion of Center activities. The council has contributed in numerous ways to image development and the communication of the Center's purpose and programs for older adults.

The Aging Services Committee

In the spring of 1986 the former president of Swedish Medical Center formed an aging services committee that included representatives from many of the affiliates, departments, and hospitals of Swedish Medical Center. Two physicians served on this 25-member committee. The objectives of the committee were as follows:

1. To identify issues and concerns pertaining to the health and welfare of older adults and to determine how these issues and concerns should best be handled

2. To disseminate new information from the field of aging to committee members
3. To develop linkages/cooperative relationships among departments and other components of Swedish Medical Center
4. To advocate for quality senior services at Swedish Medical Center

The committee's first order of business involved preparing a systematic inventory of existing resources and services currently in operation throughout Swedish Medical Center.

The second item of business involved holding a planning retreat, whereby the tasks and activities of the committee could be established. The planning retreat was held in Spring 1986 at the Swedish Gerontology Center, with the director of the center serving as facilitator for the day's activities. Participants role-played as older adults and identified opportunities and services necessary for an aging market. These needs were discussed in small groups and later represented on large sketch pads placed at convenient points around the room. A film entitled *Aging* was shown, portraying positive adaptive styles of aging. A discussion followed, comparing film portrayals and participant self-expectations concerning the aging process. After three weeks, a consensus was derived for discussion purposes and planning.

A Delphi methodology was used as a planning tool. The director of the planning department at Swedish explained to the committee that basically the Delphi process consists of having three knowledgeable individuals compose 20 to 25 questions to which professionals at Swedish could respond. Persons were expected to respond each week to a refined list of questions prepared by these composers. The committee had in its possession a descriptive inventory of existing services and resources and a document indicating what professionals currently within Swedish perceived to be the most important services needed by the elderly.

After the Delphi results had been reviewed, the committee divided into several groups to further document major initiatives based on the Delphi data. The goal was to provide direction for the aging services committee for their fall 1986 planning retreat. The aging services committee divided into three special task forces to define the special issues to be focused on by the strategic planning committee. The three groups and their directives included:

- *Swedish internal environment.* For example, employees, policies, and facilities
- *Existing programs.* For example, integration, cooperation and possible redirection of an existing program(s) at Swedish
- *New program development.* For example, expansion of existing programs and/or development of a new service

A planning outline was given to the three special task forces, whose recommendations were classified according to existing programs, external programs, and new programs.

Existing Programs

Recommendations for existing programs focused on two areas, educational programs and integrated case management:

- *Educational programs.* A focused gerontological educational emphasis using existing resources, including the addition of a prominent geriatrician, will promote Swedish Medical Center as a center of excellence within the field of gerontology. Fellowship/residency programs will ensue along with updating on current research activities. All employees will receive in-service education on information that will assist them with their professional responsibilities. Clientele served by Swedish Gerontology Center, including care givers, elderly, and professionals, will also be beneficiaries of these educational efforts. Educational staff will come predominately from those currently employed by Swedish.
- *Integrated case management.* Integrated case management includes coordinated care by providing preadmission assessment, discharge planning, and information resources as well as housekeeping and personal care. Many of the needed components are currently in place at Swedish. The major problem is with the external competition with private insurers and other home health agencies currently attempting the same activities within their own organizations. Needed are (a) a centralized tracking system, (b) four additional full-time positions, (c) office space, and (d) a marketing campaign.

External Programs

Recommendations for external programs included hospice care and Alzheimer's respite service:

- *Hospice care on an infrequent basis.* Hospice of Metro Denver will subcontract with Swedish Medical Center up to $300 per day for palliative, nonaggressive, intermittent care. It provides an opportunity for Swedish's physicians in Physicians Home Care to refer their patients to Swedish Medical Center without having patients lose benefits by being transferred to other hospital settings.
- *Alzheimer's respite service.* The Alzheimer's Disease and Related Disorders Association (ADRDA) of Metro Denver, Inc., has requested the use of a few existing beds for weekend respite for persons with Alzheimer's disease. Alzheimer's is a leading cause of death among

Americans over the age of 65. As the number of older Americans increases, cases of Alzheimer's disease will increase. Staff training will be conducted by both ADRDA and staff from Swedish Gerontology Center. Reimbursement will be private pay.

New Programs

New programs include the Care Givers Assistance Program and the Senior Resource Center:

- *Care Giver's Assistance Program.* By providing information and education this program focuses on the needs of families who provide care to elderly relatives. Most older adults reside in communities and at home. Most care givers of the frail older population are women. The most common need cited by care givers is for more information on how to use community resources. The new programs committee at Swedish prepared an employee survey to determine the number and the extent of the needs of care givers currently working for Swedish Health Systems.
- *Senior Resource Center.* This center would be utilized by older adults and family members. It would answer the growing need for access to practical up-to-date medical, health, and life-style information for the elderly and their families, physicians, and other health professionals. Special components would include:
  - Technical information
  - Information referral
  - Insurance counseling
  - Case management
  - Community education
  - Care-giver assistance
  - Volunteer staffing
  - Research
  - Leisure planning
  - Financial counseling

  Much of the center's staffing would be senior volunteers.

Care-Givers Survey

One of the first actions taken by the aging services committee after reviewing the recommendations presented by the three task force groups was to implement the Care Giver's Survey on Aging Services to all managers at Swedish Health Systems (see figure 20-2). This survey was to determine how many managers already had care-giver responsibilities or expected to have them in the future.

Figure 20-2. Care Giver's Survey on Aging Services

Managers' Results—November 1986

Total surveys received:	54
Current care givers:	11 (20%)
Past care givers:	7 (13%)
Expect to give care:	27 (50%)
Other Do not expect to give care, not past care givers, or do not currently give care:	9 (17%)

Criteria	Current Care Givers	Future Care Givers	Do Not Expect to Give Care
Average age	46–55	36–45	36–45
Average family income	$40,000–50,000	$40,000–50,000	$30,000–40,000
Relationships	2 spouses 4 mothers 4 others*	10 parents 2 siblings 1 spouse 1 grandmother 5 others**	

*Daughters-in-law (2), mother-in-law, grandson
**Grandfather-in-law, children (4)

Current care givers

Average age of elder	71–75
Gender of elder	8 Males, 2 Females, 1 Unspecified
Distance:	Four have persons living in home Six travel less than 20 miles

Future care givers

Average age of elder	71–75
Gender of elder	8 Males, 14 Females (6 expect to care for both males and females)

Current care givers

Living arrangements of elder
- 2 Own home with another
- 2 Own home alone
- 1 Live in with me full time/no respite
- 1 Nursing home
- 1 Congregate living
- 0 Cooperative living—part-time
- 0 Adult day care
- 0 Someone else's home

Continued on next page

Figure 20-2. (Continued)

Services provided or arranged by care giver
- 6 Errands, transportation
- 5 Home maintenance
- 4 Light housekeeping
- 4 Companionship
- 3 Financial support
- 3 Home health
- 3 Handling of finances
- 1 Lifeline services

Financial Services Used by Elder
- 5 Insurance (basic)
- 3 Insurance (long-term)
- 2 Financial planning

Other Services Used by Elder
- 1 Mental health
- 1 Day hospital
- 0 Preretirement education 0 Health screening
- 0 Socialization
- 0 Drug/alcohol units
- 0 Respite care
- 0 Adult day care
- 0 Nutrition programs
- 0 Hospice
- 0 Other

Additional Services for the Elderly
- 3 Resource Center
- 3 Wellness program
- 2 Insurance counseling
- 0 Drug/alcohol unit
- 0 Financial counseling
- 0 Hospice
- 0 Adult day care
- 0 Home modification
- 0 Other

Only Barrier Listed Was Cost by One Respondent

Services for care giver
- 3 Long-term care insurance
- 3 Financial resources
- 1 Support groups
- 1 Time out from care giver role
- 0 Hotline about care
- 0 Education

Knowledge of Swedish Gerontology Center

Care givers:	10 out of 11 are aware of the Center (91%)
Non–care givers:	37 out of 43 are aware of the Center (86%)
Overall:	47 out of 54 are aware of the Center (87%)

Of the 54 managers who responded, 11 (20 percent) were currently care givers to an older adult, 7 (13 percent) were past care givers, and 27 (50 percent) predicted they would be care givers in the future. Apparently the tasks and responsibilities surrounding care giving were and are a major concern for a significant number of managers currently employed by Swedish Health Systems. This finding supported providing education to those serving or preparing to serve in the care-giving role. Furthermore it gave impetus to the Gerontology Center, which provides day care programs for the elderly and support groups for care givers, to interpret more completely its services to the employees within the total Swedish Medical Center organization. A second survey was sent to all employees of Swedish, which verified earlier findings.

Case Management and Assessment

Case management occurs at several strategic points within Swedish's system. It occurs most prominently at discharge planning from the main hospital campus. Nursing, social services, and Swedish Home Health all assume major roles in planning for the patient's successful reentry into the community. Home Health often extends its service and consultation after the patient has left the hospital.

The Swedish Gerontology Center also provides a limited form of case management for the participants of the various programs. The social worker and other interdisciplinary team members develop an individualized care plan for each participant. The social worker, in working with the family or care giver, provides consultation on needed community resources. The social worker often works in the "broker" role, by facilitating referrals, monitoring their effectiveness, and integrating those activities into a revised care plan at the Center. By working with both the older participant and family members, the social worker can maximize the usefulness of these important components. The geriatric nurse practitioner, by working with the social worker, family, and primary physician, adds to the holistic approach. The total plan is given additional support by the geriatric nutritionist, who monitors the dietary needs of the participant, prepares special menus when needed, and counsels the family as required. The activities plan is constructed by the activities coordinator, with all of these important ingredients being kept in balance with the special needs and interests of the older individual. The care plan is revised periodically as circumstances and needs change.

To meet the requirements of the Colorado Health Department, several assessment procedures were developed. One assessment form reviews the health and medical history (including nutritional history and special dietary considerations) of the individual. Items such as medications, previous illnesses, and current diagnoses from the primary physician are care fully documented. A social history reviews important occurrences, preferences, and interests in a person's life. The activities form obtains information from the participant and care giver on the preferred activities and the special talents an individual possesses.

The involvement of both the older participant and family member at intake helps to ensure that all vital information is assessed. Participation in the program for a one-week trial period enables staff to observe if information obtained in the intake interview is supportive to observed behaviors. Periodic charting and progress notes on individualized care plans ensure that assessments are kept up to date with changing circumstances. Health monitoring by both the geriatric nurse practitioner and nutritionist helps ensure that the total person is being assessed on a regular basis.

Assessments have occurred at Swedish Gerontology Center at two important intervals. The first and most complete total assessment utilized the OARS methodology in the early beginning of the Center during the fall of 1984. The second set of assessments are those associated with the day care programs and the Thursday wellness activities.

The OARS Methodology of Assessment

The Older American Resources and Services (OARS) methodology of assessment was developed by investigators at the Duke University Center for the Study of Aging and Human Development. It has been used extensively throughout the United States during the past decade. The OARS questionnaire is divided into two sections corresponding to the first two elements of the OARS model: The Multidimensional Functional Assessment Questionnaire (MFAQ) and the Services Assessment Questionnaire (SAQ).[1]

In August 1984, the Center staff at Swedish decided to use the OARS instrument as a means of assessing the needs of the population it would be serving in the new Swedish Gerontology Center. The contention was that to serve a more elderly "at-risk" population, a fuller understanding was needed of the characteristics of that population. This understanding would allow for more effective interventions by staff as well as assisting in any future planning activities.

At the outset of the project the director of Swedish Gerontology Center sought the assistance of the Institute of Gerontology at the University of Denver. The result was development of a cooperative effort between these two institutions. The Swedish Gerontology Center hired someone from the Institute at the University of Denver to serve as research coordinator of the project. As part of this effort, the Swedish Gerontology Center sponsored the coordinator's attendance at a week-long training session at Duke University, home of the OARS project. This training allowed the Swedish Gerontology Center to be designated as an "official" training site for trainers in the use of the OARS instrument within the state of Colorado.

The research coordinator recruited graduate students from the School of Social Work at the University of Denver to assist with the project. The eight students selected and the entire staff of the Gerontology Center were then trained in the use of the instrument.

The director of the center sought out professional consultation and reviewed the literature concerning the use of OARS with persons with Alzheimer's disease. After researching the subject, it was decided to have the "significant other," or person closest to the patient, respond for the participant in those areas pertaining to activities of daily living (ADL) and social resources. It was also decided that any individuals with mental or physical limitations would have an informant or family member answer the entire assessment for them. For the Alzheimer's participants, the interviewer rated the respondents on the other dimensions of the OARS instrument. If there appeared to be discrepancies in the recorded responses, then the research coordinator checked with the Alzheimer's day care program coordinator to verify the validity of the response. In a few instances ratings were changed to render them more consistent with what was known concerning a specific individual.

The ebb and flow of students and a developing Center population resulted in this project taking considerably more time than had been anticipated. Meanwhile the research coordinator took another position and a new one had to be trained, as did additional students. Project results became available during March 1986, providing a complete profile of all the participants in the program and the opportunity to compare various program participants within the Center itself.

Financing

Financing at Swedish Gerontology Center occurs on several levels: private pay, Medicaid, foundation grants, individual donors, and operating support from Swedish Medical Center. In addition, the various programs at Swedish have different charges, and various means are used to fund them.

Private Pay

Approximately 90 to 95 percent of all participants in Swedish Gerontology Center programs are private pay. The current fee for day care participants is $30 per day (9:00 a.m.–3:30 p.m.), five days a week. It is projected that the rate may increase to $35. Respite services beyond program hours (up to 4:30 p.m.) are available on request.

Medicaid

In recent years the Colorado legislature has enacted the Senate Bill 138 program (S.B. 138, home, community-based services), which provides funding for alternative long-term care services for Medicaid-eligible elderly. The Colorado program serves only a limited number of older adults seen at the Center. Approximately 5 percent of the day care continuum at the Center has been subsidized through this program and, again, primarily through the non-Alzheimer's–related day program.

Community Circle

The Community Circle Program, a wellness program that meets on Thursdays, includes the following: community service group, exercise class, Nutrition Club, Plato Society (intellectual topics, speakers, and so forth), and spiritual fitness. The day includes a nutritious noon meal and a speaker. Presentations usually include health promotion topics, information on community resources with an emphasis on independent living and self-help. The noon program costs $3.50.

Educational Programs

Key components of Swedish Gerontology Center have been the educational programs pertaining to community-based, long-term care. National authorities in the field of gerontology (including Elaine Brody, Stanley Brody, and the late Richard Kalish) have spoken to community groups in behalf of Swedish Gerontology Center. Professionals at the Center have given workshops for professionals and volunteers on issues of aging. Staff have also gone to skilled nursing homes to provide in-service training on the care of residents and on Alzheimer's disease. The Center has provided meeting space for the Older Women's League of Denver and for the Alzheimer's Association and Related Disorders Association of Metropolitan Denver. Health Maintenance Organization of Colorado has rented the facility for community presentations. Teleconferences on aging sponsored by the American Hospital Association, shown via satellite at Swedish Medical Center, have been open for community participation. In the spring of 1986, a six-week series, *Giving and Receiving of Care,* was offered to care givers. A number of authorities in the service area were involved in this series. Most of the educational programs have generated revenue or have included the rental of the gerontology building.

Transportation

In late October 1986, a transportation system emanating from the Swedish Gerontology Center was established to serve older adults living within a few miles of the Center. The Helen K. and Arthur E. Johnson Foundation provided the Center with approximately $6,000 in 1985 to 1986 to help establish a transportation system to serve persons who need to come to the Center, go to medical appointments, shop, visit spouses in nursing homes, and so forth. The Center was successful in raising money from local businesses and Rotary Clubs to acquire a 15-passenger van. A driver/dispatcher especially trained in caring for the elderly has been hired for this service. The total costs associated with operating this service, including driver, insurance, maintenance, fuel, office supplies, pager, and publicity, are projected to be $1,600 per month.

Financing a transportation system takes several forms. The program currently subcontracts with Arapahoe County Transportation Services (ACTS), which is authorized to provide Medicaid reimbursement and Title III monies from the Older Americans Act. Trips subsidized by ACTS include medical appointments or medical-oriented activities, senior adult day care, shopping, meetings, and important personal needs. This reimbursement is restricted to persons residing in Arapahoe County. Arapahoe County Transportation Services screens the prospective ridership on the basis of economic levels and social need. Approved persons are then referred to the Center for transportation services. More affluent elderly or persons residing outside Arapahoe County pay a standard fare. Federally supported reimbursements encourage riders to give a donation, which in turn is given back to ACTS for documentation of participant giving. When Title III monies are running low in a given month, the participant donation pattern assists the ACTS technicians in determining who should be given priority for certain rides. The Center also suggests a small standard donation for persons coming to its Thursday wellness program. This is considered to be most appropriate because many participants are on fixed incomes and reside in subsidized housing.

During 1989–1990 (to date) the hospital has purchased two vans for the Center to transport people to hospital and nonhospital appointments, Center activities, and so forth. Service is also available to persons not associated with the Center but who need transportation for checkups, discharge from the hospital, and so forth.

Other Financing Mechanisms

Over the past several years, Swedish Medical Center has been able to secure charitable support from many different philanthropic foundations, both locally and nationally. A partial list includes the Union Pacific Foundation, Safeco Insurance, the Arthur E. and Helen K. Johnson Foundation, the Hill Foundation, the Denver Foundation, the A. E. Hunter Trust, and the Molner Foundation.

Moreover, the Swedish Medical Center Foundation has supported the gerontology program from its general revenue from investments. The Center's prospects for the future look promising.

Continuing Services

Over the years at Swedish, there was a shift from a medically oriented model for gerontology to a more socially oriented one. The current model has shifted back to a more medically oriented one. The hospital has now developed a Senior Health Plus clinic for older adults that has a multidisciplinary staff, including a medical director who performs geriatric assessments. Referrals are now made from the clinic to various departments within the hospital. Referrals are also made to the Swedish Gerontology Center, which is still basically a "social model" program. However, the current program administrator of the Center is a registered nurse, and the program population has become increasing frail, necessitating more medical support and procedures for this at-risk population. The emphasis back to a more medically oriented approach has resulted in minimal conflict between the surrounding community and the Gerontology Center. In fact the community has been enthusiastic about this newer revision, having come full circle from its attitude in 1984. The trauma associated with the relocation of a hospital-based program to a community setting is the basis for this case study.

Several program areas were explored in order to reduce the trauma, especially for employees. A survey was conducted among all Swedish employees to determine the care-giver needs that persons are now confronting and are projected to confront in the very near future. The Center has helped facilitate employee-based participation in both day care programs and educational activities pertaining to care giving. Discounts have been provided to family members of Swedish, and a variety of educational programs have been offered for employees and the community-at-large.

Conclusions

Several lessons can be gleaned from Swedish's experience in developing gerontological services. First, community involvement and education are required because hospital community outreach services are often misunderstood at the outset. Some feel that the profit orientation is what generates a hospital's desire to become more community service-oriented. Time has to be spent in advance of project implementation, discussing with members of residential groups and with organizations and professional entities the reasons behind the new social programs. Elderly groups need to be part of the planning process, especially those affected by the change. Assistance in the actual design of the building, staffing, and program development ensures more tranquility and acceptance when actual implementation begins. It is hoped that this process will provide support in the acceptance of fee structures and the general financing of the programs. Hospitals have tended not to use citizen groups in program development, emphasizing more remediation than reciprocity in the planning process. When hospitals venture out into community turf, however, both community groups and participant groups must be involved in significant ways to minimize friction during the implementation of the new program.

The final note concerns the ongoing dilemma of financing social programs. Federal legislative initiatives concerning Medicare support for Alzheimer's day care and for other forms of older adult day care programs will go a long way toward relieving the financial stress that many day care programs experience across the country. In the meantime, administrators concerned about supporting such programs, including wellness-oriented activities, must be entrepreneurs in order to survive. Developing sound relationships with foundations, business groups, donors, and volunteers is necessary to subsidize the modest fees that are charged members. This becomes especially necessary when a center maintains premium-quality staffing. High-quality personnel, along with volunteers and student interns from every major university in the state, have developed a progressive forward-thinking set of programs for Swedish Gerontology Center. Institutional support for an aging population and its care givers is critical if hospitals are to succeed in the development of social programs for the elderly and their families.

Reference

1. *The Older Americans Resources and Service Methodology.* Durham, NC: Duke Center for the Study of Aging and Human Development, 1978.

Chapter 21

A Hospital System's Approach to Continuum of Care for the Elderly

Susan Taylor

Introduction

The Health One Corporation, based in Minneapolis, is a unified system of primary, secondary, and tertiary care hospitals and related health service programs serving the Minneapolis–St. Paul metropolitan area and the Upper Midwest. It was formed in 1987 by a merger of two Twin Cities–based health care organizations: Health Central, which had 9 owned and 11 managed hospitals, predominately rural institutions split across 6 midwestern states; and the original Health One, operator of 3 large metropolitan special care hospitals and one smaller outlying facility. Combined, the two organizations have 3,182 acute-care and 621 long-term care beds. Currently $599 million in assets and $550 million in revenue are under the management of Health One. More than 11,000 employees are organized into four separate divisions, which focus on acute care, medical affairs, managed care, and diversified businesses.

Since the mid-1970s, the Health Central organization had developed a wide range of services for the elderly, with the Center for Aging Services serving as the hub and clearinghouse for these activities, as described in *Hospitals and the Aged: The New Old Market*.[1] Today, within the diversified businesses division of Health One, services for older adults continue to have a focal point for the operations of corporate-based programs and the development of new programs coordinated throughout the organization. Currently, services for older adults within Health One span the continuum of care for the elderly as shown in figure 21-1. These programs include those based from the hospital (for example, rehabilitative care) as well as those based from the corporate offices (for example, home care and housing). They were all developed individually based on the unique circumstances of their setting. Guided by the corporate

Figure 21-1. Health One Corporation: Continuum of Care for Older Adult Services

Hospitals—Nursing Homes	Housing	Home Care	Transportation	Membership Program
• Inpatient hospital care	• Subsidized housing	• Skilled nursing visits	• Emergency medical services	• Free transportation
• Primary and specialty medical care	• Rental units	• Durable medical equipment	• Scheduled rides	• Case management
• Diagnostic services	• Condominium units	• Homemaker services		• Information and referral
• Rehabilitative services		• IV therapy		• Private room
• Skilled/intermediate custodial care		• Hospice		• Free parking
• Transitional care units				• Hospitality center
• Swing beds				• Financial counselor
• Day care				
• Alzheimer's disease care unit				
• Home-delivered meals				
• Geropsych unit				
• Free Medicare clinic				
• Volunteer program				

initiative to develop as broad a range of all types of health-related services as possible, individual efforts were guided generally by strategic planning but occurred sporadically over several years with many different players involved.

External Environment

The Twin Cities is a highly competitive marketplace for Health One flagship hospitals. It is an area where over 90 percent of the physicians belong to one or more of nine health maintenance organizations (HMOs); over one-half the population is enrolled in HMOs; and approximately 60 percent of more than the 200,000 older adults have assigned their Medicare benefits to HMOs. Further, average hospital occupancy has dropped below 50 percent, and 75 to 80 percent of the local hospitals' business is on a fixed-payment schedule of some kind.

Other Health One hospitals are located in rural midwestern communities where the proportion of older adults (13 to 18 percent) is considerably higher than the national average. Correspondingly, Medicare inpatient days are higher, with 45 to 50 percent of total hospital days attributed to the elderly.

Planning/Development Process

As a direct result of these competitive forces, combined with increased demand and advances in technology, "senior" services within Health One were developed. Initially the services that evolved were based on both an altruistic and financial philosophy. By balancing the two motives it was thought that innovative needed and revenue-producing programs could be offered. For example, housing, home care, and specialized transportation were developed to promote noninstitutional health care alternatives, generate revenues from diverse sources, and decrease patient lengths of stay in the hospital. The individual hospital's programs for the elderly, such as nursing home activity, emergency transportation services, and membership programs, were designed to increase both market share and market loyalty to the hospital. Experimentation led to the development of innovative programs such as Senior Health Plan, a Medicare HMO demonstration program that was created as a joint effort with two other Twin Cities health services organizations to meet the needs of older adults and to encourage the use of noninstitutional alternatives.

Services and programs for the elderly were a natural evolution for rural Health One hospitals as well, where a high percentage of elderly encouraged the development of diverse services. Swing beds, specialized units for patients with Alzheimer's disease, transportation, and housing were developed under a "campus" approach with the hospital serving as the catalyst for program development.

As each of these programs was considered for development, a planning process was put into place to identify the benefits of the program to the organization. In addition to validating the program's strategic "fit" into the organization and ensuring that it was in keeping with the stated values of Health One, a business plan was developed for each program that included the following components:

- *Demographic analysis* of size and projected growth of the population who will use the program; age distribution, gender, and educational attainment; income estimates for households by age and poverty status; housing and rent values and types of housing units; and health status indicators (birth, morbidity, and mortality rates)
- *Economic trends* in the marketplace, including number and type of industries, employers, and employees; unemployment rate trends and pension programs; and general economic trends where the program will operate
- *Competitive analysis* focusing on features, pricing, and differentiation; market share; utilization and financial comparative data of competing programs
- *Qualitative market research,* including focus groups of target markets and key informant interviews (especially important for rural areas) to ascertain consumer response to programs
- *Quantitative market research,* which is done through mail and telephone survey to further analyze the consumer's response
- *Operations audit* of staffing, organizational structures, space and facility planning necessary to manage the program properly
- *Financial performance hurdles and projections,* including a five-year operations and capital budget

This planning framework is applied to a new program to guide decision making and implementation. Then each program is reviewed annually against these criteria for continued strategic fit and financial strength. If the program continues to meet both of these parameters, little might be done to modify it. However, if a program no longer fits strategically—it does not support the base operations of Health One or does not meet the financial hurdles previously set in the financial performance section of the business plan—then divestiture is considered.

Organization and Staffing

As mentioned previously, services for older adults are coordinated from the general central offices of the Health One Corporation. The Senior

Services and Home Care division manages housing and home care and provides strategic planning and consulting support throughout the organization. Emphasis is placed on using the synergy of each hospital's programs to enhance all programs within the system. Outside consultants are used for general counsel or for specific tasks such as market research.

Each hospital within Health One serves as the hub for a wide variety of services for older adults. The staff designated to manage these programs are linked to the general offices in several ways. The Nursing Home Council, for example, brings nursing home administrators together to share information, solve joint problems, and deal with state legislative issues. Also, the membership program, Serving Seniors, is offered by the two hospitals located in Minneapolis and St. Paul, and uniformity of these programs is coordinated by the corporate office. Further, each hospital has a designated "senior services" liaison working with the office in a team approach.

Financing

The financing of Health One's services and products is diverse. The public housing complexes and the Senior Health Plan experiment were partly funded by government sources; remaining funding is in the form of privately paid rent and premiums. Private condominium housing is funded on a private pay basis. Several services have received grants provided by national and local foundations and the Area Agency on Aging.

Medicare, private insurance, and managed care contracts pay for most hospital and home care services. The nursing homes within the organization are funded either on a fee-for-service basis or through the Medicaid program. Most of Health One's services for older adults were originally capitalized by the corporation but are now financed through operating revenues.

Conclusions

Each product or service is responsible for its own financial liability, customer satisfaction, and quality evaluation. Despite the constant challenge by competitors and new regulations, inpatient and outpatient hospital care, nursing homes, housing management, and consulting services have been profitable. On the other hand, although for many years such programs as home health care were not profitable, because they are seen as essential to continuity of care for the hospitalized patients, they meet the strategic fit requirements of Health One's evaluation. Most of the programs designed specifically for the older adult market within Health

One have achieved the goal of developing innovative and cost-effective services, complementing other hospital or corporate activity, and demonstrating favorable financial results. It is expected that Health One's successful experiences and services for the elderly, combined with the magnitude of service options within Health One, will enable this new organization to continue to offer high-quality, diverse, and competitive options for older adults.

Reference

1. Brody, S. J., and Persily, N. A., editors. *Hospitals and the Aged: The New Old Market*. Rockville, MD: Aspen Publishers, 1984.

Chapter 22

Extensions and Partnerships in the Community

Elyse Salend, Marie Bolduc Liston, and John C. Beck, M.D.

Introduction

In 1979, the University of California at Los Angeles (UCLA) School of Medicine and the UCLA Medical Center made a major commitment to the development of innovative geriatric education, research, and service models. The goal was to establish nationally recognized exemplary programs that would train a variety of health and social services professionals to care for the elderly and, ultimately, to improve health care delivery to older adults.

The Multicampus Division of Geriatric Medicine (Multicampus Division) was established in 1979 by the UCLA Medical Center Department of Medicine. The purpose was to improve the well-being of the elderly by educating appropriate health professional personnel, conducting research, and providing high-quality health care services in demonstration settings. To achieve this, the Multicampus Division sought to foster coordination, program development, monitoring, evaluation, and decision making, in cooperation with other institutions and organizations.

Internal/External Environment

Many factors led to the Multicampus Division's programmatic thrust toward improved eldercare. At that time, the commissioner of the federal Administration on Aging (AoA) advocated improved geriatric/gerontologic research, education and training, and more effective service delivery as key components in the development of a continuum of care. In response to these needs, AoA created long-term care gerontology centers whose mission was to build new bridges between universities and the community on a regional basis. The UCLA was successful in becoming a designated site for a long-term care gerontology center, and in 1980, in a partnership with the University of Southern California (USC), the UCLA/USC Long-Term Care Gerontology Center was established within UCLA's Multicampus Division of Geriatric Medicine and the USC Andrus Gerontology Center.

The UCLA/USC Long-Term Care Gerontology Center focused on five defined project areas: (1) information dissemination, (2) education and training, (3) community-based demonstrations, (4) research, and (5) technical assistance. As one of its model service programs, UCLA developed a partnership with Jewish Family Services of Los Angeles (JFS) in 1980 for the purpose of providing a neighborhood-based system of quality health and social services.

The community-based service delivery component of UCLA's entire program will be described here.

In 1983, when Medicare instituted a prospective payment system to reduce hospital costs, the impetus for developing a continuum of community and posthospital services was even greater. Under this new payment system, hospitals had incentive to discharge patients as quickly as medically possible.

Faced with a myriad of challenges imposed by the government and private sector as well as the changing needs of the elderly, UCLA viewed these issues as a new opportunity for innovation. In 1983, UCLA received a Robert Wood Johnson Foundation (RWJF) grant, *Hospital Initiatives in Long-Term Care.* The grant provided a catalyst for making geriatrics /gerontology one of the Medical Center's priority areas. In fact, UCLA Medical Center matched the foundation grant dollar-for-dollar, and senior administration was closely involved in the development of the geriatric program.

The University of California at Los Angeles was committed to a major effort in geriatric medicine. Through its Multicampus Division, the Department of Medicine replaced the traditional concept of a primary teaching hospital linked to satellites with a consortium of equal partners under the UCLA umbrella. This partnership included the Veterans Administration Medical Center, West Los Angeles (Wadsworth and Brentwood divisions); the Veterans Administration Medical Center, Sepulveda; and UCLA Medical Center. In addition, formal associations between UCLA and the Health Science Program of the Rand Corporation, the Jewish Homes for the Aging, and JFS have developed.

Goals

The Medical Center's aim was to provide older adults with a coordinated system of high-quality health and social services. It sought to achieve this aim by testing the feasibility of a multisite, vertically integrated model of care.

The RWJF grant provided the vehicle for the Multicampus Division and the UCLA Medical Center to enhance community services and to develop a wide array of step-down services. The resources of an academic medical center were combined with established community agencies to serve elderly persons of the Beverly-Fairfax area in a model project. The philosophy of the Hospital Initiatives Program was in complete harmony with the goals and long-range plans of UCLA Medical Center.

Seven objectives were identified as being critical to the overall success of the Multicampus Division program:

1. The establishment of high-quality, community-based, and comprehensive clinical care services, including a system of and procedures for the comprehensive assessment of physical and psychosocial health and the economic and environmental status of elderly persons
2. The development of collaborative and coordinated efforts with other institutions and organizations in the community
3. Continuing professional education for a variety of service providers, including efforts at improvement and community-based long-term care services and service-systems management
4. The development of multidisciplinary educational programs to enhance the capabilities of professionals to understand and treat the elderly
5. The provision of technical assistance to service providers and to decision makers to enhance their capacity to meet and serve the needs of the elderly
6. The development of strategies for disseminating information about care of older adults to them and their families so they can be better consumers and make more informed decisions about health care
7. Clinical, biomedical, and health services research on issues related to the development and management of model systems of care for the elderly

Planning/Development Process

To meet its objectives, the Multicampus Division needed to develop community-based affiliations and have a base of operations that extended beyond the walls of the academic Medical Center. Nine criteria were developed for selecting potential community agencies:

1. The agency had to be a well-established community organization.
2. The agency had to have a proven track record in providing community-based care to the elderly.

3. The board of directors and senior administration of the agency needed to be strongly supportive of a UCLA community care component.
4. The agency had to have the capacity to raise funds for enhancing the program.
5. The agency staff needed to be willing to develop a multidisciplinary team approach to caring for the elderly.
6. The agency had to be within a radius of 5 to 10 miles from the Medical Center.
7. The agency needed to have a volunteer corps that would be willing to work on joint projects.
8. The need for community-based health services to older adults had to be documented.
9. Successful components of the program developed with the agency needed to be replicable in other community sites.

The project was fortunate to find Jewish Family Services, a progressive agency in Los Angeles interested in developing a comprehensive model of health and social services for the elderly. In 1980, an associate agreement was signed by JFS and the Regents of the University of California.

A private, not-for-profit family service agency, Jewish Family Services is the oldest social services agency in Los Angeles. Both its senior services and volunteer programs have received local, statewide, and national recognition as models of excellence and cost-effective service delivery. Jewish Family Services provides nonsectarian social services to individuals and families coping with the problems and crises of daily living, with a major emphasis on services to the frail elderly.

The Freda Mohr Multiservice Center (FMMC) was established in 1970 as a JFS outreach effort. A storefront located in the Beverly-Fairfax area was chosen as a setting for a model of service delivery responsive to the needs of elderly clients. The Freda Mohr Multiservice Center had a wealth of social services but lacked comprehensive health care services. The site met all the criteria for partnership with the Multicampus Division, except that the need for health services perceived by the board and staff of JFS had not yet been documented. Thus in 1979 it became necessary to conduct a community-based needs assessment to define the target population. The Freda Mohr Multiservice Center ultimately became the primary entry point for this portion of the program. Once this was accomplished, various internal and external factors contributed to the development.

Needs Assessment

Institutional change is a lengthy process. Plans for UCLA Medical Center have been periodically reviewed and revised; changes in personnel, environment, resources, and policies have all shaped the course of program development. Both internal and external factors contributed to the process.

The Beverly-Fairfax area of Los Angeles has a high percentage of older people; 40 percent of the residents are over age 60. Three populations were identified as potential users of services: the general elderly population in the area, current users of the FMMC, and residents of board-and-care facilities in the neighborhood. Based on these demographics and the needs perceived by FMMC staff, a comprehensive needs assessment instrument was developed by Multicampus Division staff and administered by a group of older volunteers affiliated with JFS and the USC Andrus Gerontology Center. The survey, conducted in 1980, primarily assessed the current health status and access to services by area residents.

Design of the survey instrument involved several factors: inclusion of necessary data, reliability of responses, and ease of administration (especially by volunteer interviewers). Information was collected on population characteristics such as cognitive dysfunction, life satisfaction, opinions on medical care, illnesses and medications, activities of daily living, supportive networks, and potential use of health services. Selected demographic findings are presented in table 22-1.

Among the survey findings that indicated a need for health services were these: 17 percent of the FMMC population had not seen a physician in more than one year, 22 percent had not had their eyes checked in two or more years, 29 percent had not been to a dentist in two or more years, and 19 percent indicated difficulty with foot problems. A large number, 36 percent, had been hospitalized within the year before the survey was conducted; 5 percent had been admitted to a nursing home within that period.

When this information was correlated with that describing the elderly population around the country, the results were disclosed:

- A much higher hospitalization rate (36 percent versus 17 percent nationally) for elderly in this area
- A higher median number of visits to the doctor in the year preceding the survey (5.2 versus 3.4 nationally)
- A higher median number of illnesses per year (3.1 versus 1.8 nationally)
- A greater number regionally who had difficulties in performing the usual activities of daily living

In response to the health and social services needs of this frail elderly, low-income population, the Freda Mohr Health Center was established in January 1981, as a collaborative project of UCLA and JFS. The Freda Mohr Health Center was later renamed the Sylvia Olshan Health Center (SOHC). The site trains a variety of professionals in the care of the elderly in a nonacute setting; provides health and social services to elderly people in their own neighborhood; and serves as a model for other teaching hospitals interested in developing community-based programs.

A second survey was conducted in 1984 to provide information to enhance health care delivery at the SOHC and to collect planning data for the initial phase of the Hospital Initiatives grant.

Surveys of three distinct groups were necessary: (1) current SOHC patients, (2) former SOHC patients, and (3) board-and-care residents who did not use SOHC. The objectives of the study were to collect descriptive and demographic data on all three groups, determine current patient satisfaction with SOHC, identify new needed services, and assess receptivity to nurse practitioners. Nurse practitioners are used in combination

Table 22-1. 1980 Demographic Summary of the Beverly-Fairfax Area

Criterion	Community	Freda Mohr Multiservice Center	Board-and-care
Sex			
Female	72%	93%	92%
Male	28%	7%	8%
Age (median)	74.9 years	74.9	79.7
Length of residence (median)	10 years	3	2
Nativity			
Native-born	43%	28%	48%
Foreign-born	57%	72%	52%
Marital status			
Married	39%	28%	15%
Widowed	45%	65%	67%
Separated/Divorced	5%	7%	4%
Single	10%	0%	15%
Living arrangements			
Alone	52%	59%	38%
With spouse	38%	28%	11%
Other	0%	14%	50%
Education (median) (3 = completed 8th grade) (4 = completed 12th grade)	3.6	3.1	2.8
Income (median) (3 = $334–416/month) (4 = $417–499/month)	3.7	2.9	3.3
Insurance			
Covered by Medicare B	73%	78%	84%
Covered by Medi-Cal	16%	32%	31%
Other insurance	70%	41%	15%

with physicians as primary care providers at the Health Center. The use of nurse practitioners initially raised some concerns because people were used to relating to physicians, and it was unclear how they would respond to nurse practitioners as providers of primary care.

An updated needs assessment instrument was developed (see the appendix at the end of this chapter) and again administered by volunteers from JFS. A summary of the salient demographic findings compared with data from the 1980 survey is shown in tables 22-2 and 22-3. Highlights of the survey included information on demographics, patient satisfaction, use of nurse practitioners, and other needed services.

Demographics

Three-quarters of SOHC patients were 75 years or older. Knowing the proportion of patients in this group was important in evaluating their needs for health and social services. Care for chronic conditions continues to be the major component of health care delivery at the Health Center. Four-fifths of the board-and-care population were 75 years of age or over: more than half were age 85 or over. Given the association of chronic disease and functional impairment with age, it was likely that the board-and-care residents required more health services and assistance with activities of daily living than SOHC patients.

Patient Satisfaction

Sylvia Olshan Health Center patients were generally satisfied with all five categories addressed to measure patient satisfaction: continuity of care, finances, access, physician conduct, and general satisfaction. Finances scored lowest overall—not surprising, given this population's average annual family income of $4,000 to $6,000. Many patients incurred expenses beyond what Medicare would reimburse.

Use of Nurse Practitioners and Other Needed Services

Nurse practitioners appeared to be acceptable providers of health care for this group, especially in combination with a physician. Additional needed services identified by the survey included drugs, dental services, and eyeglasses. Even though these services and items accounted for only 12 percent of the total cost of health care for the elderly, Medicare did not cover them.

Internal Factors

Although it is easy to articulate organizational goals from central administration, translating these goals into reality takes time. Thus UCLA's

Table 22-2. UCLA Comparison of Population Health Care and Services Data

Subject	1980 Survey		1984 Survey		
	Community	Board-and-care	All SOHC Patients	SOHC B&C Patients	Board-and-care residents
Problems getting medical care?	—	—	21% Yes	0% Yes	10% Yes
Help when sick?	29% None	15% None	50% None	38% None	16% None
Have emergency help?	—	—	28% No	17% No	12% No
When last saw doctor?	7% > 1 year ago (FMMC users: 17% > 1 year ago)	7% > 1 year ago 81% < 3 months ago	4% > 1 year ago 83% < 3 months ago	17% > 1 year ago 70% < 3 months ago	6% > 1 year ago
MD visits per year	4.0 visits (median) —	4.1 visits (median) —	6.0 visits (median) 9.0 visits (mean)	5.0 visits (median) 12.3 visits (mean)	4.0 visits (median) 7.5 visits (mean)
Hospital visits per last year? Rate	64% No visits —	58% No visits —	70% No visits 0.51 (mean) hospitalizations per patient	63% No visits —	69% No visits 0.76 (mean) hospitalizations per patient
Emergency room visits last year? Rate	— —	— —	69% No visits 0.41 (mean) visits per patient	71% No visits —	72% No visits 0.80 (mean) visits per patient

Table 22-3. UCLA Comparison of Population Demographics and Descriptive Information

	1980 Survey		1984 Survey		
Subject	**Community**	**Board-and-care**	**All SOHC Patients**	**SOHC B&C Patients**	**Board-and-care residents**
Sample size	95	27	95	8	51
Age	74.9 years (median) — — —	79.7 years (median) — — —	77 years (median) 78.1 years (mean) 74% aged 75+ 30% aged 85+	85 years (median) 84.1 years (mean) 91% aged 75+ 59% aged 85+	84 years (median) 82.4 years (mean) 82% aged 75+ 43% aged 85+
Race	—	—	97% white	100% white	98% white
Sex	72% female	92% female	82% female	100% female	86% female
Marital status	45% widowed 39% married	67% widowed 15% married	63% widowed 20% married	100% widowed 0% married	76% widowed 8% married
Living siutation	52% alone	38% alone	74% alone	75% alone	—
Income	$392 per month (median)	$358 month (median)	—	—	—
Insurance	73% Medicare 16% Medi-Cal —	84% Medicare 31% Medi-Cal —	72% Medicare only 5% Medi-Cal only 22% both	62% Medicare only 4% Medi-Cal only 31% both	82% Medicare 50% Medi-Cal — both
Mobility from abode	—	—	59% almost daily 7% < once monthly	38% almost daily 25% < once monthly	10% almost daily 55% < once monthly
SOHC referral source and publicity	—	—	Referrals 46% FMMC 30% Friend/relative 8% media 11% UCLA/MC 13% Other	—	Told of— 63% FMMC 25% SOHC

ambitious agenda has had to be deliberate and politically acceptable to many groups and organizations – including the University of California bureaucracy. Following are some reasons for this:

- The sheer size and complexity of UCLA Medical Center makes change a long process. To implement the various components of a coordinated system of care, an adequate number of health and administrative professionals with appropriate skills, knowledge, and attitudes must be in place. Middle management, faculty, and staff need training and an understanding of the new and/or expanded goals. Although cooperation and support for UCLA's program has been good, this limitation has caused some delays. Because UCLA recognizes that similar problems exist across the nation, it also recognizes a need for a national commitment to geriatric/gerontologic training to ensure that resources allocated to acute-care and long-term care services are efficiently utilized.
- Although surrounded by a number of other hospitals (both for-profit and not-for-profit) that have aggressively entered into entrepreneurial enterprises, UCLA Medical Center is proceeding with caution in this area. Some internal discussion focused on the role of a university teaching hospital and diversification.
- UCLA Medical Center's decision to apply for a RWJF grant was the catalyst for reexamining long-range plans. Although aging services development was already a goal of the Medical Center, the grant made it a priority. Resources from the director's office and associate directors were made readily available. Computer facilities, financial services, public information, marketing, social work, nursing, geriatrics, medicine, geropsychiatry, volunteer, emergency room, and patient services personnel all began to work together in identifying gaps and planning for new ways to serve older adult patients.

External Factors

With the exception of some bureaucratic delays and external factors beyond UCLA's control, the process has proceeded according to plan. In fact, in some instances outside factors have helped further program development activities, including the following:

- UCLA Medical Center has continued to strengthen its relationship with community agencies and other hospitals. In association with JFS, UCLA has cosponsored two major foundation proposals, one of which includes Cedars-Sinai Medical Center, located about a mile from the JFS site. The process of preparing the proposals has more closely integrated JFS with other departments of UCLA Medical Center and increased the visibility of aging services with the hospital. The cooperative efforts of two

major, often competing, medical centers is an important organizational accomplishment as well.
- The Medical Center deliberately chose not to provide on-site adult day health care services but rather to develop those services through working with another community agency. Proposal-writing resources were provided by UCLA Medical Center that successfully helped the agency secure grants from the state of California and a private foundation.

The UCLA Medical Center is located in West Los Angeles, surrounded by a highly affluent residential community. Property values in this area are among the highest in the nation, and the private rental market is prohibitively expensive. To date the proposed community-based day care center has been unable to secure space adjacent to the Medical Center. The UCLA Medical Center is exploring the feasibility of developing a day hospital itself, which would potentially address some of the same client base.

The site location problems were complicated by several political factors as well. Administrators at the first site, a senior center, had second thoughts about reallocating space on an ongoing basis for the program. A secondary, unarticulated factor may have been the older adults' fears and anxieties about being faced with the daily presence of frail elderly people. A local church then agreed to house the adult day health care center. However, neighborhood homeowners vehemently objected for fear of increased traffic and the potential use of the area by other "less desirable" groups. These developments have caused the Medical Center to reexamine the issue of adult day health care.

Case Management and Assessment

From the beginning UCLA Medical Center's premise was that neighborhood-based, ambulatory health and social services centers provide the best model of care to the frail elderly. In keeping with that hypothesis, case coordination and management begins in the community with the Freda Mohr Multiservice Center (FMMC)/Sylvia Olshan Health Center (SOHC) multidisciplinary team.

An assessment enables practitioners to provide for care planning. Using a proven system of volunteer social services aides as client advocates (with social workers directly supervising each case aide), FMMC provides a vast array of supportive social services to elderly clients through a coordinated case management approach.

As the client moves through either the social services or medical components of the system, various members of the multidisciplinary team (case aide, community social worker, gerontologic nurse practitioner, physician, psychiatrist) manage a particular problem for a period of time.

However, the overall coordination rests with the social worker and case aide. Weekly team case conferences include discussion of a care plan for each client (see figure 22-1 for the client pathway).

Social work staff at UCLA Medical Center are responsible for maintaining case coordination between the Medical Center and the community site. Specific activities include coordinating and facilitating patient admissions to the Medical Center, daily record surveillance at the UCLA Emergency Medicine Center and other services, case management and discharge planning for enrollees admitted to the Medical Center, and

Figure 22-1. Case Coordination Client Pathway at Sylvia Olshan Health Center/Freda Mohr Multiservice Center, Los Angeles

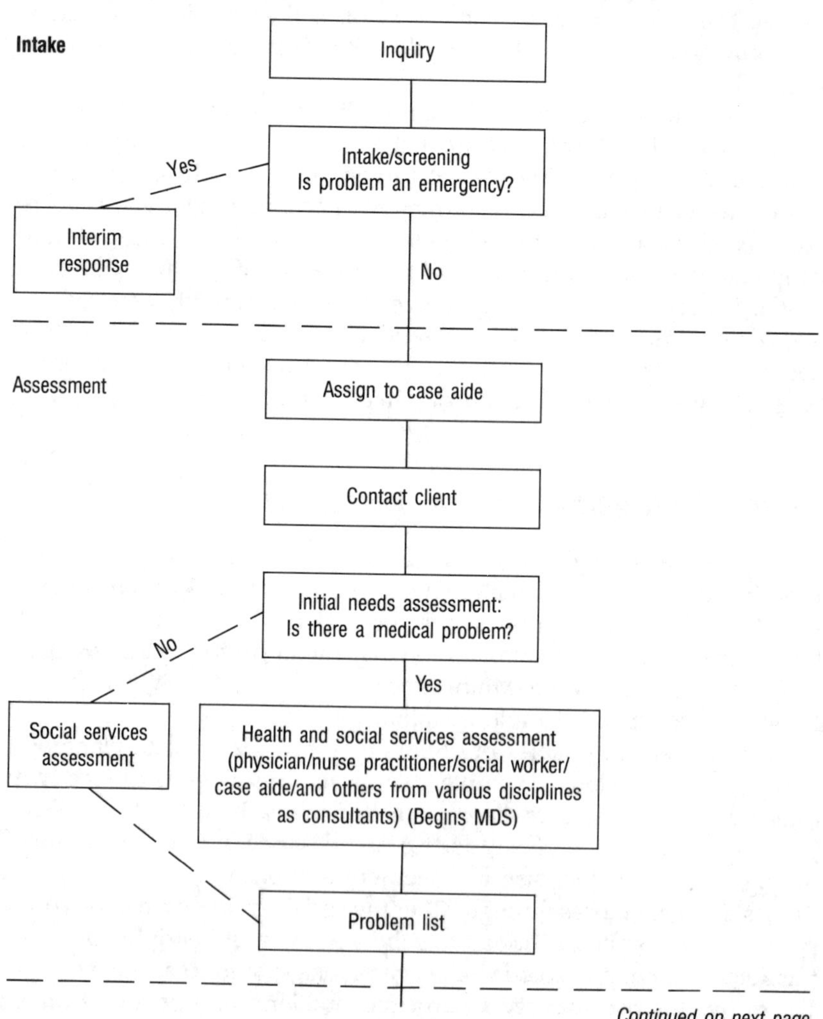

Continued on next page

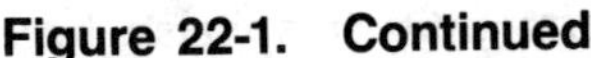

Figure 22-1. Continued

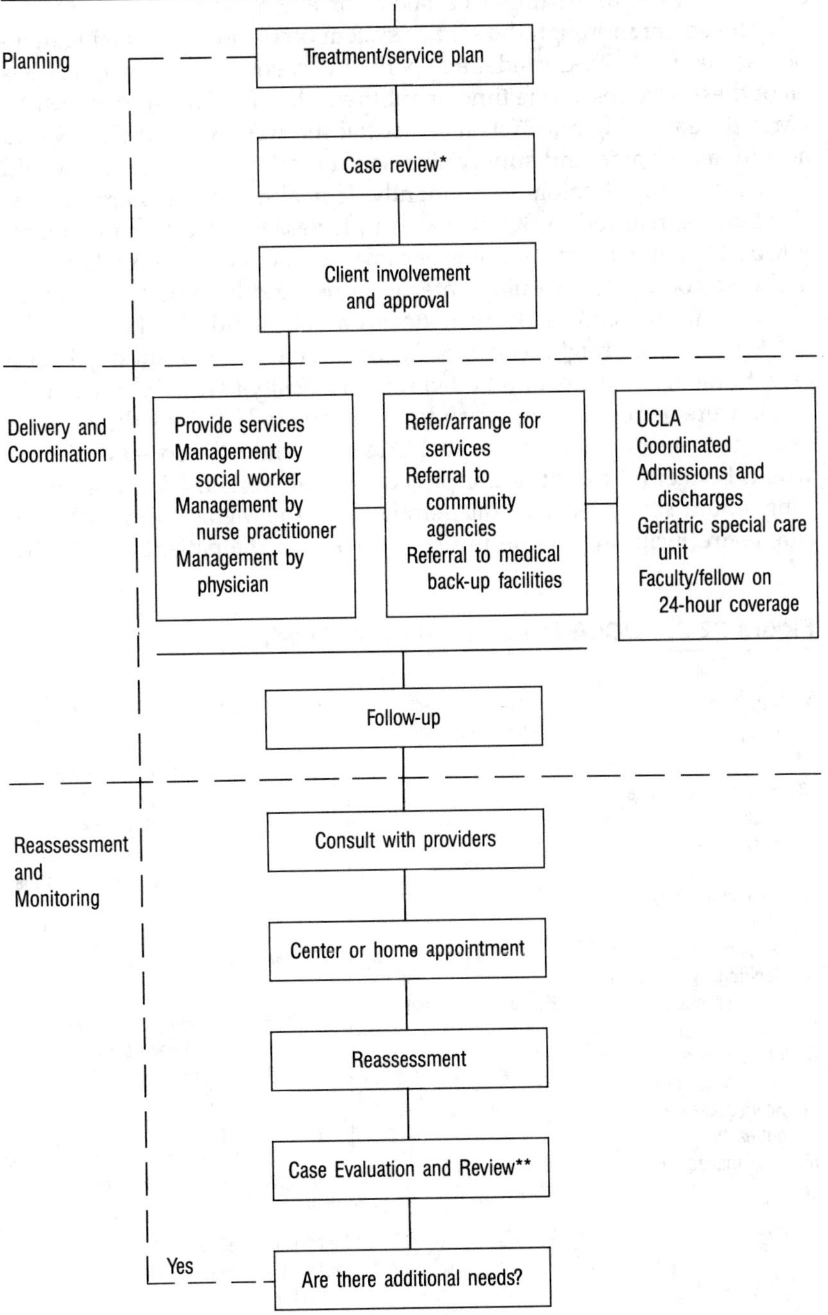

Planning

Treatment/service plan

Case review*

Client involvement and approval

Delivery and Coordination

Provide services
Management by social worker
Management by nurse practitioner
Management by physician

Refer/arrange for services
Referral to community agencies
Referral to medical back-up facilities

UCLA
Coordinated
Admissions and discharges
Geriatric special care unit
Faculty/fellow on 24-hour coverage

Follow-up

Reassessment and Monitoring

Consult with providers

Center or home appointment

Reassessment

Case Evaluation and Review**

Are there additional needs?

Yes

*All primary clients will have regular chart review by physician.

**Clients will be reassessed yearly.

serving as liaison to social workers at other community hospitals where an Initiatives enrollee might be taken for emergency care.

Movement thorough the service system occurs in the following manner (see figure 22-2). Consider a hypothetical client, Mrs. T., who requires all of these services at one time or another. Mrs. T. might start at FMMC (Area B) requesting one of its many social services (Area A). She would acquire a case aide and supervising social worker who together would be her case coordinators permanently. If health problems arose, Mrs. T. would be referred to SOHC (Area B) for assessment and treatment. If Mrs. T.'s ability to stay at home became questionable, the medical staff and case coordinator would confer with her and her family and reach a decision, for example, to refer her to a board-and-care facility.

Similar steps might lead Mrs. T. to be referred for adult day health care, home health care, or a skilled nursing facility (Area C). If hospitalization were required, Mrs. T. would usually go to UCLA Medical Center or to the Neuropsychiatric Hospital (Area D), where the social work staff would be alerted to notify the project's social worker. Discharge planning would be carried out collaboratively by the Medical Center health care team (including the project social worker), the patient and family,

Figure 22-2. UCLA Medical Center Network

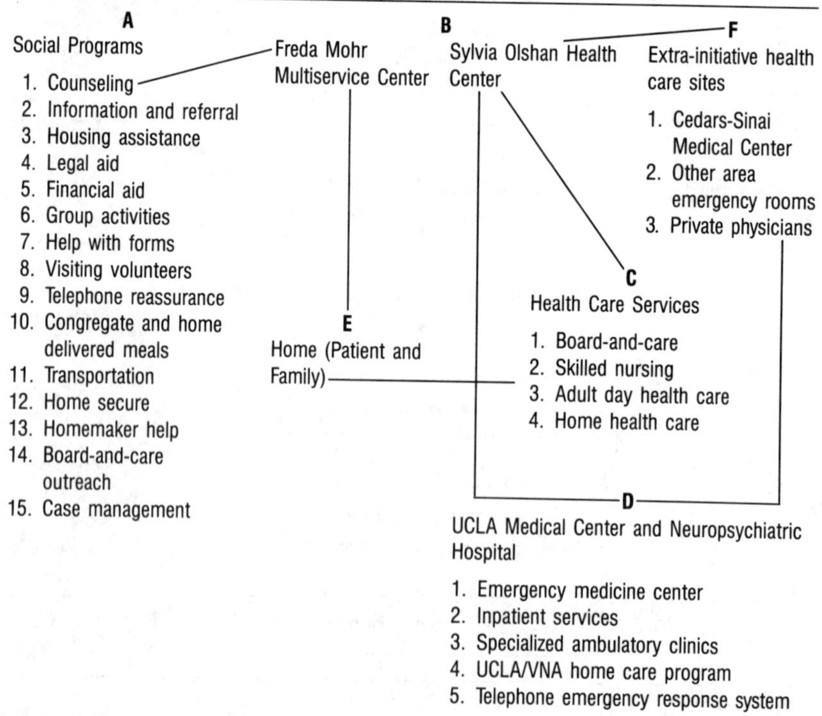

and the FMMC/SOHC case coordinator. Upon discharge, Mrs. T. would return to the case coordinator, except in the case of short-term admission to a skilled nursing facility, where the Medical Center social worker would continue to help her. If she suffered an emergency, Mrs. T. might be taken to Cedars-Sinai Medical Center or, a rare occurrence, to other emergency rooms in the area (Area F). UCLA Medical Center has made arrangements to track patients and for the FMMC/SOHC case coordinator to participate in discharge planning in collaboration with the Department of Social Work at Cedars-Sinai. With the exception of Area F, the project's medical, nursing, and social work staff are either responsible for or closely affiliated with every entity shown in figure 22-2 so that patients will receive continuous, well-coordinated care.

The FMMC services are available to people age 60 and over who meet four criteria for becoming an SOHC patient:

1. The person must be age 65 or over, or a disabled Medicare recipient between ages 60 and 64.
2. The person has no primary physician or is dissatisfied with his or her current physician.
3. The person needs ongoing medical care, including maintenance care for chronic conditions.
4. The person has initially been enrolled as an FMMC client and assigned a case coordinator.

The primary sources of referral to the Health Center are FMMC staff, printed material received through the mail, UCLA Medical Center physicians, and family members and friends. All SOHC patients are enrolled as participants in the RWJF Program and reassessed at yearly intervals. In conjunction with RWJF directives to Hospital Initiatives grantees nationwide, a Minimum Data Set was developed to coordinate patient care and social services activities between the FMMC/SOHC site and UCLA Medical Center, and to centralize collection and storage of data about Initiative participants for use by management and service providers. During the three-year Initiatives program, the goal was 600 participants, and 567 were enrolled. A client profile appears in table 22-4.

Implementation of the Minimum Data Set has aided in the sharing of information and has encouraged communication and case coordination planning between the two primary project sites, FMMC/SOHC and UCLA Medical Center. The assessments are conducted at FMMC/SOHC by Initiatives staff and trained volunteers, and assessment information is accessible to UCLA. A comprehensive how-to manual was developed that enables new staff and volunteers to understand and use the system easily. Case aides and social workers from FMMC; Medical Center social workers, faculty, and clinicians; and Health Center faculty, clinicians, and personnel have subsequently increased their contacts for the purpose of scheduling program enrollments. This has promoted a concomitant coordination of services and exchange of information.

Innovative Services

The UCLA Medical Center has developed an array of services for the frail elderly and is exploring a number of new service initiatives.

Current Services

Among the numerous current services available to older adults are a geriatric special care unit, geriatric consultation service, a geriatric ambulatory assessment center for outpatients, mental health services, social work

Table 22-4. Client Profile for UCLA Medical Center's *Hospital Initiatives in Long-Term Care* Program

The following are descriptive statistics of selected variables from the Initial Assessment Instrument for the 567 persons enrolled from 1985 through 1987. All percentages are the percent of the total enrolled.

Demographic Data		
Sex	Female	71%
Age	75–99 years	83%
Race	White/Caucasian	93%
Marital status	Widowed	57%
Education	< high school graduate	67%
Yearly income	$5,000–$10,999	58%
Housing	Apartment	58%
Health insurance	Medicare	97%
	Medi-Cal	32%
	Other	45%
Medical Data		
Five most frequent medical conditions experienced in the past	Arthritis	53%
	Cataracts	47%
	Depression	46%
	High blood pressure	37%
	Heart disease	30%

	Mean + standard deviation	**Median**	**Minimum**	**Maximum**
Number of major surgeries	1.6 ± 1.6	1	0	9
Number of hospitalizations	0.9 ± 1.0	1	0	7

services, supportive services, home care, board-and-care, emergency response system, access and transportation, public information, and a geriatric resource center.

Geriatric Special Care Unit

The geriatric special care unit has 12 beds designated for the care of frail elderly patients. Specialized nursing services, social services, and medical and psychiatric care as well as rehabilitative services are available for all patients on the unit. The unit treats frail older adult patients with multiple problems such as confusion, incontinence, decubitus ulcers, failure to thrive, and immobility. The goals of treatment are to enhance or maintain function while minimizing the negative effects associated with hospitalization. Future plans call for enlarging the unit.

Geriatric Consultation Service

A geriatric consultation service is available on a 24-hour basis to provide advice throughout the hospital. Assistance in medical care, discharge planning, and follow-up care are provided by a team that includes a geriatrician, a social worker, a nurse-clinician, and a home health nurse.

Geriatric Ambulatory Assessment Center for Outpatients

A multidisciplinary team, including a geriatrician, a social worker and a geropsychiatrist, provides comprehensive evaluation and assistance in the care of elderly patients and their families in the geriatric ambulatory assessment center. Special services for patients with dementia and urinary incontinence are available.

Mental Health Services

Consultative and supervisory mental health services are now provided by UCLA geropsychiatrists to FMMC/SOHC geriatric medicine teams and to FMMC social workers and case aides. This service is coordinated with the existing 20-bed inpatient geropsychiatric unit and outpatient geropsychiatric services in the Neuropsychiatric Hospital. Findings from the community surveys (especially regarding depression) documented the need for mental health services (see table 22-4). These services are now an integral part of SOHC and have proven that when mental health services are accessible to older adults, they readily make use of them.

Social Work Services

Case coordination and discharge planning are provided by the Department of Clinical Social Work. As the workload has increased, new social work staff with gerontology expertise have been employed by the department.

Supportive Services

The emphasis of the FMMC/SOHC is on the integration of health and social services. The FMMC offers a wide range of supportive services, including counseling, information and referral, a project for the homeless, advocacy, financial aid, group activities, help with forms, visiting volunteers, telephone reassurance, nutrition-congregate and home-delivered meals, transportation, home security, aides to the elderly, board-and-care outreach, conservatorship/durable power of attorney, and case management.

The SOHC provides comprehensive ambulatory assessment and management for common as well as complex problems in the elderly. Health promotion, ambulatory care and follow-up, psychiatric consultations, physical and speech therapy, and a complete range of social services are provided by a multidisciplinary team of specialists from UCLA. Special clinics have been developed for assessment of vision, foot disorders, blood pressure, arthritis, and incontinence. When the needs arises, patients are referred to UCLA Medical Center for inpatient care and specialized procedures. Transportation is available to UCLA Medical Center from Jewish Family Services.

UCLA Home Care Program

UCLA Medical Center entered into a joint venture with a community-based home health agency to deliver home health services to area elderly. Housed at the Medical Center, special nurse coordinators act as liaisons between the Medical Center and FMMC/SOHC to provide information on patients' discharge and follow-up home care and to work with the medical team on the UCLA Medical Center geriatric special care unit. Specialized training in the care of the elderly is emphasized.

Board-and-Care Services

The FMMC/SOHC serves as one of two test sites for the Community Care Facilities for the Elderly Program, a three-year, state-supported demonstration project designed to test the hypothesis that by providing case-managed, supplemental personal care programs, board-and-care residents can avoid transfer to a skilled nursing facility. Staffs of the Multicampus Division of Geriatric Medicine and JFS and a local assemblyman developed the legislation. In conjunction with the state-funded program, in 1984 Multicampus Division and JFS developed a program to systematically expand the provision of primary care services to board-and-care facilities for frail elderly not requiring medical supervision.

Emergency Response System

Funding from the UCLA Medical Center auxiliary made possible the purchase of 20 emergency response system units to be placed in people's homes. The pilot project provides a link between frail older adults living in the community and access to emergency care. It also serves as a marketing device and a means of collecting information about additional types of needed services. Volunteer services administers the program. If the pilot is successful, additional units will be purchased.

Access and Transportation

Measures to improve physical access to UCLA Medical Center and to render its interior environment more attractive to elderly patients have been introduced. Daily transportation services from the Beverly-Fairfax area to the Medical Center are available through JFS. Volunteer services, patient escorts, and information and referral services have been increased and made more responsive to the needs of elderly users. Emphasis is placed on the identification and tracking of elderly patients as they move from the Emergency Medicine Center through inpatient and ambulatory services.

Public Information Activities

Dissemination of information on findings and innovations in the field of aging is vital to program planning for the needs of older adults and to enhancing the ability of the elderly to maintain their well-being. The UCLA has undertaken a number of information dissemination activities, including distributing the following:

- "How to Talk to Your Doctor" provides information on how older people can better communicate with their physicians.
- "Managing Continence" provides information on causes, treatment, aids and devices, and techniques for managing this problem.
- "On Aging," the Center's newspaper column syndicated nationally through the *Washington Post* Writers Group, appears in 120 newspapers from Sarasota, Florida, to Seattle, Washington, reaching more than 15 million households.

Geriatric Resource Center

The passage of California Assembly Bill 2614 provided the Multicampus Division with additional funds for educational training activities and dissemination of information. These activities include:

- *Interdisciplinary colloquia.* The purpose of these sessions is to capture the attention and interest of faculty throughout the UCLA campus as a means of attracting attention to aging-related education and research.
- *Public lecture series.* In conjunction with the monthly colloquia for faculty, a free public lecture series is offered on health-enhancing behavior for the elderly, their special care needs, and resources available to meet those needs.
- *Intensive Course in Geriatric Medicine.* This annual five-day course enables participants to build a foundation of basic science information as it applies to geriatrics, to increase their clinical knowledge and skills, and to understand some of the problems surrounding long-term care.

New Service Options

UCLA Medical Center is exploring several new service options. Three under consideration are:

- *Adult day health care.* UCLA Medical Center is working with a community agency to develop an adult day health care center.
- *Nursing home services.* UCLA Medical Center issued a Request for Information (RFI) for a joint venture Academic Teaching Nursing Home. A number of leading nursing home care providers have expressed interest in joining with the Medical Center. This joint venture will match the management and operational capabilities of the nursing home industry with the academic reputation and geriatric expertise of UCLA.
- *Senior membership program.* UCLA Medical Center is studying various models of packaging health and social services for the elderly. The purpose is to make the myriad of available services more understandable to older consumers and to encourage use of the Medical Center. The hospital is interested in maintaining and increasing its market share of elderly patients.

Financing

Until a universal federal entitlement and/or private insurance program for long-term care is established, any group providing long-term care services will need to be resourceful in developing a number of funding sources to address the problems. UCLA Medical Center has employed a number of strategies to support the geriatric program. Funding sources include the state of California, foundations, private companies, the federal government, and individuals. Although each source may be primarily interested in only one particular aspect of the problem, the aggregate of these resources can be impressive and provides for some important components of the continuum of care.

The Multicampus Division and UCLA Medical Center have employed the following strategies to fund the program:

- *Strategy 1.* Core faculty and staff support is available on an annual basis from the Department of Medicine. Core faculty support has been vital in having a nucleus of faculty who—in addition to patient care, research, and teaching responsibilities—have, as central to their mission, proposal development and fund-raising activities. In fact, everyone employed in a professional capacity by the Multicampus Division understands the need to generate extramural funds and programs their time accordingly.
- *Strategy 2.* In 1983, UCLA Medical Center was approached by the Multicampus Division about submitting a proposal to the Robert Wood Johnson Foundation *Hospital Initiatives in Long-Term Care* program. Those at the Medical Center were enthusiastic because the goals of the Initiatives were in close harmony with the Center's own evolving long-range plans. Also, whereas UCLA has many foundation and governmental grants in specialty areas, this was perceived as a joint grant of hospital administration and the Multicampus Division, thus giving hospital administration a real role and stake in the outcome.

  As a sign of its commitment to geriatrics/gerontology and the RWJF Program, UCLA Medical Center agreed to match the RWJF grant dollar-for-dollar. As the program has developed, the hospital has more than matched the grant. The grant activity has spurred interest in developing other components of a vertically integrated health care delivery system. Studies of rehabilitation services, nursing homes, capitated care, marketing, and transportation have been supported by additional Medical Center resources. The UCLA Medical Center auxiliary provided start-up funds for equipping an emergency response system for the frail elderly in the community.

  UCLA Medical Center agreed to provide funding for the project for an additional two and one-half years beginning January 1, 1988. The support will ensure the continuation of SOHC, the RWJF major component, and allow for partnerships between UCLA and the community to be strengthened. A not-for-profit corporation has been developed to raise funds on an ongoing basis for the SOHC.

- *Strategy 3.* Foundation and government grants have been another important component of the overall program development activities. Success in attracting grants over the last five years has provided for much of the training, education, and community service delivery components. Additionally, JFS has been successful in raising funds that support community social services. As much as possible, the different funding services are integrated into a comprehensive program.
- *Strategy 4.* In addition to grant and Multicampus Division support, SOHC collects Medicare, Medi-Cal, and other third-party health insurance reimbursements. Podiatry, rheumatology, and physical and speech therapy services also pay for some SOHC expenses.
- *Strategy 5.* Another source of support has been the state of California, which provides funding for educational activities through the Academic Geriatric Resource Program and core funding for adult day health care services. In cooperation with JFS, legislation was drafted for the Community Care Facilities Bill. With the passage of this bill, appropriations were made for additional services to board-and-care residents.
- *Strategy 6.* As mentioned earlier, UCLA foresaw the ability to do joint fund-raising with a community agency as a key ingredient to determining the success of the program. Thus over time UCLA has joined with JFS in several fund-raising endeavors. The principal fund-raising activity became the rehabilitation and renovation of the Health Center, co-located with the FMMC. Through a foundation proposal, UCLA raised $50,000 of the $150,000 needed, and, through joint fund-raising with JFS, a case aide at the FMMC and her husband donated the additional $100,000. In recognition of this significant contribution, the FMMC was renamed the Sylvia Olshan Health Center.

  In July 1986, JFS and UCLA received a grant, Family Friends, from the Robert Wood Johnson Foundation. This grant is an example of how the partnership of UCLA and JFS is working to increase opportunities for older adults and provide needed services to families.
- *Strategy 7.* There is a small but growing number of individuals who donate money to the Multicampus Division in memory of an individual, in appreciation of care, or because of an interest in aging. These funds support the overall program activities as well.
- *Strategy 8.* Private companies have provided resources, principally for educational endeavors. The nationally recognized Intensive Course in Geriatric Medicine is one example of an educational program supported in part by several private companies. The university, through the Multicampus Division, has a contract with the *Washington Post* Writers Group to prepare a weekly nationally syndicated newspaper column called "On Aging."
- *Strategy 9.* UCLA Medical Center is currently exploring a number of different options to finance new components of its service delivery

system. Discussions are under way to develop a joint venture teaching nursing home. Also, a marketing study was completed using focus groups to test the feasibility of a special health care program for older adults. A number of administrative, policy, and practical decisions will determine future directions in these areas.

- *Strategy 10.* As an outgrowth of the work of the Jewish Federation Council Committee on Aging, a new organizational entity has been formed consisting of JFS, Cedars-Sinai Medical Center, Jewish Homes for the Aging, and UCLA Medical Center. The coalition is called Jewish Services for the Aging. Each founding agency designated two steering committee members who are part of the board of directors. Additionally, each agency made an initial $60,000 investment to cover the cost of the first year's planning operations. The organization seeks to deliver and coordinate services to middle- and upper-income elderly and use the profits to address the needs of low-income elderly.
- *Strategy 11.* Seventy-eight percent of the population served by SOHC is 75 years of age or older. Caring for these often very frail elderly is time-consuming and a personnel-intensive task. These people come to the Health Center with a myriad of health and social problems. Providing high-quality services to this population is costly, and the funds generated from Medicare, Medi-Cal, other third-party insurance, and laboratory services provided in-house do not cover the costs of providing care on-site. Grant support, private fund-raising, and the UCLA Medical Center make up the difference. Adequate funding for community-based health centers, such as SOHC, is a constant concern and source of anxiety. The service is needed and appropriate, given the patient characteristics; however, reimbursement falls often short of the target need.

To become economically viable, UCLA needs to market SOHC to a younger age cohort and thus acquire a greater case mix. At the same time, reimbursement policies must take into account the fact that most 85-year-olds consume more health resources than 65-year-olds. Until some meaningful recognition of age differences among the over-65 group is recognized, health care programs that serve the frail elderly will be a risky venture. The care of the very frail raises important societal questions about the allocation of resources and the access to high-quality care.

In summary, in the absence of a comprehensive federal and/or private insurance program, a variety of funding sources must be developed.

Conclusions

The past five years have given UCLA the opportunity to work with a variety of professionals and organizations at federal, state, and local levels to examine health and social policy issues. At the local level, efforts have been instrumental in promoting organizational change and client advocacy. Additionally, through the clinical activities of the Multicampus Division of Geriatric Medicine, UCLA has worked with thousands of patients and their families. The lessons that follow are but a few of the many learned:

1. Community-based long-term care services are costly to deliver. The federal government and/or private insurance companies need to establish a long-term care program that is available universally and provides adequate reimbursement.
2. Until such a program is established, it is important to be creative in pulling together programs that meet the needs and goals of multiple funding sources and that can provide services to a variety of audiences.
3. In working with community agencies, relationships take time to develop. The respect and trust of senior staff of both the community and academic components is crucial.
4. Choosing established leaders for the project who have high visibility and access to hospital administration and resources is vital to moving the program along.
5. The placement of the project high in the Medical Center administrative hierarchy served it well. (Had the project been placed in a Department of Social Work, for example, its impact would have been lessened, although in fact social workers in large measure provide the leadership and coordination of the project.)
6. Hospitals need to look at ancillary services and patient hospital days as a way of measuring the financial viability of off-site ambulatory care.
7. In a hospital, or most other organizations, one is always competing for resources. Be prepared to spend time educating hospital personnel and listening to their needs.
8. When possible, pick a winner to work with. The UCLA strategy for choosing a community agency has worked out extraordinarily well. It has access to volunteers, has done joint fund-raising, and has recently developed two new proposals for joint projects.
9. Marketing and public information efforts are useful in creating public awareness about the program. It is important to be clear what you have to market and who is in the driver's seat: the professional geriatric staff or the marketers.
10. The UCLA public lecture series and syndicated newspaper column have been successful in reaching older adults and have had an additional unanticipated benefit of referrals to the geriatric program.
11. Externally mandated, computerized and standardized assessments may be of interest to funding sources; however, some practitioners may find them of little practical use.

12. Hospital administrators generally know little about community-based eldercare organizations (for example, Area Agencies on Aging, multipurpose senior centers). The movement of hospitals into community care provides an opportunity for innovative collaboration to the benefit of older adults.
13. Finally, a little well-placed seed money can go a long way in creating a critical mass needed for program development. This has been the experience at the Multicampus Division and UCLA Medical Center.

The future of health care organizational development will be colored by the reality of restricted resources. We will have to carefully choose the uses to which limited resources will be put, which raises a number of serious questions. Within the context of the national health care budget, what choices will society make between research and treatment? Between restorative therapy for those already ill and preventive measures for those at risk? Among different age groups and disease and treatment models? The answers to these resource, ethical, and value-laden questions will determine the future of program development activities for the frail elderly.

Appendix. Robert Wood Johnson—UCLA Medical Center, 1984: Sylvia Olshan Health Center Patient Satisfaction Survey

User-Phone

Coding

Interviewer ________ Edit date/time ________

Date ________

Geographic code ________

Subject name ________ ID number ____ Phone number ________

Time began ________

It is very important to the UCLA Medical Center, the Sylvia Olshan Health Center, and all the elderly living in the area that you are helping us with our survey. I think you'll find the questions interesting and hope you will answer each as best you can.

(IF FROM A SCREENING PHONE CALL)

What is your first and last name, please? (*Fill in above.*)

First, I'd like to ask you some general questions.

1. (*Fill in*) ______ Male ______ Female

2. What race would you classify yourself as?

   ______ Caucasian/white ______ Hispanic ______ Other (specify)
   ______ Black ______ Oriental ________

3. How would you best describe your type of housing?

   ______ Single family
   ______ Duplex or triplex
   ______ Small apartment complex, less than 10 units
   ______ Apartment building with 10 or more units
   ______ Independent housing for the elderly
   ______ Residential hotel, with no kitchen
   ______ Board and care
   ______ Other (specify)
   ____

4. How old are you?

   ______ (Skip to Q. 5) ______ Don't know

   IF DON'T KNOW—

   a. In what year were you born?
   ______ ______ Don't know

5. Have you ever been married?

   ______ Yes ______ No (Skip to Q. 6)

   a. Are you presently:
   ______ Married ______ Separated
   ______ Widowed ______ Divorced

User-Phone Coding

6. What language are you most comfortable speaking?

______ English ______ Russian ______ Other (specify)
______ Yiddish ______ Hungarian ______________ ________

7. Does anyone live with you?

______ Yes ______ No (Skip to Q. 8)

IF YES—

What is their relationship with you?

______ Husband/wife ______ Children ______ Other (specify)
______ Roommates ______________ ________

8. What was the last year of school you completed?

______ No formal education
______ 1st to 7th grade (some grade school)
______ 8th grade (completed grade school)
______ 9th to 11th grade (some high school)
______ 12th grade (completed high school)
______ 1 to 3 years of college (some college)
______ 4 years or more of college (college graduate) ________

The next set of questions concerns tasks that we face in our daily life.

9. About how often do you get out of your house or apartment for any reason?

______ Almost every day (Skip to Q. 10)
______ A few times a week (Skip to Q. 10)
______ Several times a month
______ About once a month
______ Never or almost never except for emergencies ________

IF ONCE OR SEVERAL TIMES A MONTH or ALMOST NEVER—

a. Would you say you don't got out as much as you would like because it is very difficult for you physically?

______ Yes ______ No ______ Not sure ________

10. Are you prevented from going places because you don't have transportation?

______ Yes ______ No ________

11. When you get out, how do you usually get around?

______ Walk ______ Taxi
______ Drive ______ Other (specify) ________
______ Have someone drive you ______ Don't go anywhere
______ Bus ________

12. Is there someone who helps you with such things as shopping, housework, bathing, dressing, and getting around?

______ Yes ______ No ________

User-Phone Coding

13. Taking everything into consideration, how would you describe your satisfaction with life in general at the present time? Would you say it is good, fair, or poor?

    ______ Good ______ Fair ______ Poor

Now I'd like to ask you some questions about medical care and your health.

14. Do you have any problems getting enough medical care?

    ______ Yes ______ No ______ Not answered

15. If you were sick, is there someone you could call on to help around the house or to help take care of you (for example, if you had the flu or needed someone to bring meals)?

    ______ Yes ______ No (Skip to Q. 16)

IF YES—

a. Who would that be?

    ______ Spouse (wife or husband)
    ______ Child
    ______ Relative
    ______ Friend
    ______ Neighbor
    ______ Social services agency
    ______ Other (specify) ______________

16. In an emergency, is there someone you could call to get help for you right away?

    ______ Yes ______ No

17. Where do you *usually* go when you want to see a doctor?

    ______ Doctor's office (Not at SOHC) (Skip to Q. 19)
    ______ Hospital (name) ______________
    ______ Clinic (name) ______________
    ______ Emergency room (hospital) ______________
    ______ Other (specify) ______________
    ______ Doctor visits home (Skip to Q. 19)
    ______ Sylvia Olshan Health Center

18. Do you have a *particular* doctor that you usually go to?

    ______ Yes ______ No (Skip to Q. 20) ______ Don't know

19. When was the last time you saw your doctor?

    ______ Less than 3 months ago
    ______ 3 to 6 months ago
    ______ 6 months to 1 year
    ______ 1 to 2 years
    ______ 2 or more years

20. How many times in the past year did you see a doctor?

    ______ times

21. In the past year, on the average how often have you visited a clinic, including visits to community health centers and hospital outpatient clinics?

    ______ At least once a week
    ______ 3 to 4 times a month
    ______ 1 to 2 times a month
    ______ 6 to 12 times a year
    ______ Less than 6 times a year

User-Phone

Coding

22. Have you been hospitalized in the last year?

    ______ Yes ______ No (Skip to Q. 23) ______

IF YES—

a. How many times were you hospitalized?

   ______ times

b. How many of these were at UCLA?

   ______ times ______

23. In the past year, how many times have you gone to or have you been taken to an emergency room?

    ______ times (If "0", skip to Q. 24)

a. How many of these were at UCLA?

   ______ times ______

Next, I'd like to ask a few questions about nurse practitioners.

24. Do you know what a nurse practitioner is?

    ______ Yes (Skip to Q. 25) ______ No ______ Not sure ______

IF NO or NOT SURE, EXPLAIN—

A nurse practitioner is a nurse who has had extra training and education in managing health care problems. Nurse practitioners have often gained a lot of practical experience working with doctors in clinics, hospitals, and in doctor's offices. They are often able to spend more time with patients, teach patients about their diseases, and help an office run more efficiently. If a nurse practitioner needs help, there is always a doctor nearby to consult with.

Now back to the questions.

25. If you had your choice would you rather be seen by a nurse practitioner, a doctor, or does it matter to you?

    ______ Nurse Practitioner (Skip to Q. 26) ______ Doctor
    ______ Either (Skip to 26) ______ Don't know ______

IF DOCTOR or DON'T KNOW:

a. Would you mind being seen by a nurse practitioner if a doctor was not available?

   ______ Yes ______ No (Skip to Q. 26) ______ Not sure ______

IF YES or NOT SURE—

b. Would it still bother you if a doctor came in to see you after the nurse practitioner finished?

   ______ Yes ______ No ______ Not sure ______

c. If you were to be seen only by a nurse practitioner on some of your Sylvia Olshan Health Center visits, would it cause you to seek health care somewhere else?

   ______ Yes ______ No ______ Not sure ______

Now I am going to read some sentences about medical care. Think about the medical care you are receiving now at Sylvia Olshan Health Center or what you would expect if you needed care there today. After each statement I will ask you if you strongly agree, agree, are not sure, disagree, or strongly disagree. Remember, think of how you *feel* about the Sylvia Olshan Health Center.

	Strongly Agree	Agree	Not Sure	Disagree	Strongly Disagree
26. I'm very satisfied with the medical care I receive.					
27. If I have a medical question, I can reach someone for help without any problem.					
28. The fees doctors and nurse practitioners charge are too high.					
29. In an emergency, it's very hard to get medical care quickly.					
30. The amount charged for medical care services is reasonable.					
31. Doctors and nurse practitioners are very careful to check everything when examining their patients.					
32. I think my doctor's and nurse practitioner's office has everything needed to provide complete medical care.					
33. It's hard to get an appointment for medical care right away.					
34. Medical insurance coverage should pay for more expenses than it does.					
35. It takes me a long time to get to Sylvia Olshan Health Center.					
36. I hardly ever see the same doctor or nurse practitioner when I go for medical care.					
37. Doctors and nurse practitioners do not spend enough time with their patients.					
38. Sylvia Olshan Health Center is very conveniently located.					
39. Doctors and nurse practitioners cause people to worry a lot because they don't explain medical problems to patients.					
40. Most people could receive better medical care.					
41. Sylvia Olshan Health Center lacks some things needed to provide complete medical care.					

	Strongly Agree	Agree	Not Sure	Disagree	Strongly Disagree
42. The medical problems I've had in the past are ignored when I seek care for a new medical problem.					
43. Doctors and nurse practitioners don't advise patients about ways to avoid illness or injury.					
44. I am happy with the coverage provided by medical insurance plans.					
45. People are usually kept waiting a long time when they are at Sylvia Olshan.					
46. I see the same doctor or nurse practitioner just about every time I go for medical care.					

I am going to read you a list of possible Sylvia Olshan health services. As I read each one, you tell me Yes, meaning I think it is offered; No, meaning I don't think it is offered; or I'm not sure.

47. Do you believe the Sylvia Olshan Health Center offers:

	Yes	No	Not Sure	
a. Physical examinations	______	______	______	______
b. Dental evaluations	______	______	______	______
c. Podiatry—for most foot problems	______	______	______	______
d. Flu and pneumonia vaccinations	______	______	______	______
e. Hearing checkups	______	______	______	______
f. Blood pressure screening	______	______	______	______
g. Urinary problem evaluations	______	______	______	______

Now I'd like to ask a few questions about Sylvia Olshan Health Center.

48. How did you find out about the Sylvia Olshan Health Center?

______ Friend (Skip to Q. 50) ______ Freda Mohr Multiservice Center
______ Relative (Skip to Q. 50) ______ Other (specify) ______________
______ Media—newspaper, TV, etc. ______

49. When you first started coming to Sylvia Olshan, did you have any friends or relatives who were also using the Center?

______ Yes ______ No ______ Don't know or not sure ______

50. Do you have any friends or acquaintances who have stopped coming to Sylvia Olshan?

______ Yes ______ No (Skip to Q. 51) ______ Not sure (Skip to Q. 51) ______

IF YES—How many?

a. ______ (number) ______ Not sure ______

User-Phone Coding

b. Do you know why they stopped coming?

______ Died ______ Got own doctor ______ Moved ______ Not sure
______ (number) ______ (number) ______ (number) ______ (number) ______
______

______ Other (specify)
______ (number)

51. Given the present services and that you continue to live where you are now, do you think you are likely to continue using Sylvia Olshan Health Center?

______ Yes (Skip to Q. 52) ______ No ______ Not sure ______

IF NO or NOT SURE—

Why? ____

52. If you wanted, could you get the care you are receiving at Sylvia Olshan somewhere else?

______ Yes ______ No (Skip to Q. 53) ______ Not sure (Skip to Q. 53) ______

IF YES—

a. Then why do you choose to come to Sylvia Olshan?

______ Cheaper ______ Closer ______ Other (specify) ______
______ Good doctors ______ Friends use it ____________ ______

53. Are there any additional services that you would like to see offered and that you would use at Sylvia Olshan?

______ Dental services
______ Hearing tests
______ Exercise classes
______ Drug and prescription information
______ Satisfied, no other
______ services desired
______ Other (specify)
____

______
______
______
______

54. About how long have you lived at your present address?

______ Years/months ______

This completes the interview. Thank you very much for your help. Would you like me to send you some information about the Sylvia Olshan Health Center and the Freda Mohr Multiservice Center?

______ Yes ______ No

IF NO—

OK, thanks again.

IF YES—

Is the address you have in your file here at Sylvia Olshan correct?

______ Yes ______ No ______ Not sure

IF YES—

OK, thanks again.

	User-Phone
	Coding

IF NO or NOT SURE—

May I have your present address?

____

____

Thanks for your help.

Time ____________________

(Fill in after interview)

Questions have been asked of:

55. ______ Respondent ______ Surrogate ______ Both ______

Relationship of informant to respondent:

56. ____ ______

57. Do you believe the information obtained is:

______ Completely reliable ______ Reliable on some items ______
______ Reliable on most items ______ Completely reliable ______

58. Did the informant/respondent seem to find the interview too long?

______ Yes ______ No ______

(Now please go back and check your marks for accuracy, neatness, and completeness. Make sure all the information on the first page is filled in.)

Sylvia Olshan Health Center Ex-Users—1984 Survey

Interviewer ____________________ Interviewee ____________________

Date ____________________ ID number ____________________

Telephone number ____________________ Geographic code ____________________

Address ____________________ Corrected address ____________________

____________________ ____________________

Age ____________ Sex ____________

1. Why did you stop coming to Sylvia Olshan Health Center?

____

____

____

2. When was the last time you went to Sylvia Olshan Health Center? ____________

3. Where do you usually go now to get medical care? ____________

(Do for Sylvia Olshan Health Center, then for present provider. Change tense as is necessary.)

	Yes	No	Not Sure
4. Are you generally satisfied with the care you receive at:			
Sylvia Olshan Health Center	1	2	3
Present Provider	1	2	3
5. Do you receive complete and comprehensive medical are at:			
Sylvia Olshan Health Center	1	2	3
Present Provider	1	2	3
6. Do you have difficulty getting appointments at:			
Sylvia Olshan Health Center	1	2	3
Present Provider	1	2	3
7. Is ___(place)___ conveniently located?			
Sylvia Olshan Health Center	1	2	3
Present Provider	1	2	3
8. Are you happy with the people who treat you at:			
Sylvia Olshan Health Center	1	2	3
Present Provider	1	2	3
9. Do you believe they are knowledgeable?			
Sylvia Olshan Health Center	1	2	3
Present Provider	1	2	3
10. Do you think they spend enough time with you?			
Sylvia Olshan Health Center	1	2	3
Present Provider	1	2	3
11. Do you think ___(place)___ charges too much?			
Sylvia Olshan Health Center	1	2	3
Present Provider	1	2	3
12. Do they keep you waiting too long at:			
Sylvia Olshan Health Center	1	2	3
Present Provider	1	2	3
13. Did you stop coming to Sylvia Olshan Health Center because you wanted your own doctor?	1	2	3
14. Did you like the nurse practitioners at Sylvia Olshan Health Center?	1	2	3
15. Did you stop using Sylvia Olshan Health Center because you felt UCLA Medical Center was too far?	1	2	3
16. Did you stop using Sylvia Olshan Health Center because you had some billing problems?	1	2	3
17. If ___*(fill in and note below)*___ were changed, would you start using Sylvia Olshan Health Center again?	1	2	3

NOTES: ______________________________

____

____

Bibliography

Bowers, B., and Musser, K. Changing home health care marketplace in Wisconsin. *Home Health Services Quarterly* 8(4):5–23, Winter 1987–88.

Branch, L. G. Continuing care retirement communities: self-insuring for long-term care. *Gerontologist* 27(1):4–8, Feb. 1987.

Brody, S. J. Strategic planning: the catastrophic approach. *Gerontologist* 27(2):131–38, Apr. 1987.

Brody, S. J. Geriatrics and rehabilitation: common ground and conflicts. Conference presentation, "Rehabilitation and Geriatric Education: Perspectives and Potential." Philadelphia, Dec. 4–7, 1988.

Brody, S. J., and Magel, J. S. *DRGs: the second revolution in health care for the elderly. Journal of the American Geriatric Society* 32(9):676–79, Sept. 1984.

Brody, S. J., and Persily, N. A., editors. *Hospitals and the Aged: The New Old Market*. Rockville, MD: Aspen Publishers, 1984.

Buglass, K. The business of eldercare. *American Demographics* 11(9):32–34, 38, Sept. 1989.

Fackelmer, K. Hospitals reserving nursing home beds. *Modern Healthcare* 15(9):68, Apr. 26, 1985.

Fast facts. *Mature Market* 3(7):7, Aug.–Sept. 1989.

Florida Hospital Association. *Florida Hospitals 1989*. Orlando, FL: FHA, 1989.

Francese, P. Today's trends, tomorrow's markets: demographic outlook. *American Demographics* June 1, 1988.

Friedman, E. Problems plaguing public hospitals: uninsured patient transfers, tight funds, mismanagement, and misperception. *Journal of the American Medical Association* 257(14):1850–57, Apr. 1987.

Ginsburg, J. A., Eisenberg, J. M., and others. Financing long-term care. *Annals of Internal Medicine* 108(2):279–88, 1988.

Graham, J. Diversified hospitals review plans after some bumpy rides. *Modern Healthcare* 17(17):30–40, Aug. 14, 1987.

Health Care Insurance Association of America. *Sourcebook of Health Insurance Data.* Washington, DC: HCIAA, 1989.

Hospital Research and Educational Trust. *The Hospital's Role in Caring for The Elderly: Leadership Issues.* Series on Aging and Long-Term Care. Chicago: American Hospital Association, 1982.

Hospital Research and Educational Trust. *Caring for the Elderly: New Directions for Hospitals.* Chicago: American Hospital Association, 1986.

Jensen, J. Health care alternatives. *American Demographics* 8(3):36–38, Mar. 1986.

Jensen, J., and Sherman, J. F. Payment, rules are top strategic issues. *Modern Healthcare's Eldercare Business,* Jan. 15, 1990, pp. 22–24.

Jette, A. M., and Zielstorff, R. D. *Comprehensive Functional Assessment.* 1989. Unpublished material.

Johnsson, J. Providers link health with human services. *Hospitals* 64(1);34–39, Jan. 5, 1990.

Jones, E., and others. *Patient Classifications for Long-Term Care: Users Manual.* Rockville, MD: U.S. Health Resources Administration, Nov. 1974.

Kane, R. D., and Kane, R. L. *Long-Term Care: Principles, Programs, and Policies.* New York City: Springer Publishing Co., 1987.

Koff, T. H. *New Approaches to Health Care for an Aging Population: Developing a Continuum of Chronic Care Services.* San Francisco: Jossey-Bass, 1988.

Koska, M. T. RN shortage puts experience in forefront. *Hospitals* 63(9):22, May 5, 1989.

Lappa, K. Hiring standards: high quality still top priority. *Hospitals* 63(18):89, Sept. 20, 1989.

Lazer, W. Inside the mature market. *American Demographics* 7(3):23–25, 48–49, Mar. 1985.

Lee, E. D. Firms begin support for workers who look after elderly relatives. *Wall Street Journal,* July 6, 1987.

Liang, J., and Jow-Ching Tu, E. Estimating lifetime risk of nursing home residency: a further note. *Gerontologist* 26(5):560–63, Oct. 1986.

Longino, C. F., Jr. A state by state look at the oldest Americans. *American Demographics* 8(11):38–42, Nov. 1986.

Lund, D. S. Caregiving plans seen as boon to worker productivity. *HealthWeek* 2:12, Feb. 1, 1988.

Lutz, S. Ambulatory care keeps patients, hospitals on the move. *Modern Healthcare* 19(48):20–24, 28–42, Dec. 1, 1989.

McConnel, C. E. A note on the lifetime risk of nursing home residence. *Gerontologist 24(2):193*–98, Apr. 1984.

McMorran, W. C. Activities of daily living trigger broader benefits. *Contemporary Long-Term Care* 12(12):40, Oct. 1989.

Meiners, M. R. The case for long-term care insurance. *Health Affairs* 2(2):55–79, Summer 1983.

Minkler, M. Gold in gray: reflections on business' discovery of the elderly market. *Gerontologist* 29(1):17–23, Feb. 1989.

Most day care recipients pleased with care. *Aging Action Alert* No. 89-12, Washington, DC, Dec. 7, 1989, p. 6.

Myers, B. A. *A Guide to Medical Care Administration*. Vol. 1, *Concepts and Principles*. Washington, DC: American Public Health Association, 1972.

Naisbitt, J., and Aburdene, P. *Megatrends 2000*. New York City: William Morrow & Co., 1990.

National Center for Health Statistics. *The National Nursing Home Survey: 1985 Summary for the United States*. Series 13, No. 97. Hyattsville, MD: NCHS, Jan. 1989.

Newald, J. Hospitals and nursing homes: tying the knot. *Hospitals* 60(10): 91–92, May 20, 1986.

Opinion Research Corporation for AARP and the Travelers Foundation. *National Survey of Caregivers Final Report*. Opinion Research Corporation for AARP and the Travelers Foundation, Nov. 1988.

Ostroff, J. An aging market. *American Demographics* 11(5):26, May 1989.

Persily, N. A. Opinion. *Florida Medical Business Journal* 2(3):4, Jan. 31, 1989.

Peters, T. *Thriving on Chaos*. New York City: Harper & Row Publishers, 1987.

Peters, T. J., and Waterman, R. H., Jr. *In Search of Excellence: Lessons from America's Best-Run Companies*. New York City: Harper & Row Publishers, 1982.

Research on Alzheimer's disease holds hope for the future. *Alzheimer's Association Newsletter* 9(4):1, 7, Winter 1989.

Sabatino, F. G. The diversification success story continues: survey. *Hospitals* 63(1):26–32, Jan. 5, 1989.

Schorr, B. Senior backlash over Medicaid stymies Congress. *Medical Business, South Florida Edition* III(I):13, Jan. 2, 1990.

Seigner, C. A. Economics forces hospital 'players' to assume new, complementary roles. *Modern Healthcare* 15(25);60–61, Dec. 6, 1985.

Slowly, perhaps inevitably, Congress faces rural aging. *Networks [National Council on the Aging, Inc.]* NCOA, 1(2):1, Dec. 15, 1989.

Spivack, S. A challenge to survival. In: S. J. Brody and N. A. Persily, editors. *Hospitals and the Aged: The New Old Market*. Rockville, MD: Aspen Publishers, 1984.

Spotts, H. E., Jr., and Schewe, C. D. Communication with the elderly consumer: the growing health care challenge. *Journal of Health Care Marketing* 9(3):33–44, Sept. 1989.

U.S. Department of Health and Human Services. *Health Care Financing Extramural Report Evaluation of Community Oriented Long-Term Care Demonstration Projects.* Baltimore, MD: DHHS, Health Care Financing Administration, #03242, May 1987.

U.S. Department of Health and Human Services. *Secretary's Commission on Nursing.* Vol. I. Washington, DC: DHHS, Dec. 1988.

U.S. Senate Special Committee on Aging. *Aging America: Trends and Projections.* Washington: U.S. Government Printing Office, 1989.

Wagner, L. Hospitals seeing benefits in offering long-term care. *Modern Healthcare* 19(12):40–43, Mar. 24, 1989.

Waldo, D. R., and others. Health expenditures by age group, 1977 and 1987. *Medical Benefits* 6(18):2–3, Sept. 30, 1989.

Weissert, W. G., Elston, J. M., Bolda, E. J., Cready, C. M., Zelman, W. N., Sloan, P. D., Kalsbeek, W. D., Mutran, E., Rice, T. H., Koch, G. G. Models of adult day care: findings from a national survey. *Gerontologist* 29(5):640–49, Oct. 1989.

Wennberg, J., and Gittelsohn, A. Small area variations in health care delivery. *Science* 182(4117):1102–8, Dec. 14, 1973.

Wessel, D. One sure fact: baby boomers are aging. *Wall Street Journal,* Jan. 3, 1989.

Winklevoss, H. E., and Powell, A. V. *Continuing Care Retirement Communities: An Empirical, Financial, and Legal Analysis.* Homewood, IL: Richard D. Irwin, 1984.

Wolfe, D. B. The ageless market. *American Demographics* 9(7):55–56, July 1987.

Wolfson, J., and Levin, P. Linking health care for the poor to health care for profit. *Health Affairs* 6(1):129–35, Spring 1987.

Zubkoff, W. Telephone interview, Jan. 11, 1990.